Textbook of Orthopedic Infections

Prasoon Kumar • Siddhartha Sharma
Sameer Aggarwal
Editors

Textbook of Orthopedic Infections

A Comprehensive Guide to Diagnosis and Management

Springer

Editors
Prasoon Kumar
Department of Orthopedics
PGIMER
Chandigarh, India

Siddhartha Sharma
Department of Orthopedics
PGIMER
Chandigarh, India

Sameer Aggarwal
Department of Orthopedics
PGIMER
Chandigarh, Chandigarh, India

ISBN 978-981-95-5028-9 ISBN 978-981-95-5029-6 (eBook)
https://doi.org/10.1007/978-981-95-5029-6

This Springer imprint is published by the registered company Springer Nature Singapore Pte Ltd.
The registered company address is: 152 Beach Road, #21-01/04 Gateway East, Singapore 189721, Singapore

To my parents, Brajesh and Rani,

for their endless love, wisdom, and the values that guide every step of my journey.

To my wife, Tanu,

for her unwavering support, patience, and belief that make every challenge worthwhile.

To my son, Kiyaan,

whose curiosity and laughter remind me of the joy of learning and discovery.

To my dear friends,

for their companionship, encouragement, and inspiration through every phase of life.

And to the Orthopedic community,

whose dedication to healing, innovation, and excellence continues to transform lives and inspire generations

—Prasoon

Foreword

Orthopedic infection remains the single greatest threat to the otherwise transformative advances of modern reconstructive surgery. In revision arthroplasty, in particular, where the pursuit of durable function meets the reality of fragile biology, infection represents not simply a complication but a potential catastrophe. It challenges the surgeon's skill, the patient's resilience, and the healthcare system's capacity to deliver both cure and restoration.

It is remarkable, though not surprising, that in 2025, an era defined by robotics, navigation, patient-specific implants, and precision biologics, our most formidable adversary remains microbial. The complexity lies not only in the virulence of organisms but in the subtleties of host response, the nuances of host-biomaterial interactions, and the ever-present rise in comorbidities. No algorithm alone can untangle these variables; instead, success rests upon a surgeon's capacity to integrate evolving evidence with seasoned judgement, often in collaboration with a truly multidisciplinary team.

The *Textbook of Orthopedic Infections: A Comprehensive Guide to Diagnosis and Management* makes its timely arrival. Dr Prasoon Kumar, Dr Siddhartha Sharma, and Dr Sameer Aggarwal, together with Springer Nature, have curated a work of impressive breadth and depth. Their vision is clear: to unite fundamental science with pragmatic clinical application, and to do so in a way that reflects the realities of global practice.

The structure of this volume combines 19 chapters progressing from essential principles of historical, microbiological, and immunological processes through the full spectrum of diagnostic strategies and therapeutic interventions. Particular attention is given to periprosthetic joint infection and fracture-related infection: two domains where the stakes are highest and the innovations most rapid. Equally this volume discusses spinal infections, diabetic foot disease, and soft tissue involvement, each an area where clinical pathways are often clouded by diagnostic ambiguity and therapeutic complexity.

What distinguishes this textbook is its commitment to multi-disciplinary and real-world applicability. It captures not only the evidence but also the lived experience of experts across orthopedics, infectious disease, microbiology, and rehabilitation. It acknowledges that managing infection is not an isolated act of surgical adversity but a coordinated endeavour that extends from the laboratory bench to the bedside and beyond.

This work will serve as a foundational resource for postgraduate trainees and early-career surgeons seeking clarity in a challenging field. For the seasoned specialist, it provides both confirmation of established practice and illumination of the controversies and frontiers that will shape our discipline in the coming decade. For researchers, it maps out the unanswered questions that continue to demand rigorous investigation.

Most importantly, this book stands as a testament to our patients. Their courage in the face of the uncertainty and hardship of orthopedic infection inspires our relentless pursuit of better solutions. Every algorithm refined, every technique advanced, and every collaboration fostered is, ultimately, in service to them. Each patient does not fleetingly pass through our care but rather we have the privilege of stepping into their lives to taken on this challenge.

Anant N. Mahapatra, MS (Orth.), FRCS, MCh (Orth.)
Consultant Orth
Dublin North-East, Ireland
Visiting Prof
PGIMER
Chandigarh, India

Preface

Orthopedic infections continue to be among the most formidable challenges in musculoskeletal practice. They not only complicate surgical outcomes but also profoundly affect patient recovery, function, and quality of life. Despite remarkable advances in diagnostics, antimicrobial therapy, and surgical techniques, managing these infections often requires a nuanced understanding of diverse factors—ranging from microbiology and host response to surgical decision-making and long-term rehabilitation.

The *Textbook of Orthopedic Infections: A Comprehensive Guide to Diagnosis and Management* was conceived with the aim of bridging fundamental principles with contemporary clinical practice. Edited by Dr Prasoon Kumar, Dr Siddhartha Sharma, and Dr Sameer Aggarwal, and published by Springer Nature, this volume brings together leading experts to present a comprehensive overview of the field.

Structured into 19 chapters, the book spans the spectrum of orthopedic infections. It begins with core concepts, history, and microbiological foundations, before progressing to the intricacies of diagnosis and the principles of medical and surgical management. Dedicated chapters address soft tissue infections, spinal infections, and diabetic foot—conditions that are frequently encountered yet notoriously complex. Special emphasis has been given to periprosthetic joint infections and fracture-related infections, both of which represent rapidly evolving areas with significant clinical and research interest.

Our intent has been to provide not only evidence-based knowledge but also practical guidance that can be directly applied in day-to-day clinical scenarios. While the book will serve as a dependable reference for postgraduate students and early-career trainees, it is equally designed to support practicing orthopedic surgeons, infectious disease specialists, and allied professionals in their decision-making.

We remain deeply grateful to all contributing authors for sharing their expertise, and to the editorial and production teams at Springer Nature for their invaluable support. Above all, we acknowledge our patients, whose struggles with orthopedic infections continue to inspire our pursuit of better understanding and improved care.

It is our hope that this textbook will serve as both a trusted reference and a catalyst for ongoing innovation in the diagnosis and management of orthopedic infections.

Chandigarh, India

Prasoon Kumar
Siddhartha Sharma
Sameer Aggarwal

Contents

1 **Bone and Joint Infection: Introduction and Core Concepts** 1
Raunak Kotian, Sandeep Patel, Sameer Aggarwal, and Ankit Dadra

2 **Bone and Joint Infections: *Historical Perspective*** 13
Prasoon Kumar, Mehar Dhillon, and Sameer Aggarwal

3 **Microbiological Aspects of Bone and Joint Infections** 23
Rajendra Gudisa and Parakriti Gupta

4 **Biofilms in Osteoarticular Infections: A Hidden Challenge** 45
Ankit Dadra, Siddhartha Sharma, and Prasoon Kumar

5 **Diagnostic Approaches and General Principles of Management of Orthopedic Infections** 59
Vivek P. Ksheerasagar and Vijay G. Goni

6 **Antimicrobial Therapy** 75
K. Niveditha, Nusrat Shafiq, and Ankit Dadra

7 **Surgical Principles of Management of Orthopedic Infections** 89
Rakesh John, Tarkik Thami, and Prasoon Kumar

8 **Pediatric Osteomyelitis** 103
Ankit Dadra, Karthick Rangasamy, Nirmal Raj Gopinathan, and Jasmine Kaur

9 **Paediatric Septic Arthritis** 117
J. P. Khatri, Akash Kumar Ghosh, and Pebam Sudesh

10 **Adult Osteomyelitis** 135
Shahnawaz Khan and Sujit Kumar Tripathy

11 **Septic Arthritis of the Native Joint** 159
Avinash Kumar and Swayam Prakash Das

12 **Periprosthetic Joint Infection: Lower Limb** 173
Rajesh Kumar Rajnish, Sandeep Kumar Yadav, and Nitesh Gahlot

13 Prosthetic Joint Infection: Upper Limb 185
Inese Breide, Dace Vīgante, and Dmitrijs Grigorjevs

14 Fracture-Related Infections 195
Ansh Gupta, Prasoon Kumar, Benjamin Petry, Markus Süß, and Rohit Arora

15 Spinal Infections: Understanding, Diagnosis, and Treatment 209
Aditya Gupta and Vishal Kumar

16 Diabetic Foot Infection 221
Uttam Chand Saini, Singh Akashdeep, and Ashu Rastogi

17 Bone and Joint Tuberculosis 235
Arjit Bansal, Siddhartha Sharma, and Mandeep Singh Dhillon

18 Masquelet Technique 257
Dhruv Maini and Lalit Maini

19 Necrotizing Soft Tissue Infections (NSTI) 269
Yashwant Raj Sakaray and Maninder Singh

About the Editors

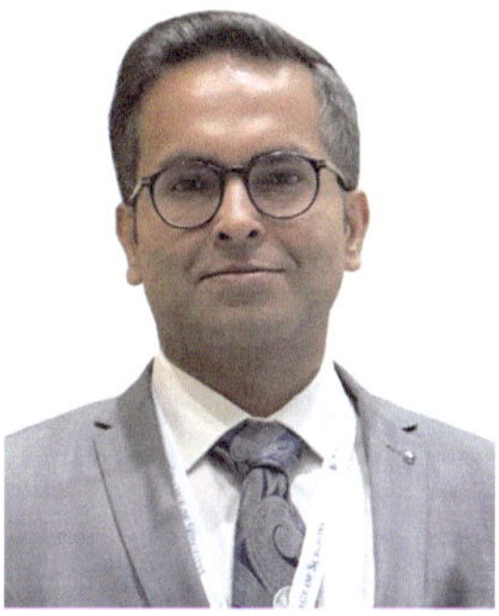

Prasoon Kumar is Associate Professor of Orthopedics at PGIMER, Chandigarh. A versatile trauma surgeon, his primary expertise lies in elbow and wrist surgeries, along with hip and knee arthroplasty. He has authored over 100 research papers and book chapters in reputed journals. Notably, he edited a book on Avascular Necrosis of the Hip in collaboration with Springer Nature in 2023. His extensive work in orthopedic infections spans both diagnostic and therapeutic domains.

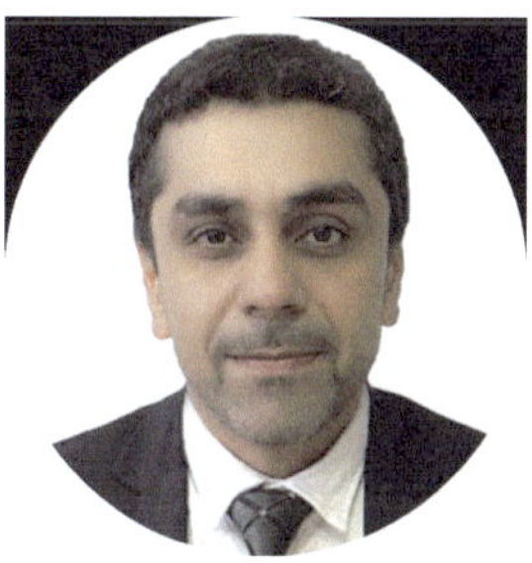

Siddhartha Sharma serves as Additional Professor of Orthopedics at PGIMER, Chandigarh. A specialist in foot and ankle surgery, he is also proficient in deformity correction procedures. He holds a PhD focused on talus malunions and has received advanced training at MGH and FARIL, Boston, USA. With nearly 120 research papers and book chapters to his credit, he recently authored a book on Foot and Ankle Surgery in collaboration with Springer Nature.

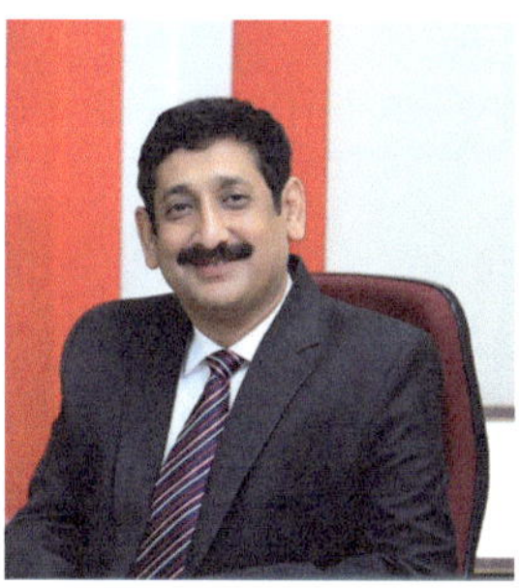

Sameer Aggarwal is a distinguished figure in the field of trauma surgery and has served as the Nodal Officer of the Advanced Trauma Centre at PGIMER, Chandigarh. With over 200 publications to his name, he is internationally recognized as an authority in trauma management.

Bone and Joint Infection: Introduction and Core Concepts

1

Raunak Kotian, Sandeep Patel, Sameer Aggarwal, and Ankit Dadra

Abstract

Bone and joint infections, including osteomyelitis, septic arthritis, prosthetic joint infections, and spinal infections, represent a significant challenge in clinical practice due to their complex pathophysiology, diagnostic difficulties, and potential for serious complications. This chapter provides a comprehensive overview of the mechanisms of infection spread—hematogenous, contiguous, and direct inoculation—and outlines the varied clinical presentations across different patient populations. Emphasis is placed on a multidisciplinary approach for diagnosis using imaging, microbiology, and molecular techniques such as sonication and PCR. Treatment strategies include long-term antibiotic therapy, surgical debridement, and the use of local antibiotic delivery systems. Emerging therapies, including hyperbaric oxygen therapy, calcium sulphate beads, genomic tools, and bacteriophages, are also discussed. Through illustrative case examples and recent advancements, the chapter underscores the importance of timely, collaborative, and individualized patient care.

Keywords

Osteomyelitis · Septic Arthritis · Prosthetic Joint Infection · Biofilm · Multidisciplinary Management

R. Kotian
Manipal Northside Hospital, Bengaluru, India

S. Patel (✉) · S. Aggarwal · A. Dadra
Department of Orthopedics, PGIMER, Chandigarh, India

P. Kumar et al. (eds.), *Textbook of Orthopedic Infections*,
https://doi.org/10.1007/978-981-95-5029-6_1

Learning Objectives
By the end of this chapter, readers will be able to:

1. *Understand the Pathophysiology of Bone and Joint Infections*: Describe the mechanisms of infection spread to bones and joints, including hematogenous, contiguous, and direct inoculation routes.
2. *Identify Clinical Manifestations*: Recognize the clinical signs and symptoms of different types of bone and joint infections, such as osteomyelitis, septic arthritis, and prosthetic joint infections.
3. *Implement Diagnostic Methods*: Explain the diagnostic techniques, including clinical evaluation, imaging studies, and microbiological testing, used to identify bone and joint infections.
4. *Apply Treatment Strategies*: Outline the treatment options, including antibiotic therapy, surgical intervention, and adjunctive therapies, and understand the importance of a multidisciplinary approach in managing these infections.

1.1 Introduction

Bone and joint infections include septic arthritis, prosthetic joint infections, osteomyelitis, spinal infections (discitis, vertebral osteomyelitis, and epidural abscess) and diabetic foot osteomyelitis [1]. These infections can occur in any age group and can result from a variety of pathogens, typically bacteria, but also fungi and mycobacteria. It poses significant clinical challenges due to its complex diagnosis, prolonged treatment, and potential for severe complications.

These infections can lead to substantial morbidity and require a multidisciplinary approach for effective management. This chapter aims to provide a comprehensive overview of the pathophysiology, clinical manifestations, diagnostic techniques, and treatment strategies for bone and joint infections.

1.2 Pathophysiology [2, 3]

Bone and joint infections can occur through three primary mechanisms: hematogenous spread, contiguous spread from an adjacent infection, and direct inoculation.

Hematogenous Spread It is the most common route in children, often involving the long bones due to the rich vascular supply in the metaphysis. In adults, hematogenous spread typically affects the vertebrae. The initial infection often stems from a bacteremia that seeds the bone or joint (Fig. 1.1).

Contiguous Spread It occurs from an adjacent infected tissue, such as skin or soft tissue infections, which can extend into the bone. This is commonly seen in patients with chronic ulcers, particularly those with diabetes or peripheral vascular disease.

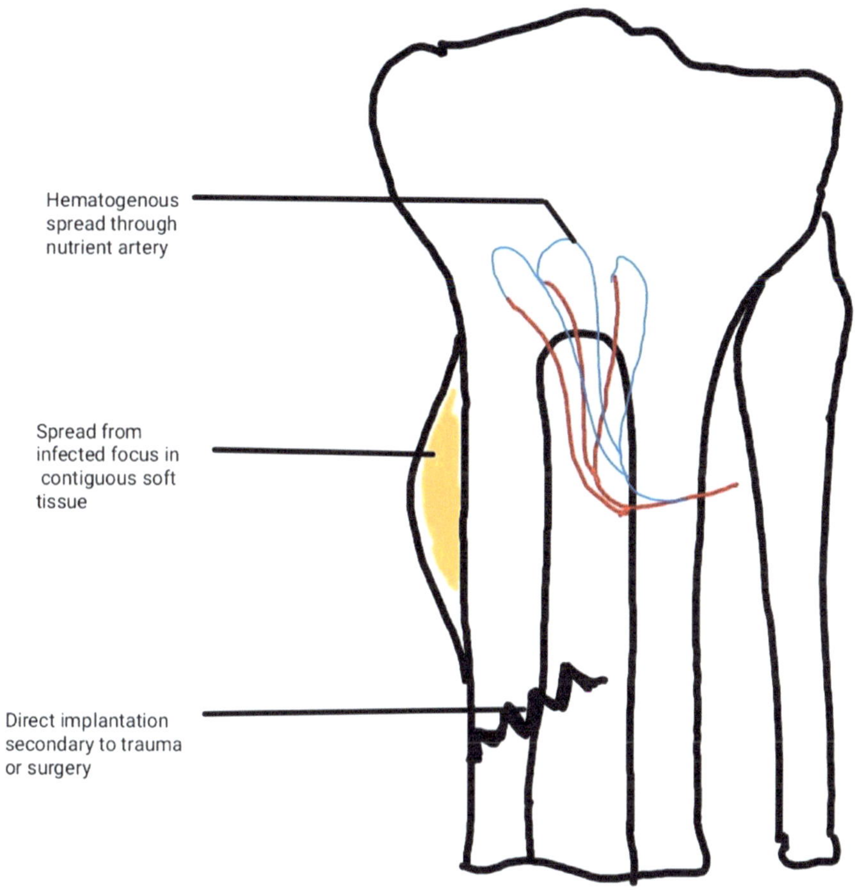

Fig. 1.1 Different routes of spread of osteomyelitis in bone and joint

Direct Inoculation It can result from trauma, surgical procedures, or injections that introduce pathogens directly into the bone or joint [4]. This mechanism is especially relevant in prosthetic joint infections, where bacteria can be introduced during implantation.

1.3 Clinical Manifestations

The clinical presentation of bone and joint infections can vary widely based on the type and location of the infection, as well as the patient's age and underlying health conditions.

A. *Osteomyelitis*: It can be acute or chronic. Acute osteomyelitis presents with localized pain, fever, and erythema. Chronic osteomyelitis often manifests with more subtle symptoms such as persistent pain, drainage from sinus tracts, and occasional fever. If untreated, chronic infections may also present with local bone destruction and systemic symptoms.

B. *Septic Arthritis*: It is characterized by the acute onset of joint pain, swelling, warmth, and restricted range of motion, often accompanied by fever [5]. The knee is the most commonly affected joint, followed by the hip, shoulder, and other large joints.
C. *Prosthetic Joint Infections*: It is classified based on the time of onset post-surgery: early (within 3 months), delayed (3–12 months), and late (more than 12 months) [6]. Symptoms include joint pain, swelling, instability, and sometimes systemic signs of infection such as fever and malaise.

1.4 Diagnostic Methods

Accurate diagnosis of bone and joint infections involves a combination of clinical assessment, imaging, and microbiological testing [7, 8].

A. *Clinical Evaluation*

   A thorough history and physical examination are critical. Important aspects include the duration and onset of symptoms, recent infections or surgeries, trauma, and underlying conditions such as diabetes or immunosuppression.

B. *Imaging Studies*

   - X-rays: Useful for detecting chronic osteomyelitis and prosthetic joint infections.
   - MRI: Highly sensitive for early detection of osteomyelitis and assessment of soft tissue involvement.
   - CT Scan: Helpful in identifying sequestra and involucrum in chronic osteomyelitis.
   - Ultrasound: Can detect joint effusions and guide aspiration in suspected septic arthritis.

C. *Microbiological Testing*

   - Blood Cultures: Particularly important in hematogenous osteomyelitis and septic arthritis.
   - Joint Aspiration and Bone Biopsy: Crucial for obtaining samples for culture and sensitivity testing to guide antibiotic therapy.
   - Molecular Methods: Techniques like PCR can be used to identify fastidious organisms that are difficult to culture.

D. *Sonication*

   - The use of low-intensity ultrasound for the disintegration of biofilm on extracted implants and the subsequent culture of the sonication fluid.
   - More sensitive than conventional periprosthetic tissue cultures.

1.5 Treatment

Treating bone and joint infections involves medical and surgical approaches, aiming to eradicate the infection, alleviate pain, and restore function. A multidisciplinary team, including infectious disease specialists, orthopedic surgeons, radiologists, and microbiologists, is essential for the optimal management of bone and joint infections. This approach ensures comprehensive care and improves patient outcomes.

A. *Antibiotic Therapy*

- Empirical antibiotic therapy should begin based on the most likely pathogens and be adjusted according to culture results.
- Prolonged courses of antibiotics, often 6 weeks or more, are typically required to ensure eradication of the infection.

B. *Surgical Intervention*

- Surgical debridement is often necessary to remove infected tissue, drain abscesses, and in some cases, remove or replace infected prosthetic joints.
- The choice of surgical procedure depends on the extent of infection and the patient's overall health.
- For PJI, a two-stage intervention is sometimes warranted wherein, in the first stage, Debridement plus Implant Removal along with insertion of antibiotic spacer is done (Fig. 1.2) which is followed by oral antibiotics for 6–8 weeks.
- In the second stage, definitive surgery is performed.

C. *Adjunctive Therapies*

- Hyperbaric Oxygen Therapy: May benefit patients with chronic, refractory osteomyelitis.
- Local Antibiotic Delivery: The use of antibiotic-impregnated beads or spacers can provide high local concentrations of antibiotics, enhancing the eradication of infection.

D. *Emerging Therapies and Research*

- Use of calcium sulphate beads to control bone and joint infection.
- New antimicrobial agents, advanced diagnostic methods, and innovative surgical techniques continue to enhance the management of bone and joint infections.
- Areas of interest include the development of biofilm-resistant materials for prosthesis, and understanding the role of the microbiome in these infections.

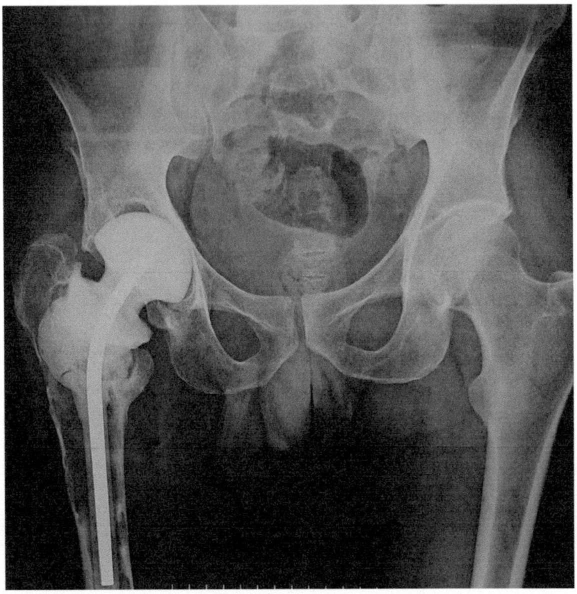

Fig. 1.2 Postoperative radiograph of a 47-year-old male diagnosed with periprosthetic joint infection (PJI), planned for a staged revision procedure. The image shows the immediate post-stage 1 surgery X-ray with a monoblock antibiotic-loaded cement spacer in place

1.6 Case Example (Figs. 1.3, 1.4, 1.5, 1.6, 1.7, 1.8, and 1.9)

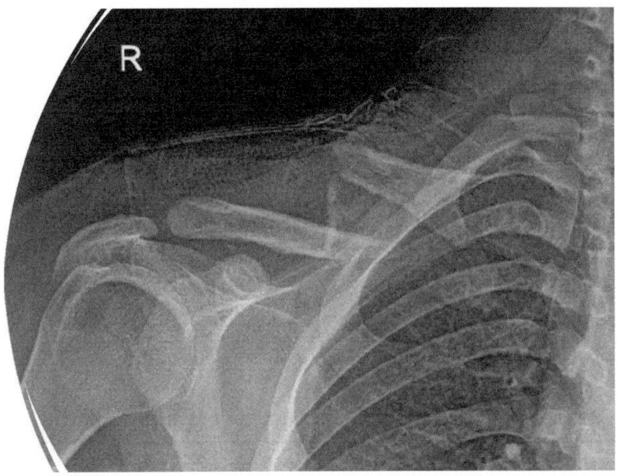

Fig. 1.3 Preop radiograph depicting a 27-year-old female with a closed right clavicle fracture following an alleged roadside accident

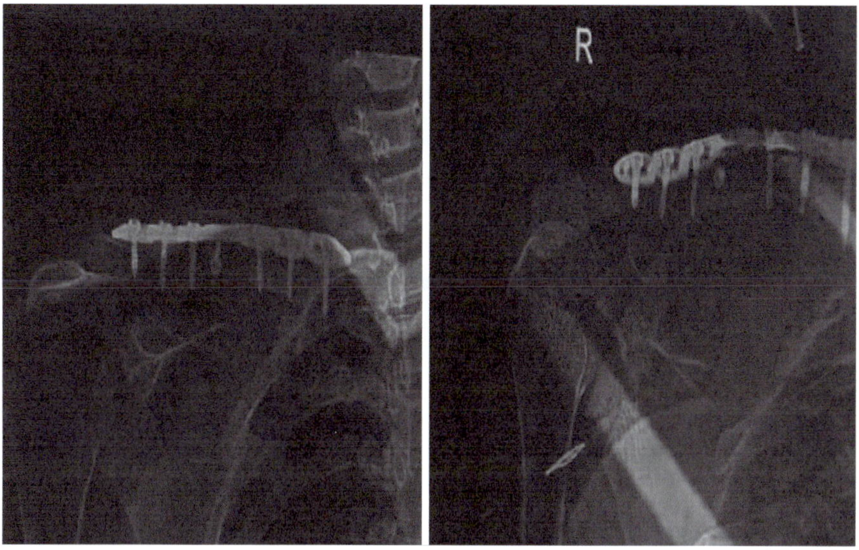

Fig. 1.4 Postoperative radiograph after initial fixation with clavicle anatomical plate

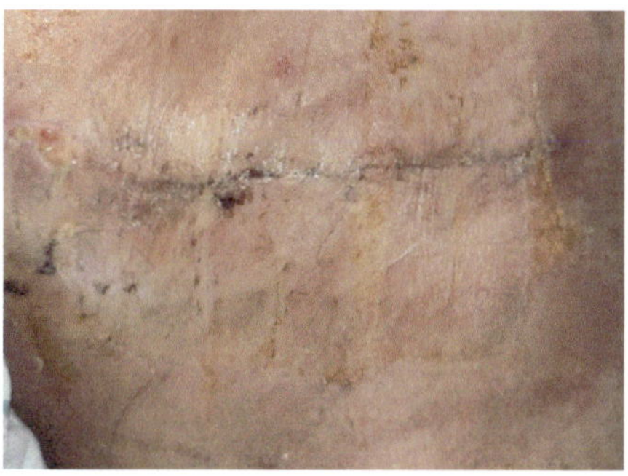

Show growth of	**Staphylococcus**	
Species	aureus	
Culture shows	-	
	Antibiotics/Organism	**Staphylococcus aureus**
Antimicrobial Susceptibility	Ciprofloxacin	R
	Clindamycin	R
	Linezolid	S
	Erythromycin	R
	Vancomycin	S
	Cotrimoxazole	S
	Oxacillin	R
	Doxycycline	S
	Interpretation	

Fig. 1.5 Clinical picture of postoperative day 10 with serous discharge and wound dehiscence at the suture site. Culture and sensitivity results depicting Staphylococcus aureus as the causative organism

Fig. 1.6 Postoperative image at day 14 after debridement, followed by initiation of iv Vancomycin

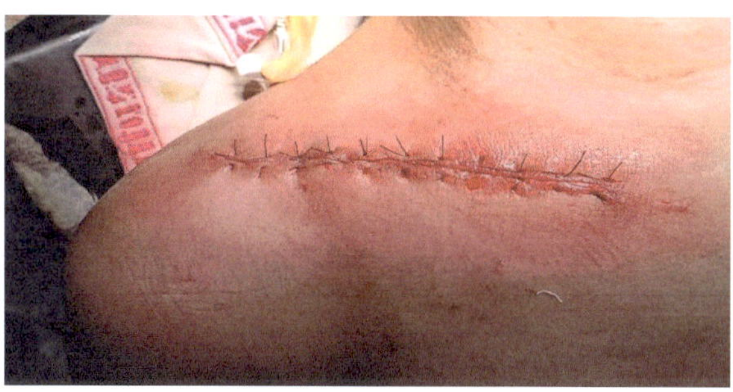

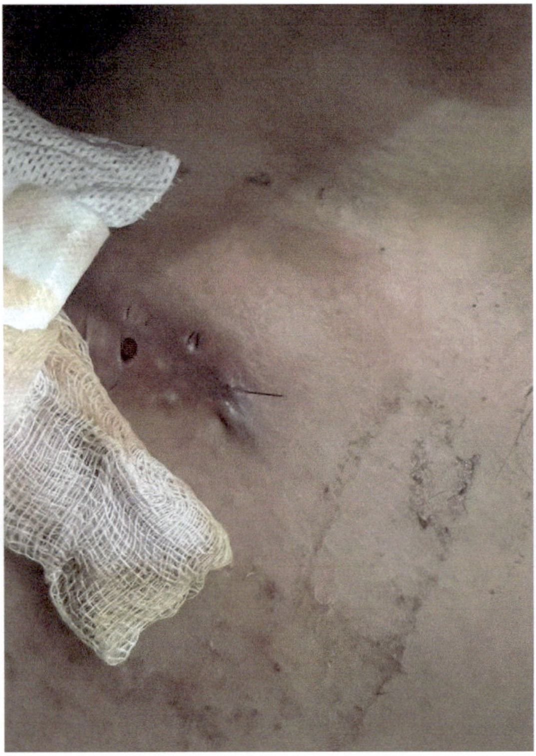

Fig. 1.7 On postoperative day 16 following the second surgery, the patient presented with an exposed implant due to non-compliance with IV antibiotic therapy

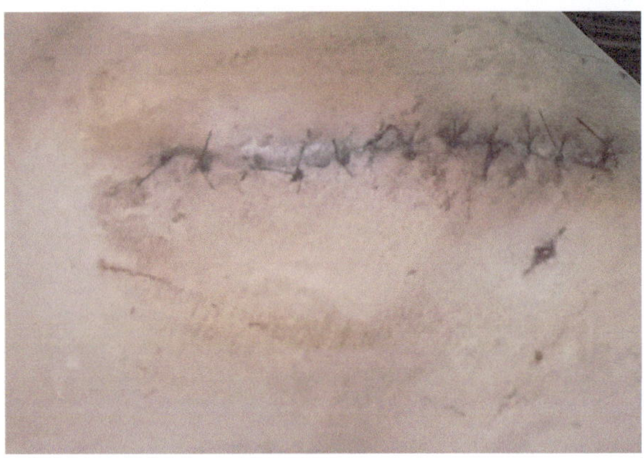

Fig. 1.8 Debridement and implant removal were performed on postoperative day 16 of the second surgery. The wound was closed using Ethilon 2–0 sutures, and the limb was supported with an arm pouch

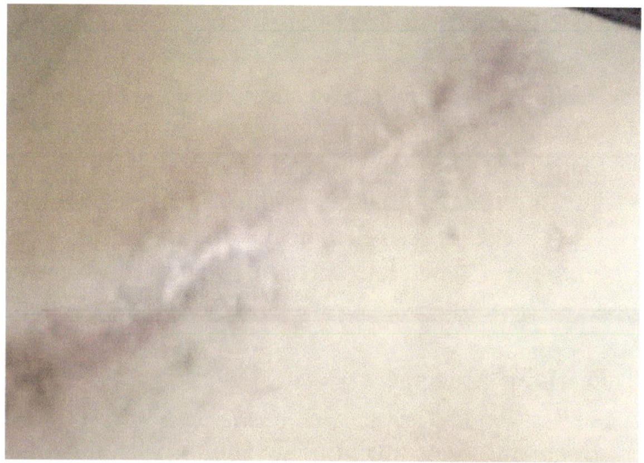

Fig. 1.9 At 2 months follow-up, the patient had a healed surgical site and infection under control

1.7 Core Concepts

1.7.1 Multidisciplinary Approach

A multidisciplinary team, including infectious disease specialists, orthopedic surgeons, radiologists, and microbiologists, is essential for the optimal management of bone and joint infections. This approach ensures comprehensive care and improves patient outcomes.

1.7.2 Monitoring and Follow-Up

Regular monitoring and follow-up are crucial to ensure the resolution of infection and to detect any recurrence early. This involves clinical assessments, laboratory tests, and imaging studies as needed.

1.7.3 Prevention

Preventive measures are crucial in minimizing the incidence of bone and joint infections. Some key strategies include:

1. *Sterile Surgical Techniques*: Ensuring proper asepsis during surgical procedures, particularly in orthopedic surgeries, significantly reduces infection risk.
2. *Early Management of Open Fractures*: Prompt debridement and appropriate antibiotic use can prevent infections following trauma.
3. *Vaccination*: Pneumococcal and meningococcal vaccines may reduce the risk of septic arthritis caused by these organisms.

1.7.4 Emerging Therapies

- Machine learning to drive surgical decision.
- Genomic sequencing to understand the pathophysiology.
- Outpatient subcutaneous antimicrobial therapy.
- Use of dithiothreitol (anti-biofilm chemical agent) as an alternative to sonication.
- Use of bacteriophages to deal with implant-associated infections and other difficult-to-treat infections involving multidrug-resistant bacteria.

Take-Home Message

1. Bone and joint infections, including osteomyelitis and septic arthritis, require prompt diagnosis and treatment to prevent severe complications and disability.
2. A multidisciplinary approach remains the cornerstone of effective management, emphasising the importance of collaborative care.
3. Advances in diagnostic techniques and treatment options continue to improve the management and outcomes for patients affected by these infections.
4. Calcium sulphate beads are a promising option for controlling bone and joint infections without significant side effects.
5. Acute bone and joint infections in children are serious and require careful evaluation to avoid misdiagnosis and ensure proper treatment.

References

1. Colston J, Atkins B. Bone and joint infection. Clin Med. 2018;18(2):150–4.
2. Frigui S, Chebbi Y, Achour W. Pathophysiology of bone and joint infections. In: Histopathology of bone and joint infections. Cham: Springer Nature Switzerland; 2024. p. 1–17.
3. Chebbi Y, Frigui S, Achour W. Microbiology of bone and joint infections. In: Histopathology of bone and joint infections. Cham: Springer Nature Switzerland; 2024. p. 19–39.
4. Klontzas ME, Vassalou EE, Spanakis K, Karantanas AH. Bone and soft tissue infection.
5. Nair R, Schweizer ML, Singh N. Septic arthritis and prosthetic joint infections in older adults. Infect Dis Clin. 2017;31(4):715–29.
6. Gomez-Urena EO, Tande AJ, Osmon DR, Berbari EF. Diagnosis of prosthetic joint infection: cultures, biomarker and criteria. Infect Dis Clin. 2017;31(2):219–35.
7. Temesgen Z, Baddour LM, Rizza S. A rational approach to clinical infectious diseases: a manual for house officers and other non-infectious diseases clinicians. 1st ed. Elsevier, Inc.;2021.
8. Ferry T, Lodise TP, Gallagher JC, Forestier E, Goutelle S, Tam VH, Mohr IIIJF, Roubaud-Baudron C. Outpatient subcutaneous antimicrobial therapy (OSCAT) as a measure to improve the quality and efficiency of healthcare delivery for patients with serious bacterial infections. Front Med. 2020;7:585658.

Further Reading

9. Evangelopoulos DS, Stathopoulos IP, Morassi GP, Koufos S, Albarni A, Karampinas PK, Stylianakis A, Kohl S, Pneumaticos S, Vlamis J. Sonication: a valuable technique for diagnosis and treatment of periprosthetic joint infections. Sci World J. 2013;2013(1):375140.
10. Bernard L, Arvieux C, Brunschweiler B, Touchais S, Ansart S, Bru JP, Oziol E, Boeri C, Gras G, Druon J, Rosset P. Antibiotic therapy for 6 or 12 weeks for prosthetic joint infection. N Engl J Med. 2021;384(21):1991–2001.
11. Pirnay JP, Ferry T, Resch G. Recent progress toward the implementation of phage therapy in Western medicine. FEMS Microbiol Rev. 2022;46(1):fuab040.
12. Pham TT, Lazarevic V, Gaia N, Girard M, Cherkaoui A, Suva D, Schrenzel J. Second periprosthetic joint infection caused by streptococcus dysgalactiae: how genomic sequencing can help defining the best therapeutic strategy. Front Med. 2020;7:53.
13. Kolenda C, Josse J, Batailler C, Faure A, Monteix A, Lustig S, Ferry T, Laurent F, Dupieux C. Experience with the use of the MicroDTTect device for the diagnosis of low-grade chronic prosthetic joint infections in a routine setting. Front Med. 2021;8:565555.
14. Parvizi J, Gehrke T, Chen AF. Proceedings of the international consensus on periprosthetic joint infection. Bone Joint J. 2013;95(11):1450–2.
15. Rajput V, Meek RM, Haddad FS. Periprosthetic joint infection: what next? Bone Joint J. 2022;104(11):1193–5.
16. Parvizi J, Shohat N, Gehrke T. Prevention of periprosthetic joint infection: new guidelines. Bone Joint J. 2017;99(4_Supple_B):3–10.
17. Baldan R, Sendi P. Precision medicine in the diagnosis and management of orthopedic biofilm infections. Front Med. 2020;7:580671.
18. Ward SA, Habibi AA, Ashkenazi I, Arshi A, Meftah M, Schwarzkopf R. Innovations in the isolation and treatment of biofilms in periprosthetic joint infection: a comprehensive review of current and emerging therapies in bone and joint infection management. Orthop Clin. 2024,55(2).171–80.

2 Bone and Joint Infections: *Historical Perspective*

Prasoon Kumar, Mehar Dhillon, and Sameer Aggarwal

Abstract

Early history: Evidence of osteomyelitis dates back to more than *250 million years ago* in the fractured spine of *dimetrodon Permian reptile.* From the time of *Hippocrates* (460–370 BC), infection after fracture of the bone has been reported, although the clinical aspects of these post fracture infections were reported much later. *Pathology*: Nelaton coined the term "osteomyelitis," describing it as inflammation of the bone caused by an infectious agent. It can be due to trauma, surgery, or secondary to any vascular insufficiency. The cause of osteomyelitis remained obscure until *Louis Pasteur* described the causative agents for infection.

Evolution of treatment: Early treatment consisted of a combination of conservative and radical approaches in the form of excision and immobilization primarily. 1948 a paper from the Royal Hospital for Sick children in Glasgow first illustrated the benefits of penicillin in osteomyelitis. In 1980, the introduction of Fluoroquinolones revolutionized the treatment for infective cases. Rowling et al. by 1959 reported a positive approach to treat chronic osteomyelitis, requiring surgery to improve the blood supply over the scarred and affected bone. The involved bone requires excision of the affected soft tissue and scarring to improve recovery for adequate delivery of antibiotics over the bone that is chronically affected. *Conclusion*: The management principles like extensive debridement, dead space management, and antibiotic therapy still hold true in current times. The introduction of antibiotics revolutionized the treatment strategy leading to the transition from a highly fatal condition to a treatable disease.

P. Kumar · M. Dhillon (✉) · S. Aggarwal
Department of Orthopedics, PGIMER, Chandigarh, India

P. Kumar et al. (eds.), *Textbook of Orthopedic Infections*,
https://doi.org/10.1007/978-981-95-5029-6_2

Keywords

Osteomyelitis · Sequestrum · Bone necrosis · History · Evolution · Brodie's abscess

Learning Points

- To gain knowledge about the evolution of various terms related to osteomyelitis over the past centuries
- To understand the basic pathology of osteomyelitis that was described by various physicians, from all parts of the world that ultimately led to the development of various treatment principles
- To learn how the World War I and II had an impact on understanding the progression and management of the disease
- To understand how infections of the bone were managed before introduction of antibiotics
- To learn about the evolution of antibiotics and antibiotic-related resistance for management of osteomyelitis
- To understand the evolution of the treatment principles for management of chronic osteomyelitis and their relevance in today's era

2.1 Introduction

2.1.1 Early History

Evidence of osteomyelitis dates back to more than *250 million years ago* in the fractured spine of *dimetrodon Permian reptile*. The presence of infection was reported in the form of inflammation and roughened bone around the fractured site. However, no histological evidence was reported [1]. From the time of *Hippocrates* (460–370 BC), infection after fracture of the bone has been reported, although the clinical aspects of these post-fracture infections were reported much later. The word "pus" has been described in the Edwin-Smith Papyrus as the word "*ryt*" in the earliest surgical expertise. They described cases of "*pouring ryt*" (pus) and wounds communicating with bones as osteomyelitis [2].

2.2 History of Pathological Knowledge

The Edwin-Smith surgical papyrus around 1600 BC initially translated by Breasted elaborated on ancient Egyptian methods like avoiding probing wounds to prevent pus formation. They even expected that wound over fracture may discharge pus and even lead to extrusion of bone pieces [2]. Hippocrates in the fifth century BC described infection of the skull and long bones after wounds and reported extrusion of *sequestra* and scarring of the bone [3]. Alexander Monro in 1740 described the infection of vertebral column with a fatal prognosis [4].

In 1773, William Bromfield from England described "Abscessus in medulla" as bone that *"may become carious, first in its internal parts and that from external injury, as well as from a vitiated state of the animal fluids."* They even advised that *"we cannot be too early in letting it out when we are assured of matter being under the periosteum"* [5]. In 1786, John Hunter described the mechanism of sequestrum formation. Benjamin Brodie first described *Brodie's abscess* of the long bones as a localized abscess due to previous low-grade osteomyelitis [6].

Nathan Smith in 1831, the first professor of Surgery at Yale University, in his memoirs reported that *"a very great majority of patients survive the attack, albeit with long confinement, protracted suffering and great emaciation. In a few cases, however, the disease proves fatal."* He further elaborated infection of the bone as necrosis, to indicate death of the bone [7].

In 1844, Auguste Nelaton (1807–1873), a French surgeon, first coined the term "Osteomyelitis" describing it as inflammation of the bone caused by an infectious agent. It can be due to trauma, surgery or secondary to any vascular insufficiency. The cause of osteomyelitis remained obscure until Louis Pasteur described the causative agents for infection [8] (Fig. 2.1).

Louis Pasteur in 1877 closely studied infectious diseases had described microbes as the cause of furuncles and osteomyelitis. He described it as *"a boil of the bone marrow."* He further reported *staphylococcus* to be the causative agent for furuncles and osteomyelitis and streptococcus for puerperal infections [9].

Alexander Ogston was a professor of surgery in Aberdeen and elaborated the importance of the antiseptic system and microbes as the cause of sepsis and "blood poisoning" in 1881 through an article regarding microorganisms in surgical diseases. He examined a series of 82 abscesses, which were carefully removed with antiseptic precautions. He reported two kinds of micrococci responsible for abscesses, namely, one forming chains and one forming groups like fish in clusters. Geddes, the professor of Greek, suggested to name the organisms that grew in masses of grapes as "Staphyloccocus". This was described first by Ogston from surgical pus isolated form a knee joint [10]. Theodor Bilroth, an Austrian surgeon, named the organisms that grew in chains as "Streptococci" in 1874 [11]. Furthermore, in 1884, a German physician Friedrich Julius Rosenbach differentiated bacteria on

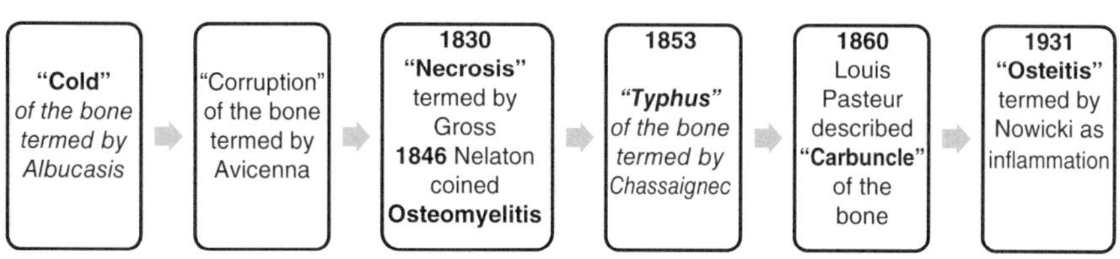

Fig. 2.1 Various terminologies describing infection of the bone over the years before osteomyelitis

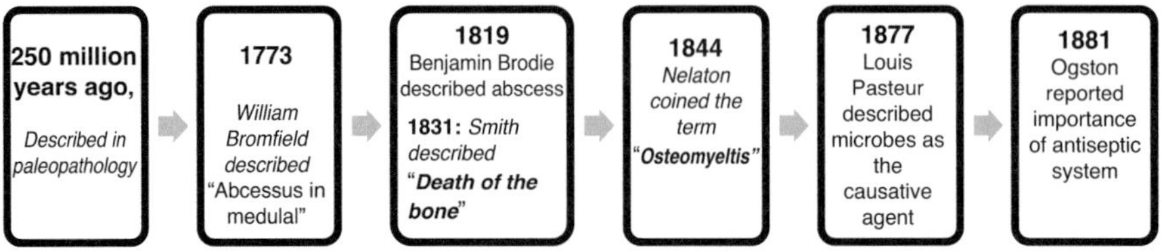

Fig. 2.2 Timeline depicting the evolution of the term "Osteomyelitis"

the basis of color of the colony growth [10, 12]. The hematogenous route of infection was proven experimentally in animals by Rodet in 1889 by injecting staphylococcus aureus intravenously in rabbits [13]. Wilensky described acute osteomyelitis as a metastatic lesion due to settlement of blood-borne organisms [14] (Fig. 2.2).

2.3 Evolution of Treatment

Ancient Chinese treated suppuration of bone by application of slow burning wood in the form of small pieces. *Rest, localized heat, and immobilization* consisted as the mainstay of treatment until Lister introduced antiseptics in 1867. However, it was soon realized that the agents could damage the surrounding tissue even though they cause bacterial cell death [15]. The World War I gave surgeons immense experience in the treatment of open fractures and osteomyelitis. Baer reported that wounds which suffered contamination by maggots healed faster and with ease compared to other wounds. Thus, *maggot therapy* was introduced for treatment of acute and chronic cases. The maggots were believed to destroy necrotic tissues along with bacteria by ingestion and release of proteolytic enzymes [16].

Before the introduction of penicillin in the 1940s, acute osteomyelitis was treated on the principles of Winnett Orr (1877–1956), an American surgeon. The treatment consisted of a combination of conservative and radical approaches.

The management required one primary operation which was performed at any stage, during which a trial to remove all the visible infection was aimed. He promoted the use of liberal incisions to expose the maximum diseased necrotic areas of the bone and promoted "saucerization" of the cavity to maximize drainage. The incision sites were left open and dressing was done with vaseline gauges. He even advocated the use of plaster to immobilize the affected limb in neutral position. The plasters were changed to prevent secondary infection and maintain hygiene. During that time, he relied on the patient's natural tissue defense mechanism to fight the disease and did not use any antiseptics. The use of braces for prolonged immobilized patients to achieve functional mobility were advocated in the later stages [17]. Trueta during the Spanish war added *sulphonamides* to the dressing of wounds and introduced the "closed plaster technique" for healing [18].

In 1948, a paper from the Royal Hospital for Sick Children in Glasgow first illustrated the benefits of *penicillin* in osteomyelitis. It elaborated that before the introduction of chemotherapeutic agents like *sulphonamides*, the mortality of osteomyelitis was very high in spite of incisional drainage as previously advocated. Patients admitted with toxemia due to infection of the bone had little improvement even after treatment of local bony focus and the infection failed to arrest. The surgical intervention previously advocated were incision and drainage of soft tissue abscesses, drilling, immobilization, and even amputation. On post-mortem of these patients, it was observed that the spread occurred in the form of lung abscesses, purulent pericarditis, and widespread pyemia [19].

It was observed that between 1936 and 1940, out of 69 patients, 23 expired with a mortality of 33% as compared to a mortality of 10% (7/70) patients from the year 1941–1945. These septicemic patients (30/70) were treated with "penicillin" and after a follow-up, 93% (28/30) depicted no signs of bony disease on radiographic imaging. During that time, continuous infusion of antibiotic was less favored compared to intermittent intramuscular injections as it was found to be more suitable in children [19].

2.4 Evolution of Antibiotic Treatment

Early twentieth century depicted clearer understanding of the difference between *acute* and *chronic osteomyelitis*. Acute osteomyelitis was found to be *bacteremic* in origin, whereas chronic cases we found to be due to the continuous spread from an *infective focus*. The earliest treatment of such cases was described by Penberthy and Weller in 1941, where 19 cases were treated with *sulfapyridine* and *sulfathiazole* [20]. In 1947, Lamphier reported the use of intramuscular *streptomycin* in chronic osteomyelitis for 5–7 days in patients suffering from injuries during the World War II, depicting promising results [21]. The major groundbreaking improvement was achieved in the 1940s due to the introduction of *Penicillin* [19]. In the 1960s, there was widespread development of *Penicillin-resistant-Staphylococcus aureus*, depicting the need for newer agents. Cullen et al. published a comparative study between tetracyclines and penicillin for treatment of osteomyelitis. The study reported lower rates of complications and higher early hospital discharges in patients treated with tetracyclines [22]. Waldvogel et al. mentioned use or adequate doses of antibiotics by parenteral route and introducing the concept of antibiotic bone penetration [23]. In 1980, the introduction of *Fluoroquinolones* revolutionized the treatment for infective cases. Studies have reported up to 70% recovery rate by the use of these agents [24]. In the 1980s, further animal studies depicted the benefits of the use of *Vancomycin* and *Rifampicin* for the treatment [25].

2.5 Acute Hematogenous Osteomyelitis

In 1951, Wilkinson stated that acute hematogenous osteomyelitis required early and adequate treatment with penicillin, which prevents it from becoming a fatal or crippling disease. He even stated that early diagnosis was imperative in preventing complications and prolonged illness. With the treatment of penicillin sequestration,

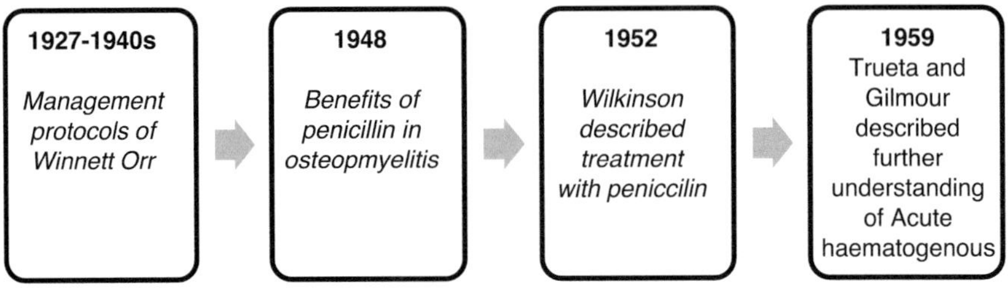

Fig. 2.3 Evolution of management of osteomyelitis over the years

flare-ups, sinus formation, and even involvement of nearly joint and bone were found to less common [26]. Furthermore, in 1983, Nade et al. stated acute osteomyelitis as a "curable disease" [27].

Josep Trueta, a Spanish surgeon, is credited for further understanding of acute hematogenous osteomyelitis in 1959. Based on the blood supply of the bone, he reported three types of forms.

He even explained that penicillin alone failed to achieve what surgery could offed the patients and thus credited surgical treatment superior and more effective [28].

Gilmour analyzed 328 cases of osteomyelitis in which from 1944 to 1950 the patients treated with penicillin gave excellent results, however, subsequently this treatment led to the development of *penicillin-resistant-staphylococci*, depicting new characteristics in the form of age incidence and severity. Increased incidence was observed in neo-natal infants and early operation did not prevent sequestrum formation and hematogenous spread; however, decompression was found to still have its benefits. The role of periosteum to provide adequate supply and prevent cortical necrosis was also understood [29] (Fig. 2.3).

2.6 Primary Sub-acute Pyogenic Osteomyelitis

In 1864, *periostitis albuminosa* was described by Ollier as a special type of bone necrosis as local cortical involvement caused by organisms of low virulence. This was further elaborated by Kuth in 66 cases [30].

It was first described by Harris and Kirkaldy-Willis in 1965 in grave detail. The primary clinical features involved a long history, ranging from weeks to months. It also involved minimal systemic features with little physical signs. Erythrocyte sedimentation rate and staphylococcal antibody titers aid in the diagnosis. Avoiding unnecessary empirical antibiotics along with use of organism-specific antibiotics is advocated [31]. Rasool Mn from Durban published findings which reinforced these observations by describing the condition in 21 children occurring due to decreased bacterial virulence and increased host resistance [32]. In the 1970s, a group of authors from Glasgow described the roles of antibiotics in such cases in the form of two papers. In a study based on 113 children, he advocated the judicious use of antibiotics with indication of surgery, where clinically pus was evident. They described the emergence of penicillin resistance in the last 10 years [33, 34]. In 2001, the further decline in acute and subacute forms of osteomyelitis from 1990 to 1997 was reported in children below the age group of 13 years. There was a fall of 44% in these forms of osteomyelitis by the judicious use of antibiotics, with only 20% patients requiring surgery. And 10% presenting with complications. Hematogenous osteomyelitis in that paper was termed as a rare entity with an annual incidence of 2.9 per 100,000 of the population as compared to the previous prevalence in 1948 [35].

Comprehensive paper by Nade in 1983 regarding this topic still holds true in the basic principles to be followed in clinical practice with regards to acute osteomyelitis [27].

2.7 Evolution of Treatment of Chronic Osteomyelitis

The differentiation between chronic osteomyelitis and tuberculosis of the bone was not understood until Koch isolated the tubercle bacillus in 1882 [36]. Rowling et al. by 1959 reported a positive approach to treat chronic osteomyelitis, requiring surgery to improve the blood supply over the scarred and affected bone. The involved bone requires excision of the affected soft tissue and scarring to improve recovery for adequate delivery of antibiotics over the bone that is chronically affected. They even advocated the use of muscle grafts, flaps over the *dead space* left after *debridement* to promote recovery [37]. Kirkcaldy and Rowling by 1970s further elaborated on the treatment with use of Fucidin, penetrating sufficiently over the bone. It was discussed that it was easier to remove the sequestrum than to tackle the remaining dead space left after excision [38]. Some dead spaces were resistant to treatment with flaps, which led to the introduction of use of *cancellous bone chips*. Introduced by De Oliveira in 120 patients gave satisfactory results and were found to be resistant to infection, with relapse in only four cases [39]. Furthermore, McNally et al. from Belfast advocated the staged treatment by reporting a series of 37 patients, in which the first stage required liberal excision of all the infected tissue and bone followed by the second stage carried out after 3–6 weeks in which grafting and bone chips from iliac crest were incorporated in the dead space [40].

The "lautenbach method" was found to be successful in the treatment of chronic osteomyelitis, reported in a series in 2004 over a span of mean 12.5 years. It involved debridement, reaming, and the insertion of intramedullary tubes with double lumina for the delivery of local antibiotics, analysis of bacterial culture, and adequate irrigation. The inner tube consisted of a central venous line for delivery of antibiotic and the outer tube contained a large suction drain. The end point of debridement was regarded as when the irrigation fluid produced three consecutive clear cultures and obliteration of volume cavity [41]. Professor Simpson and colleagues from Edinburgh reported the importance of thorough excision of infection as the primary goal to achieve elimination of the disease by *liberal debridement* by reporting a study of 50 patients treated with three forms of treatment in the form of:

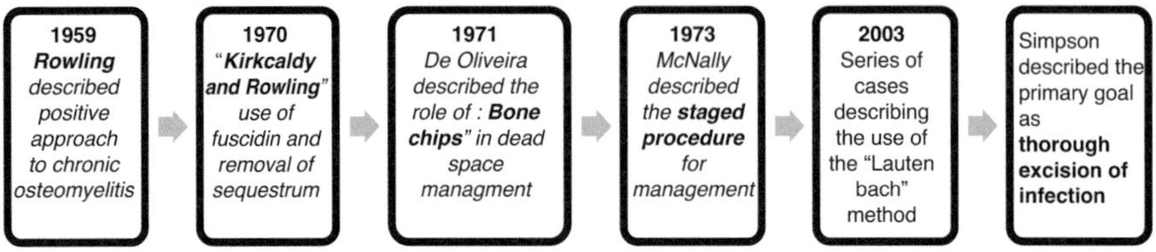

Fig. 2.4 Evolution of management of chronic osteomyelitis over the years

Group 1: wide resection, with a clear margin of 5 mm or more post-debridement
Group 2: Marginal resection, with a clearance of less than 5 mm
Group 3: Intralesional biopsy with debulking of the infected area

All patients received 6 weeks of intravenous antibiotic treatment followed by oral antibiotic delivery for another 6 weeks. No reoccurrence was found in group 1 reiterating the importance of liberal excision. The marginal resection group 8/29 (28%) had a recurrence and the group 3 involving debulking, reoccurrence was found in all patients within 1 year of surgery [42] (Fig. 2.4).

In 1963, a case report of the only example of virus infection of the bone "Osteomyelitis variolosa" due to smallpox was reported from Zimbabwe, now thankfully eradicated [43]. In 1951, Gallie and colleagues reported the first reoccurrence of osteomyelitis after 80 years in a 90-year-old woman after suffering from *brodie's abscess* at the age of 10 years, depicting the silent and dormant nature of the infection [44].

2.8 Conclusion

Infection of the bone and joint has been described since centuries. Various terms have evolved over decades describing the condition of the bone, which further led to development of various management tactics over the years for improving patient mortality. This was first initiated by better understanding of the progression of the pathology, along with etiology of the disease. The mechanism of progression of the infection in the bone proposed by various authors led to evolution of the management protocols, which have been contributed from all parts of the world over centuries. These management principles like extensive debridement, dead space management, and antibiotic therapy still hold true in current times. The introduction of antibiotics revolutionized the treatment strategy leading to the transition from a highly fatal condition to a treatable disease.

References

1. Moodie RL. Paleopathology. An introduction to the study of ancient evidence of disease, vol. 400. Urbana: University of Illinois Press; 1923. p. plate-78.

2. Breasted JH. The Edwin Smith Surgical papyrus (facsimile and hieroglyphic transliteration with translation and commentary, in two volumes). Chicago: The University of Chicago Press; 1930.
3. Chadwick J, Mann WN. The medical works of Hippocrates. Oxford: Blackwell Scientific Publications; 1950.
4. Monro A. The anatomy of the human bones. J. Balfour; 1768.
5. Bromfield W. Chirurgical observations and cases, vol. II. London: Cadall T.; 1773.
6. Brodie BC. An account of some cases of chronic abscess of the tibia. Med Chir Trans. 1832;17:239–49. https://doi.org/10.1177/095952873201700111. PMID: 20895586; PMCID: PMC2116712.
7. Smith N. Medical and surgical memoirs. Baltimore: William A. Francis; 1831. p. 97.
8. Nelaton A. Elements de pathologie chirurgical. Paris: Germer Bailliere; 1844. p. 586–595–7.
9. Cavaillon JM, Legout S. Louis Pasteur: between myth and reality. Biomolecules. 2022;12(4):596. https://doi.org/10.3390/biom12040596. PMID: 35454184; PMCID: PMC9027159.
10. Ogston A. Report upon micro-organisms in surgical diseases. Br Med J. 1881;1:369–75.
11. Majno G, Joris I. Billroth and penicillium. Rev Infect Dis. 1979;1(5):880–4.
12. Rosenbach J. In recent essays by various authors on bacteria in relation to disease. London: New Sydenham Society. W. Watson Cheyne, ed; 1886. p. 397.
13. Rodet A. Etude experimentale sur l'osteomyelite infectieuse. C R Acad Sci. 1884;99:569–71.
14. Wilensky AO. The pathogenesis of the end results of the lesions of acute osteomyelitis. Ann Surg. 1926;84(5):651.
15. Lister J. On a new method of treating compound fracture, abscess, etc.: with observations on the conditions of suppuration. Lancet. 1867;89(2272):326–9.
16. Baer WS. The treatment of chronic osteomyelitis with the maggot (larva of the blow fly). JBJS. 1931;13(3):438–75.
17. Orr HW. The treatment of acute osteomyelitis by drainage and rest. J Bone Joint Surg. 1927;9:733–9.
18. Trueta J. Principles and practice of war surgery. Postgrad Med J. 1943;19(217):279.
19. Dennison WM. Haematogenous osteitis in children. J Bone Joint Surg (Br). 1948;39-B:110–23.
20. Penberthy GC, Weller CN. Chemotherapy as an aid in the management of acute osteomyelitis. Ann Surg. 1941;114:129–46.
21. Lamphier TA, Cashman C. Treatment of chronic osteomyelitis with streptomycin; a preliminary report. N Engl J Med. 1947;236:318–21.
22. Cullen CH, Hargadon EJ. Penicillin verus tetracycline in the treatment of childhood osteomyelitis. Acta Paediatr. 1962;51:189–96.
23. Waldvogel FA, Medoff G, Swartz MN. Osteomyelitis: a review of clinical features, therapeutic considerations and unusual aspects. N Engl J Med. 1970;282:198–206.
24. Norrby SR. Ciprofloxacin in the treatment of acute and chronic osteomyelitis: a review. Scand J Infect Dis Suppl. 1989;60:74–8.
25. Norden CW, Bryant R, Palmer D, et al. Chronic osteomyelitis caused by *Staphylococcus aureus*: controlled clinical trial of nafcillin therapy and nafcillin-rifampin therapy. South Med J. 1986;79:947–51.
26. Wilkinson FR. Acute haematogenous osteomyelitis. J Bone Joint Surg (Br). 1951;33-B:6–7.
27. Nade S. Acute haematogenous osteomyelitis in infancy and childhood. J Bone Joint Surg (Br). 1983;65-B:109–19.
28. Trueta J. The three types of acute haematogenous osteomyelitis: a clinical and vascular study. J Bone Joint Surg (Br). 1959;41-B:671–80.
29. Gilmour WN. Acute haematogenous osteomyelitis. J Bone Joint Surg (Br). 1962;44-B:841–53.
30. Kuth JR. Subacute infections of bone: osteoperiostitis albuminosa ollier. Arch Surg. 1938;37(1):46–73.
31. Harris NH, Kirkaldy-Willis WH. Primary subacute pyogenic osteomyelitis. J Bone Joint Surg (Br). 1965;47-B:526–32.

32. Rasool MN. Primary subacute haematogenous osteomyelitis in children. J Bone Joint Surg (Br). 2001;83-B:93–8.
33. Blockey NJ, Watson JT. Acute osteomyelitis in children. J Bone Joint Surg (Br). 1970;52-B:77–87.
34. Blockey NJ, McAllister TA. Antibiotics in acute osteomyelitis in children. J Bone Joint Surg (Br). 1972;54-B:299–309.
35. Blyth MJG, Kincaid R, Craigen MAC, Bennet GC. The changing epidemiology of acute and subacute haematogenous osteomyelitis in children. J Bone Joint Surg (Br). 2001;83-B:99–102.
36. Die Aetiologie der Tuberculose von Dr. Robert Koch. Ausw: Berliner Klinische Wochenschrift, Band 19 (1882) [The etiology of tuberculosis by Dr. Robert Koch. From the Berliner Klinische Wochenschrift, Volume 19 (1882)]. Zentralbl Bakteriol Mikrobiol Hyg A Med Mikrobiol Infekt Parasitol. 1982;251(3):287–96. German. PMID: 6805152.
37. Rowling DE. The positive approach to chronic osteomyelitis. J Bone Joint Surg (Br). 1959;41-B:681–8.
38. Rowling DE, Kirkcaldy. Further experience in the management of chronic osteomyelitis. J Bone Joint Surg (Br). 1970;52-B:302–7.
39. De Oliveira JC. Bone grafts and chronic osteomyelitis. J Bone Joint Surg (Br). 1971;53-B:672–83.
40. McNally MA, Small JO, Tofighi HG, Mollan RA. Two-stage management of chronic osteomyelitis of the long bones: the Belfast technique. J Bone Joint Surg (Br). 1993;75-B:375–80.
41. Hashmi MA, Norman P, Saleh M. The management of chronic osteomyelitis using the Lautenbach method. J Bone Joint Surg (Br). 2004;86-B:269–75.
42. Simpson AH, Deakin M, Latham JM. Chronic osteomyelitis: the effect of the extent of surgical resection on infection-free survival. J Bone Joint Surg (Br). 2001;83-B:403–7.
43. Davidson JC, Bulawayo PE. Osteomyelitis variolosa. J Bone Joint Surg (Br). 1963;45-B:687–93.
44. Gallie WE. First recurrence of osteomyelitis eighty years after infection. J Bone Joint Surg Br. 1951;33-B(1):110–1. https://doi.org/10.1302/0301-620X.33B1.110. PMID: 14814172.

Microbiological Aspects of Bone and Joint Infections

3

Rajendra Gudisa and Parakriti Gupta

Abstract

Bone and joint infections (BJI) contribute to significant morbidity and mortality. The epidemiology has undergone several changes over last decade, following the advent of molecular diagnostics and non-culture-based methods. A plethora of commensal and fastidious organisms have been implicated in BJIs, which vary in native and prosthetic joints. Common etiological agents include *Staphylococcus aureus*, Other *Staphylococcus* sp., *Enterococcus* sp., Enterobacterales, intracellular bacteria, Mycobacteria, anaerobes, *Salmonella, K. kingae* and rarely fungi and parasites. Polymicrobial infections are common subsequent to trauma and chronic ulcers, in diabetic patients, while *Cutibacterium acnes* and Other *Staphylococcus* sp. are incriminated in prosthetic joint infections. Multiple sampling is suggested for septic arthritis, osteomyelitis and prosthetic joint infections, wherein at least five samples should be collected. Samples obtained from deeper tissues should be preferred, whenever possible. All the sampling should be performed under aseptic conditions, and sample is transported to laboratory within 2 h of collection. Microbiological diagnosis includes direct microscopy using Gram staining, Giemsa staining, potassium-hydroxide calcofluor stain and Ziehl-Neelsen staining, culture, serology, biomarkers and molecular diagnosis. Culture is usually performed on routine blood and MacConkey agar, however, chocolate agar supplemented with PolyViteX and Schaedler agar, RCM, brain heart infusion broth, Schaedler or Rosenow broth should also be inoculated to identify fastidious organisms. Automated blood culture bottles with enhanced diagnostic yield are significant in identification of common and fastidious, slow-

R. Gudisa
AIIMS Vijaypur, Jammu, India

P. Gupta (✉)
Department of Microbiology, Government Medical College & Hospital, Chandigarh, India

P. Kumar et al. (eds.), *Textbook of Orthopedic Infections*,
https://doi.org/10.1007/978-981-95-5029-6_3

growing organisms. Caution is required for extended incubation of bacterial and fungal cultures. Non-culture-based diagnosis with lesser turnaround time (TAT) integrates conventional biomarkers like interferon-gamma release assays (IGRA), IL-6, C-reactive protein, and newer biomarkers like leucocyte esterase, alpha defensin, calprotectin, presepsin and neopterin. Molecular modalities viz. conventional and real-time polymerase chain reaction (PCR), with or without multiplexing, PCR electrospray ionization mass spectrometry have less TAT and better accuracy. The evolving next-generation sequencing techniques like ion-torrent, Illumina, Applied Biosystems Sequencing by oligonucleotide ligation and detection system (SOLiD), oxford nanopore; mNGS and syndromic platforms are being increasingly used for precise identification, with less TAT. Timely precise diagnosis and management of BJIs mandates comprehensive understanding of host-microbe interactions, biofilm dynamics, pharmacokinetics-pharmacodynamics and susceptibility profile of etiological agents.

Keywords
Septic arthritis · Prosthetic joint infections · *S. aureus* · Microbiological · Diagnosis

3.1 Introduction

Bone and joint infections (BJI) constitute broad continuum of infections affecting bones, joints, surrounding soft tissue and muscles. Though considered uncommon as compared to other infectious diseases, BJI account for substantial morbidity and mortality, underlining the need for timely diagnosis and management [1]. Infection is common among children and adults, more in developing regions of Australia, Africa and Asia. The epidemiology of BJIs has evolved with time, and the agents responsible for infections have changed with the introduction of universal immunization programs, across the globe [2].

BJIs have been classified based on either the anatomical site involved (joint, bone, rachis or implant-related etc.), clinical presentation (septic arthritis or osteomyelitis etc.), pathological basis (pyogenic or granulomatous etc.), microbiological basis (pyogenic, fungal or mycobacterial etc.) or evolution (subacute, acute or chronic). Septic arthritis, osteomyelitis, diabetic foot osteomyelitis, implant-related and spinal infections are among the substantial set of infections, which require prompt diagnosis and management. With the advancement in diagnostic and preventive strategies, microbiology of BJI has evolved. Vaccination drive and inclusion of *H. influenzae* vaccination in universal immunization programs has led to drastic decline in *H. influenzae* infections. The dawn of molecular biology and non-culture-based methods has revolutionized the diagnosis of BJI, which has unveiled newer significant agents implicated in BJIs. These tests have alleviated the identification of fastidious and slow-growing bacteria, within short turnaround time (TAT). Moreover, the antimicrobial susceptibility and presence of resistance-encoding genes can be determined precisely. Despite availability of newer improved diagnostic tests, a steady increase in BJIs has been noted owing to increased life expectancy and enhanced usage of prostheses. Consequently, diagnosis of BJIs demands caution, supplemented with standard microbiological procedures, owing to the presence of biofilms and varied metabolic states of same microorganism at the same site, leading to phenotypic expression as small colony variants (SCV), with simultaneous presence of anaerobes. Furthermore, pharmacokinetics and pharmacodynamics of antimicrobials needs to be taken into account, before sampling and reporting, as few antibiotics persist in bone for longer durations [3].

3.2 Etiology of BJIs

The etiological agents implicated in BJI vary depending on host factors like age, immune status, presence of co-morbidities (human immunodeficiency virus [HIV] or tuberculosis [TB]), presence of prosthesis, history of trauma and acquisition of infection, if it's community or hospital-acquired. Majority of the microorganisms are usually members of patient's own microbiome, that is, commensals of skin or mucosal surfaces of gastrointestinal or urogenital tract, the most common agent being *Staphylococcus aureus*. Other pathogens include Gram-positive cocci like Other *Staphylococcus* sp., *Enterococcus* sp., Gram-negative bacteria of order Enterobacterales, intracellular bacteria, Mycobacteria, anaerobes and rarely fungi and parasites. *Salmonella* is predominantly implicated in patients with sickle-cell disease, while *Serratia* and *Aspergillus* are common among patients with chronic granulomatous disease [4]. Exogenous infections are common perioperatively, and are caused by skin commensals. On the contrary, Gram-negative organisms are frequently reported following instrumentation, when in close proximity to gastrointestinal or urogenital tract. Polymicrobial infections are commonly observed following traumatic open fractures and chronic ulcers, in diabetic patients, with deranged wound healing and obese patients. The etiology varies for prosthetic joint infections (PJIs), wherein *Cutibacterium acnes* and Other *Staphylococcus* sp. are also commonly incriminated.

3.3 Pathogenesis

BJIs occur as a consequence of dysregulated crosstalk between osteoblasts and osteoclasts, induced by infectious agents, hampering the bone homeostasis. Healthy bone tissue is usually resilient to invasion, however, factors like diabetes mellitus, intravenous drug use (IVDU), trauma, prosthesis, surgery, high-dose corticosteroid therapy, HIV, chemotherapy, rheumatoid arthritis and elderly age, predispose the patients to infectious pathology. The pathogens can directly colonize the bone, infecting and killing the cells, or follow an ancillary mechanism, wherein the host immune response leads to cascade of pro-inflammatory cytokines (IL-1β, TNFα, IL-6 and macrophage-stimulating growth factors), which in turn dysregulate the balance between bone formation by osteoblasts and resorption by osteoclasts.

BJIs can result either from hematogenous or contiguous spread, but can also be a direct outcome of traumatic inoculation or proceed surgical procedures. In children, hematogenous spread is more common, while traumatic or post-surgical inoculation is commonly noted among adults. Overall, hematogenous spread is the most common mode of spread for septic arthritis and acute osteomyelitis, with *S. aureus* as the most commonly implicated agent. The hematogenous spread can also occur following primary or reactivated focus elsewhere in body, like spinal infection trail the seeding from genitourinary infections and endocarditis.

Direct inoculation usually occurs following trauma, steroid infusion and open wounds (bites or penetrating trauma). Trauma might cause devascularization of the site, with perilesional hematoma, which acts as seeding site for bacterial colonization by skin and mucosal flora. Infection can also occur post-surgery and can rarely be iatrogenic, following arthroscopy and arthrography. PJIs occurring within 1 year are considered a consequence of intraoperative inoculation, either from patient's skin flora, gloves of the operating surgeon or contaminated instruments [5]. Contiguous mode is the result of spread of infection from a nearby focus, and is commonly noted in septic arthritis of infants, owing to the existing vascular anastomoses.

3.4 Septic Arthritis

Septic arthritis (SA) is an orthopedic emergency that can cause substantial damage to joints. It is reported amongst children and adults, but is more common in children <5 years of age owing to highly vascularity [6]. SA mainly involves large joints, knee joint being the principal target in adults. Hip and knee joint are almost equally affected in children. In infants, vascular anastomoses between epiphysis and metaphysis enable the contiguous spread of infection. The predominant etiology of SA is monomicrobial, with *S. aureus* trailed by *Streptococcus* as the common agents. Polymicrobial infection with Gram-negative bacilli, *S. pneumoniae*, *S. agalactiae* and *N. gonorrhoeae* has been reported. *Streptococcus pyogenes* (Group A *Streptococcus*) has been reported from patients following trauma or in patients with autoimmune disorders, chronic skin infections, while *Streptococcus agalactiae* (Group B *Streptococcus*) is noted in patients with diabetes and cirrhosis. Cases with Group C, F and G *Streptococci* have also been reported [7]. Age-wise etiological agents of SA have been depicted in Table 3.1. On the contrary, Gram-negative bacilli account for ~10–20%, and is common among IVDU and elderly patients. Of these, non-fermenting Gram-negative bacilli like *Pseudomonas aeruginosa*, *Acinetobacter baumannii*, *Burkholderia cepacia*, *B. cenocepacia*, *B. pseudomallei* and *Stenotrophomonas maltophilia* are commonly isolated from patients who have undergone any medical procedures in hospital. SA can also occur as a consequence of systemic complication following gonococcal infection in 30–90% of cases. A recent rise in SA following *N. gonorrhoeae* has been reported, owing to the unsafe sexual behavior, improved diagnostic modalities and escalating antimicrobial resistance [8]. *Salmonella* is implicated in bone and joint infections in patients with

Table 3.1 Age-wise etiological agents of septic arthritis

Age group	Etiological organisms
Neonates <2 months	*Streptococcus* sp., especially Group B Streptococci (*S. agalactiae*) Gram-negative organisms, especially *E. coli* *S. aureus*
2 months-5 years	*S. pyogenes, Kingella kingae*
>5 years	*S. aureus*
Infants	*S. aureus* *H. influenzae*
Children	*S. aureus* *Salmonella* sp., especially in patients with sickle cell anaemia *S. pneumoniae* *S. pyogenes*
Adolescents	*S. aureus* *Streptococcus* sp. *Neisseria gonorrhoeae*
Adults	*S. aureus* *Pseudomonas aeruginosa* *E. coli* *Serratia marcescens* Other *Staphylococcus* sp.
Patients with defects in cell-mediated immunity	Intracellular bacteria Fungi
Intravenous drug abusers	*S. aureus* *P. aeruginosa*
Patients with animal and human bites	*Staphylococcus* sp. *Streptococcus* sp. *Eikenella corrodens* Anaerobes (oral)

sickle cell disease, as local thrombosis following thrombotic crisis predispose intestinal mucosal injuries, which facilitate entry of gastrointestinal pathogens like *Salmonella* in bloodstream [5].

3.4.1 Diagnosis

Since SA is an orthopedic emergency, diagnosis is framed on clinical, radiological and laboratory parameters, in absence of microbiological diagnosis for prompt management. Microbiological diagnosis is, however, necessary for confirmation and to initiate specific treatment. Synovial fluid from the target joint is the sample of choice for SA. The same can be obtained by arthrocentesis, with or without ultrasonographic or radiological assistance [9]. Sample collection should be obtained before initiating antimicrobial treatment; however, treatment ought not be withheld in case of any delay in sample collection, for patients with sepsis and extensive joint damage [9]. Caution should be taken when local anesthesia is used for arthrocentesis, as lidocaine has its own antibacterial activity and can incumber the accurate interpretation of results [5]. Moreover, a small incision prior to initiation of procedure is always suggested, to prevent the introduction of skin commensals. Synovial fluid should preferably be sent in automated blood culture bottles, which can increase the yield by ~20% [9]. Two sets of blood culture should be collected prior to initiation of antimicrobial treatment and surgery. Automated blood culture systems are preferred, as they monitor the cultures continuously on a real-time basis and have better yield with shorter TAT. In cases with surgical interventions, sampling from deeper tissue is the sample of choice. Swabs are not considered appropriate samples as commensals from the swabbed region might convolute the interpretation. Samples are transported as soon as possible to the laboratory, within 2 h of collection. In case the delay is inevitable, transport media, like Robertson's cooked meat (RCM) media, should be used to preserve the anaerobes.

3.5 Osteomyelitis

Osteomyelitis encompasses heterogenous BJIs, wherein microorganisms gain entry into the bone. The same is achieved either by hematogenous route, direct inoculation or the contiguous spread. Of all these routes, hematogenous route remains the most common mode, which commonly infects long bones in prepubertal age. Hematogenous route is most commonly encountered in osteomyelitis of long bones. The progress of infection following hematogenous spread varies with age of the patient (Fig. 3.1).

Direct inoculation is a result of penetrating injury, trauma, open compound fractures or is a post-surgical event. The degree of tissue damage, bone integrity and host defense influence the extent of infection. Moreover, subsequent surgical interventions might augment the ongoing vascular injury, which indirectly hastens the spread of infection via osteonecrosis. This extends the infection to extra-osseus sites and culminates into osteomyelitis. The spread of infection and progress of acute to chronic phase of osteomyelitis has been depicted in Fig. 3.2. On the contrary, contiguous spread is common following decubitus ulcer in elderly, adjacent burn wounds and periodontal disease in adults, wherein inflammatory process destroys the articular surface, facilitating progress to the bone.

Acute infection via hematogenous route is commonly noted in children <5 years of age, with *S. aureus* as commonly implicated organism in 70–90% of cases. However, premature infants with necrotizing enterocolitis are commonly infected with pathogens of gastrointestinal tract, as they are prone to microbe translocation from the gut [5]. Agents like *S. agalactiae* are noted among infants <3 months of age, while *S. pyogenes, K. kingae* and *S. pneumoniae* are common among children of 3 months to 5 years of age. *H. influenzae* infections have declined tremendously after the introduction of Hib vaccine, however, the same doesn't hold true for *S. pneumoniae*, as strains included in vaccination vary from the ones implicated in illness. *Salmonella* is common among patients with sickle cell disease, while *Serratia* and *Aspergillus* infect patients with chronic granulomatous disease. In

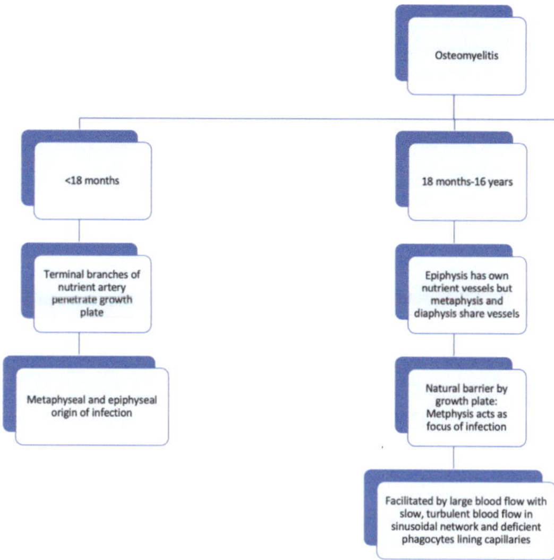

Fig. 3.1 Age-wise spread of osteomyelitis

patients with burn wounds, infection is usually polymicrobial in nature and spread is contiguous. *Staphylococcus* and *Streptococcus* are usual pathogens, while Gram-negative pathogens can also be isolated in hospitalized patients. Puncture wounds might lead to osteomyelitis in ~1.5% of soft tissue infections, with *Pseudomonas* and *Eikenella* as common pathogen (90% cases). The same might be ascribed to the presence of *Ps. aeruginosa* in spongy liner of the sneakers and the commonly used prophylaxis with mere Gram-positive coverage. *Eikenella* is a part of oral microbiota, and thereby, puncture wounds due to injury by toothpicks predispose to this infection [10]. These post-traumatic wounds can have a long course, with tendency to become chronic. The infection becomes polymicrobial during their chronic course, and common agents include *S. aureus*, *Streptococcus*, Gram-negative bacteria and rarely, anaerobic bacteria.

3.5.1 Diagnosis

Diagnosis of osteomyelitis can be achieved using aspiration from abscess, under CT-guided or ultrasonographic guidance. Samples should preferably be collected prior to the initiation of antimicrobial therapy. Samples obtained from deeper tissues are preferred, and similar to SA, at least five samples should be obtained, at the beginning of surgery. In osteomyelitis, the preferred sites include fragments of necrotic bone, fracture impact site, site of non-union, deeper tissues, necrotic tissue, sequestrum and bone-metalwork interface. Blood culture is of utmost significance in children as most of these infections are hematogenous. Automated blood culture bottles are of significance in improving yield of bacteria from other samples.

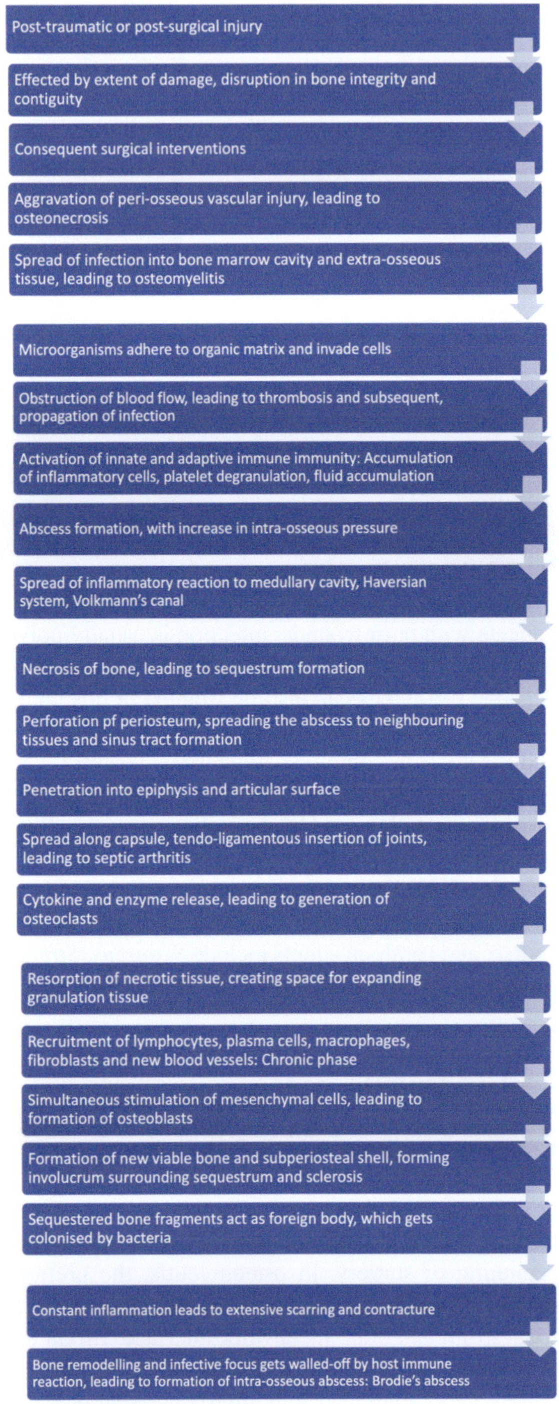

Fig. 3.2 Mechanism of osteomyelitis

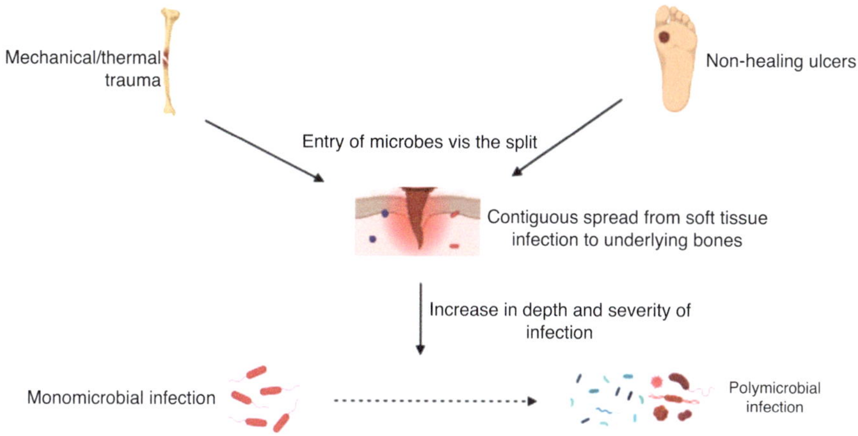

Fig. 3.3 Mechanism of diabetic foot osteomyelitis

3.6 Diabetic Foot Osteomyelitis

In diabetics, osteomyelitis of foot is encountered in ~15–50% of infections [11]. The disease commonly affects weight-bearing bones of forefoot, viz. calcaneum, fifth metatarsal head and first metatarsal head. Risk of osteomyelitis is more in ulcers >2 cm^2, when patient has persistent hyperglycemia, along with neuropathy and vasculopathy. The disease process starts with non-healing ulcer, or post-trauma. Trauma causes a nick in overlying envelope, which facilitates the contiguous spread to underlying bones (Fig. 3.3). The implicated microorganisms infect the cortex, followed by marrow. As the infection becomes chronic, initial monomicrobial nature changes to polymicrobial; and diabetic foot osteomyelitis (DFO) usually presents as polymicrobial infection. *S. aureus* is the most commonly implicated organism, trailed by *Pseudomonas*, Other *Staphylococcus* sp., *E. coli*, *Proteus*, *Enterococcus* and *Streptococcus* sp. Besides these aerobic pathogens, anaerobes like *Bacteroides* and *Peptostreptococcus* sp. have also been isolated.

3.6.1 Diagnosis

Diagnosis of DFO is commonly attained using swab culture from wound, which isn't the recommended specimen, as it gets difficult to differentiate commensals from true pathogens. The deeper tissues should be sampled whenever possible, and in cases where wound swab is the only specimen available, Levine technique should be followed [12]. Soft tissue and bone samples also fail to provide optimal results many a times, which is vital before surgical interventions and patients at high risk of progressive infections. In such scenarios, percutaneous bone biopsies obtained under CT or fluoroscopic guidance should be preferred [5].

3.7 Prosthetic Infections

With the advent of effective treatment strategies and increased life expectancy, prostheses are being increasingly used for restoring function to improve quality of life and to combat the damaged bones and joints. Once implanted, these prosthetic materials are prone to tissue interactions. This prosthesis-tissue interaction is influenced by varied factors like composition of prosthesis, surface configuration and asepsis during implantation. Few studies have noted differences between metal-to-metal hinged and metal-to-plastic hinged or cemented and uncemented prostheses, however, no conclusive evidence is available [13]. Perioperative factors viz. duration of surgery, surgical site infection, allogenic blood transfusion and presence of distant infection at the time of surgery also affect the outcome. It has been noted that an additional increase of 15 min in surgery time increases the risk of infection by 9% [13]. Post-operative wound dehiscence, hematoma formation and subsequent wound drainage pose the risk of infection, when left untreated. Host factors like gender, body mass index >35, diabetes mellitus, rheumatoid arthritis and immunosuppression, increase the risk of infection. Males are affected more than females, which has been attributed to smoking habits in males, affecting oxygenation and blood flow to bone and joints at the time of surgery [13]. In diabetic patients, there is hyperglycemia along with dysfunctional leucocytes, which enhance the biofilm formation and delays wound healing at the site of trauma or surgery. Rheumatoid arthritis might predispose the patients by disease process itself or use of biological disease-modifying anti-rheumatic drugs (DMARDs), as these drugs act by inhibiting IL-6 and TNF-α. Thereby, the American College of Rheumatology has recommended withholding these biological DMARDs drugs peri-operatively for arthroplasty or revision of the prosthesis [14]. Allogenic blood transfusion, even after leucocyte reduction upsurges the infection due to its immunomodulatory effects. Moreover, distant infections at the time of surgery lead to transient bacteremia, especially during the high-risk period, seeding the bacteria to prosthesis. Any antecedent septic arthritis or bacteremia also increase the risk of infection for ongoing event. In view of these multiple risk factors, few composite risk scores have been formulated to alleviate the decision-making for management. The National Nosocomial Infections Surveillance System includes American Society of Anesthesiologists (ASA) pre-operative score, length of procedure and surgical wound classification. On the contrary, Mayo PJI score is divided into baseline score and one-month postoperative risk score, which includes body mass index, previous surgery of index joint, immunosuppression, ASA score, length of procedure and wound drainage. The wound drainage is included only in one-month postoperative risk score, and not in baseline score [13, 15, 16].

In the advent of aseptic procedures in an otherwise healthy immunocompetent patient, host immune system gets activated soon after the introduction of prosthesis, when prosthesis interacts with host glycoproteins, following which diapedesis of inflammatory cells ensues, creating electrophysiological and ionic changes at the target site. Neutrophils and macrophages secrete IL-1, TNF-α and IFN- γ, creating a pro-inflammatory environment around the prosthesis. This inflammatory phenomenon can either subside with time in absence of any predisposing factors, assisting the integration of prosthesis in body or might persist, in cases of degradation of prosthesis. Degradation of prosthesis generates fragments, which in turn invoke inflammatory response, culminating in chronic stage. The size, number and density of generated fragments effect the inflammatory response, being more for multiple fragments <5 μm. On the contrary, larger fragments can't be internalised and, thereby, get surrounded by aggregates of inflammatory and phagocytic cells, forming the granuloma. This process further gets complicated by bacterial superinfection, and even a small inoculum is sufficient for initiating the infection. The ongoing process of inflammation leads to generation of few dysfunctional 'frustrated phagocytes', and the cycle continues. The commencement of infection can be a consequence of direct inoculation following trauma, surgery or might be contiguous spread in early infection, whereas late infections usually trail hematogenous route [5] (Fig. 3.4).

Another substantial factor playing a key role in PJIs is 'biofilm formation'. Biofilm formation initiates as mere deposition of planktonic bacteria on the prosthesis, further assisted by deposition of proteinaceous material. The initial phase is regulated by quorum sensing and gene regulation systems, in response to increased expression of autoinducing peptides. The gene expression systems activated virulence genes and other genes responsible for colonization. As the biofilm starts maturing, lysis of bone occurs and polysaccharides with nucleic acids also start depositing on the surface of prosthesis. Bacteria inside the biofilm alter in their growth rate, have slower metabolism, with more persister cells and resist the antimicrobial action. The altered slow growth rate result in small colony variants (SCV), which are commonly seen in *S. aureus* and *Salmonella*. On maturation, planktonic forms are released into environment, establishing a new biofilm elsewhere.

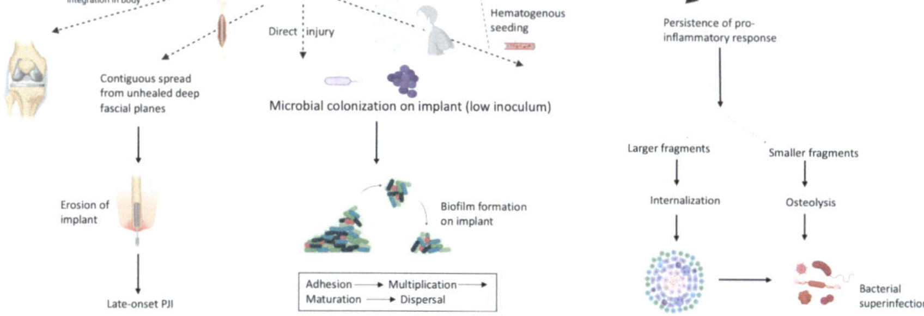

Fig. 3.4 Factors affecting the implant and progress to prosthetic joint infection

The most commonly implicated organism in PJIs include *S. aureus* and Other *Staphylococcus* species (50–60%). *S. aureus* is commonly associated with early and late prosthetic infection, and pose a great risk of prosthesis failure. Of OSS, *S. epidermidis* and *S. lugdunensis* are commonly implicated, especially post-revision arthroplasty. However, lack of automated identification systems delays the diagnosis, in absence of profuse inflammatory response. *S. epidermidis* is the most common OSS implicated in PJIs, owing to its adherence ability, along with biofilm production. *S. lugdunensis* mimics all characteristics of *S. aureus*, except its susceptibility to beta-lactams.

E. faecium and *E. faecalis* are also among common etiological agents (3–15%), however, these are more commonly a part of polymicrobial infection, frequently after hip prosthesis in early and late phases. Enterococci are mostly seeded from gastrointestinal or urinary tract.

Beta-haemolytic Streptococci viz. Group B, C and G *Streptococcus* have been isolated from PJIs (10%). An association between *S. gallolyticus sub*sp. *gallolyticus* with intestinal malignancy has been reported [13]. *S. pneumoniae* and Viridans group of Streptococci are among uncommon causes following hip and knee prostheses. Gram-negative bacteria *like E. coli*, *P. aeruginosa*, *K. pneumoniae* and *Salmonella* also account for substantial number of infections (5–60%), mainly following the hematogenous route. Of all these agents, infections caused by *S. aureus*, *E. faecium* and Gram-negative bacilli are of utmost concern, owing to the rising antimicrobial resistance. Methiciilin-resistant *S. aureus*, vancomycin-resistant Enterococci, carbapenem-resistant Enterobacterales make the treatment of these infections challenging. The treatment gets more perplexed in polymicrobial infections with anaerobes, which account for 3–6% of all PJIs. The infection caused by anaerobes is usually late, follow an indolent course, with less pronounced symptoms. *C. acnes* is among the most common anaerobes implicated in PJIs, especially in shoulder PJIs. The frequent isolation of *C. acnes* has been associated to close proximity with axilla, as *C. acnes* resides in sebaceous follicles of skin, oral cavity, gastrointestinal tract, conjunctiva and external ear. The organism gets inoculated at the time of surgery, and is more commonly isolated from males. Other anaerobes like *Bacteroides fragilis*, *Peptostreptococcus*, *Clostridium* and *Actinomyces* have also been reported from cases of PJIs, mostly as a part of polymicrobial infection. On the contrary, *Actinomyces* are implicated in monomicrobial infections, having weak association with IVDU or dental work. An association between *C. septicum* and intestinal malignancy has been reported, while *C. perfringens* is commonly noted trailing acute cholecystitis [13]. *B. fragilis* has been associated with colonic diverticulum, while *Peptostreptococcus* with periodontal infection. Other uncommon bacteria implicated in PJIs include *Corynebacterium* sp. like *C. jeikeium*, which is resistant to several antimicrobials. *Listeria*, *Brucella*, *C. burnetii* and *P. multocida* have also been isolated from rare cases of PJIs. Of these, *Brucella*, *C. burnetii* and *P. multocida* have zoonotic spread and are usually reported from endemic regions. *Mycobacterium tuberculosis* accounts for ~0.35 cases of PJIs, which increase to ~31% if patient had prior septic arthritis with *M. tuberculosis* complex. PJIs due to *M. avium* complex is noted among people living with HIV/

AIDS and post-solid organ transplant. *Candida albicans* and *C. parapsilosis* are common among fungal infections, which accounts for ~1% of all PJIs. Other fungi like *Aspergillus*, dematiaceous fungi and dimorphic fungi have also been isolated from few cases. Candida accounts for ~80% of all fungal PJIs, and concomitant bacterial infection is noted in ~80% cases.

Despite the advances in microbiological diagnostic techniques, ~7–15% cases of PJIs are still classified as culture-negative, with clinical features suggestive of PJI but recovery of no microorganism from clinical samples. The same has been ascribed to unavailability of precise advanced modalities or improper timing of specimen collection, that is, after initiation of antimicrobial therapy. Studies have revealed that culture-negative PJIs mainly contribute to late onset PJIs, occurring years later of the implant insertion [13].

3.7.1 Diagnosis

Diagnosis of PJIs is usually based on combination of clinical and laboratory parameters. Various clinical criteria have been described by the Musculoskeletal Infection Society (MSIS), the Infectious Diseases Society of America (IDSA), International Consensus Meeting and the European Bone and Joint Infection Society (EBJIS). The MSIS criteria include presence of *definitive* evidence including a sinus tract which communicates with the prosthesis OR isolation of microorganism in culture, from at least two different fluid or tissue samples obtained from affected joint OR four of the six *supportive* criteria, which include increased C-reactive protein (CRP) and erythrocyte sedimentation rate (ESR) in serum, purulence in joint, elevated leucocyte count in synovial fluid, increased neutrophil percentage in synovial fluid, isolation of pathogen in any one culture of fluid or tissue from the affected joint or >5 neutrophils per high-power field in five fields in histologic analysis of tissue. For IDSA, there are three criteria for *definitive* evidence, which includes purulence surrounding the prosthesis, along with two definitive criteria of MSIS, whereas only two *supportive* criteria are followed, that is, isolation of a virulent microorganism in culture or evidence of acute inflammation on histological examination of tissue from affected joint. On the contrary, international consensus includes the same *definitive* evidence as MSIS, while requires three out of five *supportive* criteria, which omits the presence of purulence around the prosthesis [13, 15, 16].

However, the recent PJI definition given by 2018 International Consensus Meeting (ICM) are being followed presently. There are two major and six minor criteria, out of which either of the major criteria should be present to meet the definition, and in absence of these major criteria, minor criteria are considered. The *major* criteria include two positive cultures for the same organism OR presence of sinus tract communicating with the joint or visualization of prosthesis. *Minor* criteria include increased levels of CRP or D-dimer in serum (score of 2), increased serum ESR (score: 1), increased leucocyte count or leucocyte esterase in synovial fluid (score of 3), presence of alpha-defensin in synovial fluid (score: 3), increased neutrophil percentage in synovial fluid (score of 2) and increased CRP in synovial fluid (score: 1). A score of six or more is suggestive of PJI, whereas 2–5 indicates possible PJI and 0–1 is indicative of no infection [16]. *Intraoperative* evidence includes favorable histology (score of 3), purulence (score of 3) and a single culture positive from affected joint (score of 2). A combined score (preoperative and intra-operative) of six or more is suggestive of PJI, while 4–5 is inconclusive and less than 3 indicates absence of infection [16].

Synovial fluid obtained in automated blood culture bottle is considered the most suitable sample for diagnosis of PJIs, which can be obtained under ultrasonographic or radiological guidance. The sample should ideally, be obtained prior to initiation of antimicrobial therapy, which delimits culture-negative PJI, however, the same shouldn't be withheld in cases with sepsis. Sample collection is same as from native joint in cases with septic arthritis. Periprosthetic synovial tissue and interface membrane of bone-prosthesis interface are alternative samples, when synovial fluid can't be attained. It is important to keep in mind that multiple, at least five samples are suggested when dealing with implant infections. The same is considered to enhance the sensitivity and yield of micro-organisms, which is of utmost significance for interpretation, wherein pathogens with low pathogenicity and uncommon pathogens are encountered. Multiple sampling is usually achieved aseptically from necrotic or granulation tissue, synovial tissue, interface membrane between bone and prosthesis.

Sonication can also be employed for implant material, at facilities where sonicator is available. The method is of utmost significance for prosthesis of larger three-dimensional shape, where culture of entire prosthesis isn't feasible and might yield false-positive results. It makes use of low-frequency ultrasonic waves, which help generate areas of varying pressure, which facilitates the dislodgement of biofilm with bacterial colonies present on the implant. The implants are placed in solid sterile airtight containers, along with Ringer's solution or normal saline, so that implant is immersed at least partially in it. The sonicate fluid surrounding the implant can be used for culture or can be subjected to non-culture modalities for early diagnosis. Samples should be transported to laboratory as soon as possible, without delay, preferably within 2 h.

3.8 Laboratory Diagnosis of BJIs

The diagnosis of bone and joint infections are usually based on clinical, radiological and laboratory parameters. The laboratory parameters include both histological and microbiological analysis of the samples. Besides these, peripheral blood tests like ESR and CRP are also substantial in diagnosis. The acceptable samples from bone and joint infections include synovial fluid, tissue obtained from native or prosthetic joints, deeper tissues and necrotic bone tissue. Multiple sampling is suggested for SA and PJIs, wherein at least five samples should be collected. Swabs aren't the preferred specimens, but are frequently used in cases with DFO. All the sampling should be performed under aseptic conditions, and sample is transported to laboratory within 2 h of collection. In cases with delay in transport, transport media should be considered, and RCM should always be inoculated bedside, for better recovery of anaerobic pathogens.

3.8.1 Inflammatory Markers

Serum CRP and ESR are among the frequently used inflammatory markers for diagnosis of infection, and are included among suggestive criteria for diagnosis of PJIs. Both the tests are easily available and have a rapid TAT, but lack specificity. Interleukin-6 (IL-6) is another serum marker of acute inflammation, which returns to normal rapidly after arthroplasty, and this property helps in diagnosis of early onset of infections. However, IL-6 lacks sensitivity and is presently not a part of any diagnostic algorithm. Procalcitonin is highly specific test to rule out the bacterial infections, but lacks sensitivity. It is widely used to differentiate the non-infectious causes of inflammation, in settings with elevated CRP and ESR and normal procalcitonin levels.

3.8.2 Synovial Fluid Analysis

Synovial fluid obtained perioperatively or intraoperatively is subjected to determination of cell count, along with culture. Total nucleated cell count, along with percentage of neutrophils help determine the joint infection. Threshold for the same varies in different settings, and ~1100–1700 total nucleated cells per microliter has shown high sensitivity and specificity [13, 16].

3.8.3 Histological Analysis

The histological evaluation is used to determine the inflammatory reaction, with neutrophil dominance in acute cases. This test can be used for analysis on fresh fluid and tissues, as well as frozen or fixed tissue samples. One of the major advantages of this method is that the result is unlikely to be affected by prior administration of antimicrobials. However, pathogens like Other *Staphylococcus* species and *C. acnes* don't elicit a robust inflammatory response, thereby, lessening the diagnostic utility of this test. This test is also included as supportive criteria for diagnosis of PJIs. Frozen section analysis is substantial as the results are available within half an hour, with positive and negative likelihood ratio of 12 and 0.23, respectively [17].

3.8.4 Microbiological Diagnosis

3.8.4.1 Microscopy

Direct examination of samples is performed using staining, viz. Gram stain for bacteria, potassium iodide-calcofluor staining for fungi, Giemsa for parasites and

May-Grunwald staining for demonstration and semi-quantitative assessment of inflammatory reaction. Gram staining has sensitivity and specificity of 6–30% and 99%, respectively. In septic arthritis, ~10,000 elements are noted per mm^3, of which 90% are neutrophils, however, lesser values are significant in PJIs [5, 13].

Microscopy for acid-fast bacilli is commonly performed using Ziehl-Neelsen staining. The introduction of auramine rhodamine fluorescent staining has decreased the examination time with increased accuracy. Sensitivity of direct microscopy has been noted to be 30–35%, but it fails to distinguish *M. tuberculosis* from non-tubercular mycobacteria (NTM) and gives negative results with low bacterial load [5].

3.8.4.2 Culture

Culture of synovial fluid or periprosthetic tissue is performed both aerobically and anaerobically. For diagnosis of PJIs, culture of sonication fluid has been noted to be highly sensitive, as compared to periprosthetic tissue. Threshold cut-offs vary for interpreting the CFU/ml, with 200 CFU/ml being significant for protocols using centrifugation step, while cut-off ranges from 1 to 10 or 1 to 50 CFU/ml for protocols without the centrifugation step [13]. However, this doesn't hold true for pathogens with known virulence potential like *S. aureus* and members of order Enterobacterales.

Solid media like blood and MacConkey agar are inoculated and incubated for an extended period of minimum 14 days. This is important so that none of the slowly growing and SCV, within the biofilm and lying outside are missed. Besides these routine media, chocolate agar supplemented with PolyViteX and Schaedler agar can be included in the diagnostic workup, to detect the fastidious and anaerobic pathogens. Liquid media, RCM, brain heart infusion broth, Schaedler or Rosenow broth are also inoculated. However, the recent adoption of automated blood culture bottles has shown enhanced diagnostic yield, with greater sensitivity. The method has also shown increased sensitivity for *K. kingae*, a significant agent of SA. The agar plates are read on day 1 and 2, for early reading and for late readings on day 10 and 14. The readings need to be very meticulous to identify SCV which present as microcolonies. The pathogen identified after day 1 or 2 on early diagnosis should not be considered as the sole pathogen, as polymicrobial infections are common (10–15%) and plates should be reported till 14 days of incubation. Polymorphic colonies of same organism with different susceptibility patterns might be observed, and should be interpreted with caution. Median time to detection for *C. acnes* has been noted to be 7–13 days, thereby, underlining the need for extended incubation of cultures [5, 13].

The probability of infection increases with increase in number of samples, probability increasing to 95% with three positive samples [5]. This is of utmost significance when Other *Staphylococcus* species or uncommon pathogens are isolated. Single isolation of pathogen with high virulence like *S. aureus*, Streptococci and Gram-negative pathogens with known pathogenic potential is sufficient for diagnosis.

Infections are rarely caused by uncommon bacteria like *Brucella, Gemella morbillorum, Listeria monocytogenes, Erysipelothrix rhusiopathiae, Hemophilus, Nocardia, Francisella tularensis, Yersinia enterocolitica, Pasteurella multocida, Clostridium difficile,* Actinomyces and *Coxiella burnetii.* Of all these, *Brucella, Francisella tularensis, Yersinia enterocolitica, Pasteurella multocida, Coxiella burnetiid* and *Erysipelothrix rhusiopathiae* are known to have zoonotic spread.

Brucella, being a slow-growing organism, is difficult to isolate in conventional media and takes time to grow. Automated blood culture systems are beneficial in diagnostic yield of these organisms, with short TAT in 5–7 days. The organism can be isolated on blood and chocolate agar, when grown at standard incubation conditions, supplemented with 5% CO2. The suspicion and identification of *Brucella* is of paramount significance as it is the most common zoonotic infections, and the most common laboratory-acquired infection. Any isolate with Gram-negative coccobacilli morphology on Gram-stain and small catalase and oxidase positive colonies on blood agar should be confirmed to be *Brucella* by urease and motility test. This is important not only for diagnosis but to safeguard the health of laboratory personnel, as antimicrobial susceptibility as highly discouraged for *Brucella* for its high risk of transmission.

In scenarios where osteoarticular TB is suspected, culture is performed using solid or liquid media, commonly in Lowenstein-Jensen media (LJ media). However, culture on LJ media has long TAT of 4–8 weeks, poor yield (10–30%), low sensitivity for smear-negative and extrapulmonary samples and is prone to high contamination rate. Thereby, automated Mycobacterium Growth Indicator Tube 960 (MGIT 960) system is preferred, which has shorter TAT and high diagnostic accuracy. All the positive samples are subjected to drug susceptibility testing by line probe assay, as WHO has endorsed universal DST to detect and combat the escalating resistance [18].

Sabouraud dextrose agar and brain heart infusion agar, incubated at 37 and 25 °C are inoculated when suspecting BJI due to fungal infections. The fungal cultures are incubated for a period of 4 weeks, and identified using lactophenol cotton blue preparation. Cultures which can't be identified using conventional methods are diagnosed using molecular modalities.

3.8.4.3 Serological Tests

Serological tests are not routinely performed for etiological agents of BJIs, except for brucellosis. *Brucella* can be diagnosed using standard agglutination test (SAT), IgM enzyme linked immunosorbent assay (ELISA), Rose Bengal or Coomb's test. Of all these tests, SAT is considered the gold standard serological test for diagnosis of brucellosis. A titre of ≥1:160 is considered suggestive, and all the suggestive tests are further confirmed using 2-mercaptoethanol (2-ME). 2-ME is used to differentiate acute infections from chronic ones, as 2-ME breaks the disulfide bonds of IgM, and thereby, a positive test after 2-ME suggests chronic infections. However, cross-reactivity with *Francisella tularensis, Y. enterocolitica, Vibrio cholerae, Stenotrophomonas maltophilia* and *E. coli.* Moreover, SAT fails to detect infection caused by *B. canis*. Serology is also performed for diagnosis of *Coxiella burnetiid* and *Y. enterocolitica* [5].

3.8.4.4 Biomarkers

Leucocyte esterase (LE) in synovial fluid is determined using point-of-care colorimetric strip test. A positive reading for the same has been reported to be 81% sensitive and 100% specific for synovial samples. A high correlation was noted with neutrophil count, as this enzyme is secreted by neutrophils, and this test is incorporated as minor criteria for diagnosis of PJIs, in recent 2018 ICM definition. However, the diagnostic utility of synovial LE is less as compared to positive culture or leucocyte count, but outperforms serum ESR and CRP assays. The 2018 ICM definition has incorporated synovial CRP > 6.9 mg in the minor criteria and a score of 1 is used for the same, however, its role in diagnosis is still debatable. A correlation between serum and synovial levels of CRP has been reported by studies and presently acts as an adjunct for diagnosis of PJIs [16]. Similarly, the role of synovial IL-6 is being studied by authors. Few studies have reported high diagnostic accuracy of synovial IL-6 than CRP, however, synovial IL-6 is presently not part of any PJI definition.

Interferon-gamma release assays (IGRA) were previously used for diagnosis of TB, as these are more reliable than tuberculin test. However, IGRAs lack sensitivity and specificity for the same, especially in countries endemic for TB.

3.8.4.5 Newer Biomarkers

Despite the recent changes in definition and introduction of advanced modalities in microbiological identification, diagnosis remains challenging and introduction of newer biomarkers like alpha defensin, calprotectin, presepsin and neopterin, is need of the hour. Alpha-defensin is secreted by neutrophils, upon activation. This antimicrobial peptide helps in rapid killing of microorganisms, and level of alpha-defensin in synovial fluid, with signal-to-cut-off ratio >1 is considered a minor criterion in 2018 ICM definition of PJIs. The levels of alpha-defensin can be measured by ELISA or rapid card tests, the former having more accuracy. Calprotectin is calcium and zinc-binding protein expressed by neutrophils upon activation. Calprotectin has previously been used for diagnosis of inflammatory bowel disease and *C. difficile* infection [19]. For diagnosis of PJIs, calprotectin >50 mg/l is considered significant. Both ELISA and rapid card tests are available for testing calprotectin. Study conducted by Grassi et al. divulged high sensitivity and specificity of calprotectin test by ELISA and rapid test (92.3%, 97.4%), as compared to LE (46% and 94%, respectively) [20]. A recent meta-analysis showed pooled sensitivity of 92% with specificity of 93% for diagnosis of PJIs [21]. Presepsin is the N-terminal fragment of sCD14-ST, and is released after phagocytosis. The use of presepsin in synovial fluid exhibits sensitivity and specificity of 100%. Neopterin, another biomarker, is the product of guanosine triphosphate metabolism, released by macrophages, which has revealed sensitivity and specificity of 74% and 59%, respectively, using cut-off value of 7.2 nmol/l. Study by Busch et al. showed higher sensitivity and specificity of neopterin, as compared to presepsin and TNF-α [22].

3.8.4.6 Molecular Modalities

Molecular methods have gained importance owing to their rapid TAT, ability to detect fastidious organisms and cases with prior antimicrobial therapy. The most commonly used modality is broad range PCR targeting 16S rRNA, the barcode for bacteria, owing to its ubiquitous presence in all bacteria. Previous studies used either Southern blotting or restriction endonucleases, prior to the sequencing analysis. However, this has inherent bottleneck of requisite for sequencing analysis, which becomes complex in cases of polymicrobial infection. This bottleneck is overcome by the advent of multiplexing, which increases the specificity. Another modification of conventional PCR, the real-time PCR with or without multiplexing, has overcome the problem of specificity and the user can determine the cycle threshold for positive results on real-time basis, to delineate the false-positive ones. PCR electrospray ionization mass spectrometry (ESI-MS) provides automated, high-throughput identification of the pathogen, along with addressing the query of genetic evidence of known and unknown pathogens in any clinical sample. Specific PCR is much more sensitive than broad-range PCR and have been developed for varied pathogens like *S. aureus*, *K. kingae* and *C. acnes*. Besides these advantages, PCR is of utmost significance in identification of uncommon and novel pathogens.

Commercial multiplex platforms like BIOFIRE panels have been marketed and found to be highly sensitive and specific for diagnosis of BJIs. A recent study by Schoenmakers et al. revealed BIOFIRE JI panel to be highly sensitive (83%) for patients with suspected septic arthritis of native joint and patients with PJI of late onset (73%) and early onset PJI (30%). Specificity was noted to be 100% in all patients, when compared with MSIS criteria [23]. Another study showed 95.7% or higher negative percentage agreement for antimicrobial genes, with specificity of 98.5% or more for all organisms [24]. This is advantageous over culture, in terms of sensitivity and TAT, both for identification and resistance; and are unaffected by prior antimicrobial therapy. The panel can precisely identify fastidious organism like anaerobes, *K. kingae* and *N. gonorrhoeae*, and can effortlessly ascertain polymicrobial infections. However, the panel doesn't include *S. epidermidis* and *C. acnes,* which are important etiological agents in chronic PJIs, and thereby, can't be used to rule out infection. Another commercial platform, Unyvero I60ITI, has low sensitivity and doesn't include organisms like *K. kingae* in its panel. Earlier studies have used sepsis panels for diagnosis of BJIs, and divulged 78% positivity for sonication fluid, as compared to 65% positivity in culture, using SeptiFast assay. However, *C. acnes* wasn't included in those panels, thereby, couldn't be put to use. The FilmArray panel showed lower sensitivity compared to SeptiFast panel [25].

Xpert MTB/RIF assay (GeneXpert), based on the principle of real-time PCR using molecular beacons, for simultaneous detection of *M. tuberculosis* complex and rifampicin resistance. Sensitivity of GeneXpert for diagnosis of osteoarticular TB is ~60–70%, with 100% specificity, which led to the introduction of GeneXpert MTB/RIF Ultra with improved sensitivity and low detection limit. However, the specificity of Xpert Ultra declined as compared to GeneXpert assay, for both pulmonary and extra-pulmonary samples. GeneXpert platforms can also be exploited to differentiate cases of NTM from *M. tuberculosis*, in scenarios with smear-positive and GeneXpert negative results [5].

The emerging next-generation sequencing techniques like ion-torrent, Illumina, Applied Biosystems Sequencing by oligonucleotide ligation and detection system (SOLiD) and oxford nanopore have been exploited for utility in detection of pathogens in synovial fluid. These techniques detect entire nucleic acid present in the sample, and by means of bioinformatics, the sequences are analyzed quantitatively to identify specific species. Moreover, the quantitative analysis helps distinguish true pathogens from contaminants as well. Recent studies have shown high sensitivity and specificity of metagenomic NGS (mNGS), however, the test shouldn't be used as stand-alone modality. The combination of mNGS with culture techniques is helpful in diagnosis of bone and joint infections efficiently. Moreover, Jeyaraman et al. divulged the decrease in median time to analysis from 5.2 for culture to 1.3 for mNGS, in synovial fluid and deep tissue samples [26]. A recent systematic review of NGS in periprosthetic infections showed positive and negative predictive values of 71–100% and 74–95%, respectively. The detection rate ranged from 9 to 100% for culture-negative PJIs and 74.05 to 92.31% for PJIs with prior antibiotic therapy [27]. Furthermore, NGS also imparts insights into the genetic makeup, enhances the role of microbiome in BJIs and resistance patterns of pathogens, paving way for newer biomarkers. The incorporation of NGS in routine diagnostic algorithms help in provision of personalized treatment plans for patients, thereby improving the patient care and helps in curbing the escalating antimicrobial resistance. However, incorporation of NGS in routine practice is also met by some limitations. The need for sophisticated infrastructure, high cost, personnel proficiency and complex bioinformatic analysis are among the few. The inherent tribulations of NGS include its inability to differentiate active infection from past infection or contamination, as being a molecular modality, it can detect both live and dead nucleic acids, thereby, clinical correlation is mandatory in all the cases. Despite few limitations, NGS is indispensable in management of BJIs, owing to its capability for detection of polymicrobial infections, microbial profiling, genomic characterization, identification of novel biomarkers, aid in comprehending antimicrobial resistance patterns and multifaceted genetic interactions, with less TAT, which are critical for personalized management plans.

3.9 Conclusion

Bone and joint infections (BJIs) represent a significant and evolving clinical challenge due to their complex etiology, pathogenesis and diagnostic requirements. Although advancements in diagnostic technologies, including molecular modalities and biomarker assays, have improved pathogen detection and characterization, specifically in culture-negative cases the persistent increase in BJI incidence by factors such as aging populations, comorbidities and rising use of prostheses require continuous refinement of diagnostic approaches. Extensive understanding of microbial profiles, host-pathogen interactions and biofilm dynamics is essential for timely and effective management. Integration of traditional microbiology with advanced techniques like next-generation sequencing can offer promising prospects in the future.

Conflict of Interests None.

Financial Disclosures None.

References

1. Romanò CL, Romanò D, Logoluso N, Drago L. Bone and joint infections in adults: a comprehensive classification proposal. Eur Orthop Traumatol [Internet]. 2011; [cited 2024 Jun 25];1(6):207. Available from: /pmc/articles/PMC3150792/.
2. Hunter S, Chan H, Baker JF. Global epidemiology of childhood bone and joint infection: a systematic review. Infection [Internet]. 2022; [cited 2024 Jun 25];50:329–41. Available from: https://doi.org/10.1007/s15010-021-01741-3.
3. Zimmerli W, Ochsner PE. Management of infection associated with prosthetic joints. Infection [Internet]. 2003; [cited 2024 Jun 25];31(2):99–108. Available from: https://pubmed.ncbi.nlm.nih.gov/12682815/.
4. Desimpel J, Posadzy M, Vanhoenacker F. The many faces of osteomyelitis: a pictorial review. J Belg Soc Radiol [Internet]. 2017; [cited 2024 Jun 25];101(1):1–10. Available from: /pmc/articles/PMC6032807/.
5. Histopathology of bone and joint infections. 2024;
6. Dessì A, Crisafulli M, Accossu S, Setzu V, Fanos V. Osteo-articular infections in newborns: diagnosis and treatment. J Chemother [Internet]. 2008; [cited 2024 Jun 27];20(5):542–50. Available from: https://pubmed.ncbi.nlm.nih.gov/19028615/.
7. Shirtliff ME, Mader JT. Acute septic arthritis. Clin Microbiol Rev [Internet]. 2002; [cited 2024 Jun 27];15(4):527–44. Available from: https://pubmed.ncbi.nlm.nih.gov/12364368/.
8. Moussiegt A, François C, Belmonte O, Jaubert J, Traversier N, Picot S, et al. Gonococcal arthritis: case series of 58 hospital cases. Clin Rheumatol [Internet]. 2022; [cited 2024 Jun 27];41(9):2855–62. Available from: https://pubmed.ncbi.nlm.nih.gov/35590115/.
9. Couderc M, Bart G, Coiffier G, Godot S, Seror R, Ziza JM, et al. Recommandations françaises 2020 sur la prise en charge des arthrites septiques sur articulation native de l'adulte. Rev Rhum. 2020;87(6):428–38.
10. Krogstad P. OSTEOMYELITIS. Feigin and Cherry's textbook of pediatric infectious diseases. 6th ed; 2009. [Internet]. [cited 2024 Jun 28];725–42. Available from: https://www.researchgate.net/publication/349659947_OSTEOMYELITIS.
11. Giurato L, Meloni M, Izzo V, Uccioli L. Osteomyelitis in diabetic foot: a comprehensive overview. World J Diabetes [Internet]. 2017; [cited 2024 Jun 28];8(4):135. Available from: /pmc/articles/PMC5394733/.
12. Sousa R, Carvalho A, Santos AC, Abreu MA. Optimal microbiological sampling for the diagnosis of osteoarticular infection. EFORT Open Rev [Internet]. 2021; [cited 2024 Jul 1];6(6):390. Available from: /pmc/articles/PMC8246105/.
13. Tande AJ, Patel R. Prosthetic joint infection. Clin Microbiol Rev [Internet]. 2014; [cited 2024 Jul 2];27(2):302–45. Available from: https://pubmed.ncbi.nlm.nih.gov/24696437/.
14. Ding T, Ledingham J, Luqmani R, Westlake S, Hyrich K, Lunt M, et al. BSR and BHPR rheumatoid arthritis guidelines on safety of anti-TNF therapies. Rheumatology (Oxford) [Internet]. 2010; [cited 2024 Jul 2];49(11):2217–9. Available from: https://pubmed.ncbi.nlm.nih.gov/20837498/.

15. Chang Y, Li Y, Fan T, Jiang K, Lv J, Huang J. Pathogenic bacteria characteristics and drug resistance in acute, delayed, and chronic periprosthetic joint infection: a retrospective analysis of 202 patients. Int Wound J [Internet]. 2023; [cited 2024 Jul 2];20(8):3315–23. Available from: https://pubmed.ncbi.nlm.nih.gov/37186450/.
16. Solarino G, Bizzoca D, Moretti L, Vicenti G, Piazzolla A, Moretti B. What's new in the diagnosis of periprosthetic joint infections: focus on synovial fluid biomarkers. Trop Med Infect Dis [Internet]. 2022; [cited 2024 Jul 2];7(11). Available from: https://pubmed.ncbi.nlm.nih.gov/36355897/.
17. Tsaras G, Maduka-Ezeh A, Inwards CY, Mabry T, Erwin PJ, Murad MH, et al. Utility of intraoperative frozen section histopathology in the diagnosis of periprosthetic joint infection: a systematic review and meta-analysis. J Bone Joint Surg Am [Internet]. 2012; [cited 2024 Jul 2];94(18):1700–11. Available from: https://pubmed.ncbi.nlm.nih.gov/22992880/.
18. 3.2 Diagnostic testing for TB, HIV and drug-resistant TB [Internet]. [cited 2024 Jul 2]. Available from: https://www.who.int/publications/digital/global-tuberculosis-report-2021/tb-diagnosis-treatment/diagnostic-testing.
19. Wen BJ, Te LG, Liu XX, Zhao JH. The value of fecal calprotectin in Clostridioides difficile infection: a systematic review. Front Physiol [Internet]. 2022; [cited 2024 Jul 2];13. Available from: /pmc/articles/PMC9382106/.
20. Grassi M, Salari P, Farinelli L, D'Anzeo M, Onori N, Gigante A. Synovial biomarkers to detect chronic periprosthetic joint infection: a pilot study to compare calprotectin rapid test, calprotectin ELISA immunoassay and leukocyte Esterase test. J Arthroplasty [Internet]. 2022; [cited 2024 Jul 2];37(4):781–6. Available from: https://pubmed.ncbi.nlm.nih.gov/34998909/.
21. Hantouly AT, Salameh M, Toubasi AA, Salman LA, Alzobi O, Ahmed AF, et al. Synovial fluid calprotectin in diagnosing periprosthetic joint infection: a meta-analysis. Int Orthop [Internet]. 2022; [cited 2024 Jul 2];46(5):971–81. Available from: https://pubmed.ncbi.nlm.nih.gov/35233711/.
22. Busch A, Jäger M, Engler H, Wasssenaar D, Bielefeld C, Wegner A. Diagnostic accuracy of synovial neopterin, TNF-α and Presepsin in periprosthetic joint infection: a prospective study. Z Orthop Unfall [Internet]. 2022; [cited 2024 Jul 2];160(3):299–306. Available from: https://pubmed.ncbi.nlm.nih.gov/33296945/.
23. Schoenmakers JWA, De Boer R, Gard L, Kampinga GA, Van Oosten M, Van Dijl JM, et al. First evaluation of a commercial multiplex PCR panel for rapid detection of pathogens associated with acute joint infections. J Bone Jt Infect [Internet]. 2023; [cited 2024 Jul 2];8(1):45–50. Available from: https://pubmed.ncbi.nlm.nih.gov/36756306/.
24. Esteban J, Salar-Vidal L, Schmitt BH, Waggoner A, Laurent F, Abad L, et al. Multicenter evaluation of the BIOFIRE Joint Infection Panel for the detection of bacteria, yeast, and AMR genes in synovial fluid samples. J Clin Microbiol [Internet]. 2023; [cited 2024 Jul 2];61(11). Available from: /pmc/articles/PMC10662359/.
25. Lewinski MA, Alby K, Babady NE, Butler-Wu SM, Bard JD, Greninger AL, et al. Exploring the utility of multiplex infectious disease panel testing for diagnosis of infection in different body sites: a joint report of the Association for Molecular Pathology, American Society for Microbiology, Infectious Diseases Society of America, and Pan American Society for Clinical Virology. J Mol Diagn [Internet]. 2023; [cited 2024 Jul 2];25(12):857–75. Available from: https://pubmed.ncbi.nlm.nih.gov/37757952/.
26. Jeyaraman M, Jeyaraman N, Nallakumarasamy A, Ramasubramanian S, Muthu S. Next generation sequencing in orthopaedic infections - where is the road headed? J Clin Orthop Trauma [Internet]. 2024; [cited 2024 Jul 2];51. Available from: https://pubmed.ncbi.nlm.nih.gov/38585384/.
27. Tang Y, Zhao D, Wang S, Yi Q, Xia Y, Geng B. Diagnostic value of next-generation sequencing in periprosthetic joint infection: a systematic review. Orthop Surg [Internet]. 2022; [cited 2024 Jul 2];14(2):190. Available from: /pmc/articles/PMC8867422/.

Biofilms in Osteoarticular Infections: A Hidden Challenge

4

Ankit Dadra, Siddhartha Sharma, and Prasoon Kumar

Abstract

Biofilms play a central role in antimicrobial resistance and chronic infections, particularly in orthopedics, where they contribute to periprosthetic joint infections and fracture-related infections. This chapter outlines the stages of biofilm formation—adhesion, proliferation, maturation, and dispersion—and their mechanisms of resistance, including antibiotic penetration barriers, persister cells, efflux pumps, and immune evasion. Diagnostic challenges are addressed through advanced methods like sonication, PCR, and imaging techniques. Management strategies combine surgical debridement, systemic and local antibiotics, and, when needed, implant revision. Emerging therapies such as antimicrobial coatings, nanotechnology, enzymatic agents, and photodynamic treatments show promise in disrupting biofilms. Early detection and multimodal intervention are key to improving outcomes.

Learning Points

- Understand the role of biofilms in antimicrobial resistance and their impact on infection persistence.
- Learn how biofilms form and the stages involved, from adhesion to dispersion.
- Recognize the challenges in diagnosing biofilm-related infections and the diagnostic methods available.
- Discuss briefly the current and emerging management strategies, including antibiotic therapy and novel technologies.

A. Dadra · S. Sharma · P. Kumar (✉)
Department of Orthopedics, PGIMER, Chandigarh, India

P. Kumar et al. (eds.), *Textbook of Orthopedic Infections*,
https://doi.org/10.1007/978-981-95-5029-6_4

4.1 Introduction

Biofilms play a crucial role in antimicrobial resistance (AMR) and contribute significantly to the persistence of infections, particularly in chronic and device-related conditions. A biofilm is a structured community of microbial cells embedded in a self-produced extracellular matrix composed of polysaccharides, proteins, and DNA [1]. This matrix provides physical protection against host immune responses and antimicrobial agents, making infections associated with biofilms notoriously difficult to treat. Compared to planktonic (free-floating) bacteria, biofilm-associated microorganisms exhibit up to a thousand-fold higher resistance to antibiotics, largely due to restricted drug penetration, altered metabolic states, and the presence of persister cells that can survive antimicrobial exposure [2]. This inherent resilience of biofilms contributes to prolonged infections, increased morbidity, and higher healthcare costs.

Musculoskeletal infections (MSKI), especially postoperative cases, cause significant morbidity, prolonged treatment, and poor functional outcomes. The CDC defines surgical site infections (SSI) as infections that occur in surgically treated areas [3]. In orthopedics, key SSIs include periprosthetic joint infection (PJI), which affects joint replacements, and fracture-related infection (FRI), which arises during fracture treatment [4, 5]. While consensus guidelines exist for diagnosing PJI and FRI, optimal treatment strategies continue to evolve.

The impact of biofilms on infection persistence is evident in various clinical settings, including orthopedic implants, catheters, chronic wounds, and respiratory infections such as those seen in cystic fibrosis patients. Bacteria within biofilms communicate via quorum sensing, a signaling mechanism that regulates gene expression and promotes collective behavior, further enhancing their survival and resistance [6]. Additionally, biofilms serve as reservoirs for horizontal gene transfer, facilitating the spread of AMR genes among bacterial populations [7]. This makes biofilm-related infections particularly challenging to eradicate, often necessitating prolonged or combination antibiotic therapies, surgical debridement, or device removal. Understanding the mechanisms of biofilm formation and resistance is essential for developing novel therapeutic strategies aimed at disrupting biofilms and improving infection management.

4.2 Biofilm Formation and Its Stages

Biofilms are complex, structured microbial communities encased in an extracellular matrix, allowing bacteria to adhere to surfaces and resist external threats, including immune responses and antibiotics. The formation of a biofilm follows a sequential process with four distinct stages: adhesion, microcolony proliferation, maturation, and dispersion. These stages, originally outlined by Dohlan and colleagues in 2002, have been confirmed by subsequent research [8–11].

1. *Adhesion: The Initial Step*

The first and most crucial stage in biofilm formation is bacterial adhesion to a surface. Several factors influence this process, including bacterial properties and environmental conditions. Bacteria may be introduced onto implant surfaces during surgery or through open wounds, where they encounter suitable environments for biofilm formation.

Bacterial Properties Influencing Adhesion

- Motility plays a key role in bacterial adhesion. Certain bacteria, like *Pseudomonas aeruginosa* and *Escherichia coli*, use flagellar movement to overcome repulsive forces and attach to surfaces. This movement is further enhanced by chemotaxis, allowing bacteria to move toward favorable conditions [12].
- *Staphylococcus aureus*, a major biofilm-forming pathogen, employs specific adhesion mechanisms, including sortase-attached surface adhesins, wall teichoic acids, and extracellular DNA (eDNA) production [13].

Environmental Factors Affecting Adhesion

- Surface Charge and Hydrophobicity: Proteins and bacteria adhere more to mildly hydrophobic or hydrophilic surfaces, while adhesion is reduced on highly hydrophobic or hydrophilic surfaces [14].
- pH and Gravity: Surface properties such as pH levels and gravitational forces can either facilitate or hinder bacterial attachment.

Initially, bacterial adhesion is reversible. However, as the bacteria establish a stronger hold through dipole-dipole interactions, covalent and hydrogen bonds, ionic bonds, and structural adhesion molecules (adhesins), the attachment becomes irreversible.

2. *Microcolony Proliferation*

Once securely attached, bacteria begin to multiply rapidly, forming microcolonies. This phase is critical for biofilm development, as bacteria start secreting extracellular polymeric substances (EPS), a key component of the biofilm matrix. EPS provides stability and protection to the growing biofilm [15].

At this stage, although the biofilm is still in its early phase, it remains vulnerable to disruption through physical or chemical means. Intervention during this stage may prevent full biofilm maturation.

3. *Maturation: Biofilm Development and Resistance*

As microcolonies expand, the biofilm enters the maturation phase. Bacterial colonies produce large amounts of EPS, which serves as a biological glue, strengthening the biofilm's structure.

- The biofilm develops a three-dimensional architecture with intricate networks that allow for efficient nutrient and oxygen exchange.
- Water channels form within the EPS, facilitating nutrient delivery and waste removal.
- During this phase, quorum sensing plays a critical role. Bacteria use this cell-to-cell communication system to regulate gene expression, coordinate biofilm growth, and enhance resistance mechanisms.

At this stage, bacteria within the biofilm exhibit metabolic diversity. Some cells enter a dormant state (persister cells), making them highly resistant to antibiotics and host immune responses. This is one of the primary reasons biofilm-related infections are difficult to treat.

4. *Dispersion: Biofilm Expansion and Spread*

In the final stage, the biofilm disperses, allowing bacteria to spread to new surfaces and restart the biofilm formation cycle. Dispersion can occur through both passive and active mechanisms.

Passive Dispersion

- Driven by environmental forces such as gravity, hydrodynamic flow, or shear stress.
- Fragments of the biofilm break off and colonize nearby surfaces.

Active Dispersion

- Bacteria actively escape from the biofilm matrix by downregulating EPS-related genes and upregulating motility-promoting genes.
- This allows bacteria to revert to a planktonic (free-floating) state, enhancing their ability to colonize new areas.

Once dispersed, these bacteria can initiate new biofilm formation elsewhere, perpetuating the cycle and increasing the risk of persistent infections (Fig. 4.1).

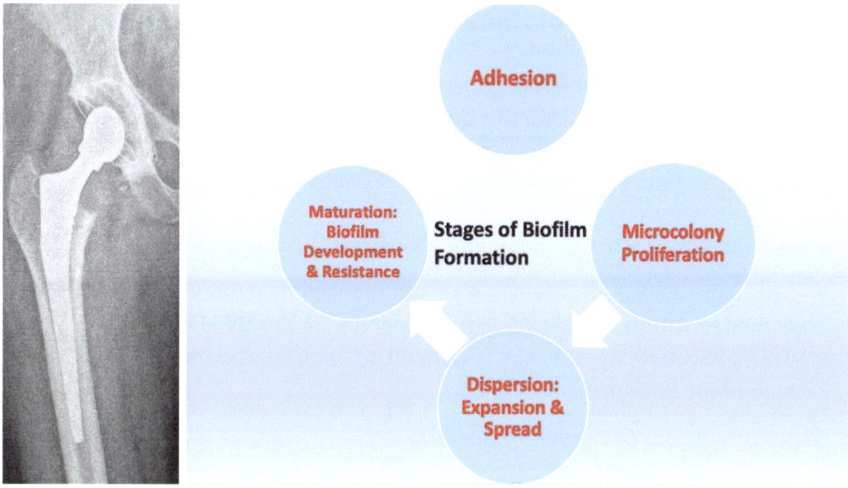

Fig. 4.1 Depicts various stages of biofilm formation

4.3 Clinical Implications of Biofilm Formation

Understanding the stages of biofilm development is critical in managing biofilm-associated infections, particularly in orthopedics, where periprosthetic joint infections (PJI) and fracture-related infections (FRI) pose serious challenges. Since mature biofilms are highly resistant to antibiotics and immune clearance, early intervention—preferably during the adhesion or microcolony stages—offers the best chance for successful treatment.

Effective Biofilm Management Includes

- *Early Detection and Intervention*: Removing bacteria before irreversible adhesion occurs.
- *Aggressive Surgical Debridement*: Removing infected tissue and biofilm-covered implants.
- *Antibiotic Therapy*: Utilizing both systemic and localized antibiotics to target biofilm-associated bacteria.
- *Emerging Anti-Biofilm Strategies*: Including biofilm-disrupting agents, antimicrobial coatings, and novel technologies like photodynamic therapy and bacteriophage therapy.

By targeting biofilms at their early stages and disrupting mature biofilms effectively, clinicians can improve outcomes for patients with biofilm-associated infections.

4.4 Mechanisms of Biofilm-Mediated Resistance

Biofilms contribute to antimicrobial resistance through multiple mechanisms, making infections significantly harder to treat. In 2003, Davies et al. demonstrated that biofilms can be up to *10,000 times more resistant* to antimicrobial action compared to planktonic bacteria [16]. Several key factors contribute to this resistance.

1. *Physical Barrier of the Extracellular Polymeric Substance (EPS)*
   - The dense *EPS matrix* acts as a shield, preventing antibiotics, immune cells, and other antimicrobial agents from penetrating deeply [17].
   - This protective layer makes it difficult to eradicate bacteria residing in the core of the biofilm.
2. *Slow Growth and Dormancy of Bacteria*
   - Bacteria within a biofilm grow more slowly than their planktonic counterparts.
   - *Limited oxygen and nutrient availability* lead to the formation of *dormant (persister) cells* in the biofilm's core [18].
   - Since most antibiotics target actively dividing bacteria, these slow-growing cells evade treatment, leading to persistent infections.
3. *Efflux Pump Activation*
   - Biofilm-associated bacteria exhibit *upregulation of multidrug efflux pump genes*, actively expelling antibiotics before they can act [19].
   - This mechanism enhances bacterial survival, particularly against a broad range of antimicrobials.
4. *Quorum Sensing and Genetic Adaptation*
   - Bacteria communicate through *quorum sensing*, coordinating gene expression to enhance resistance [6].
   - Specific genes responsible for biofilm formation and antibiotic tolerance are *upregulated*, making bacterial colonies highly resilient.
5. *Horizontal Gene Transfer (HGT)*
   - Biofilm environments facilitate *exchange of resistance genes* through plasmids and transposons [7].
   - This genetic transfer promotes the spread of multidrug resistance within bacterial communities.
6. *Immune Evasion*
   - The *EPS matrix conceals bacterial antigens*, making them less detectable by immune cells [20].
   - Neutrophils and macrophages struggle to clear biofilm-related infections, leading to chronic inflammation and persistent infection.

Table 4.1 Diagnostic Challenges in Biofilm-Associated Infections

Challenges	Description
Low Bacterial Load & Slow Growth	Dormant bacteria in biofilms are difficult to culture, leading to false-negative results.
Polymicrobial Nature	Multiple bacterial species in biofilms complicate pathogen identification.
Antibiotic Suppression	Prior antibiotic use inhibits bacterial growth, reducing culture sensitivity.
Lack of Specific Biomarkers	Common markers (CRP, ESR, WBC) lack specificity in chronic biofilm infections.
Difficulty in Sample Collection	Invasive techniques are required, with a risk of contamination.

4.5 Diagnosis of Biofilm-Related Infections

Detecting biofilm-related infections remains *challenging* due to *low bacterial loads, intermittent shedding, and resistance to standard culture methods* (Table 4.1).

Effective diagnostic strategies include:

1. *Conventional Microbial Cultures*
    - Still considered the *gold standard*, but often yields false negatives due to low bacterial counts.
    - The best results are obtained by *removing the implant*, rinsing with *phosphate-buffered saline (PBS)* to eliminate planktonic bacteria, and *swabbing multiple areas* for inoculation into growth media [21].
    - However, this method may miss biofilms on larger implants.
2. *Sonication of Implants*
    - Recommended by Shoji et al. and Trampuz et al., *sonication* involves placing an implant in a saline bath and applying *low-frequency ultrasound* to *disrupt biofilms* and release bacteria [22, 23].
    - This method significantly *increases culture yield* and diagnostic accuracy.
3. *Molecular and Genetic Methods*
    - *Polymerase Chain Reaction (PCR)* detects bacterial DNA, even in culture-negative infections.
    - *Quantitative PCR and 16S rRNA sequencing* improve specificity by identifying bacterial species and biofilm-associated genes.
    - *Next-Generation Sequencing (NGS)* offers high-resolution microbial profiling, detecting drug-resistant strains within biofilms [24, 25].
4. *Biofilm Visualization Techniques*
    - The *agar encasement method* allows for biofilm "mapping" on smaller implants like screws.

- The implant is coated with molten agar, which solidifies; bacterial colonies grow only where biofilm is present, making them visible [26, 27].

5. *Fluorescence In Situ Hybridization (FISH) and Confocal Laser Scanning Microscopy (CLSM)*
   - *FISH* uses fluorescent probes to target bacterial RNA/DNA within biofilms.
   - *CLSM* provides high-resolution imaging, revealing biofilm architecture and bacterial distribution.
6. *Methylene Blue Staining*
   - Shaw et al. demonstrated that *methylene blue staining* can identify *biofilms of S. aureus* and *P. aeruginosa* intraoperatively [28].
   - The stain selectively marks biofilms without affecting implants or human tissue.
   - While promising, further validation is needed before routine clinical use.
7. *Mass Spectrometry-Based Methods (MALDI-TOF MS)*
   - Rapidly identifies bacterial species and their antibiotic resistance profiles [29].

4.6 Clinical Implications

Biofilm-related infections require *multimodal diagnostic approaches* to ensure accurate detection. Since standard culture methods often fail, *molecular techniques, sonication, and advanced imaging* improve diagnostic accuracy. Given their high resistance, *early intervention, aggressive debridement, and targeted antibiotic strategies* are critical for effective management.

4.7 Management of Biofilm-Related Infections

Biofilm-related infections, particularly in orthopedic surgery, pose a significant challenge due to their persistence, resistance to treatment, and ability to evade immune responses. Orthopedic surgeons must maintain a high index of suspicion when dealing with implant-associated infections, as early intervention can improve outcomes. In the initial stages of biofilm formation, bacterial adhesion is reversible, and early detection may allow for implant retention. However, once biofilms mature, the infection becomes more resistant to treatment, necessitating more aggressive intervention.

The management of biofilm-related infections involves a combination of surgical and antimicrobial strategies. Standard infection control measures include thorough debridement, extensive lavage, and excision of all necrotic tissue. Implant removal is often required unless the infection is detected early, in which case debridement, antibiotics, and implant retention (DAIR) may be successful [30]. When implant removal is necessary, the decision between a single-stage or two-stage revision

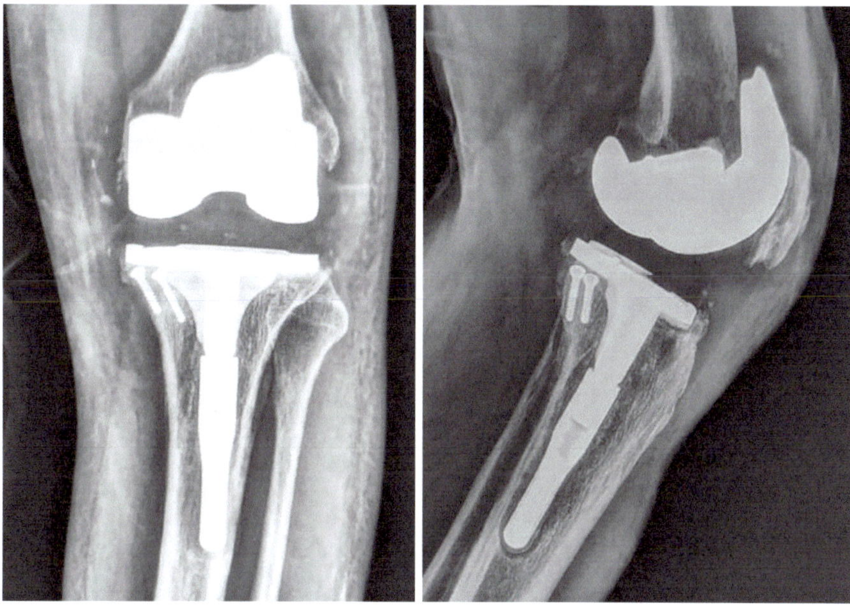

Fig. 4.2 Preoperative radiograph depicting implant loosening and osteolysis around the components

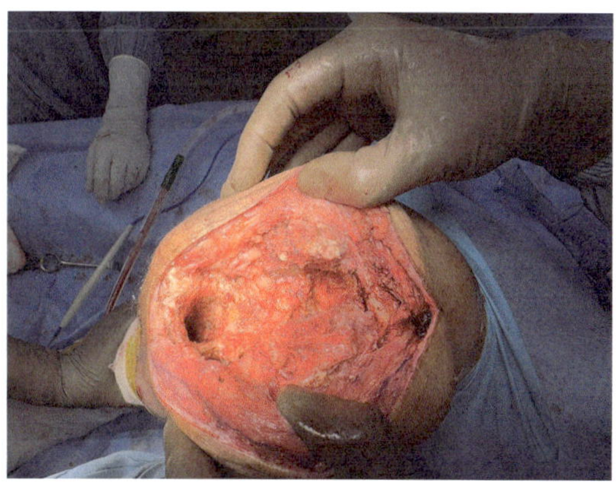

Fig. 4.3 Intraoperative image during the first stage of revision surgery after thorough debridement and implant removal

remains debated, though two-stage revision remains the preferred approach for chronic biofilm infections (Case 1 Figs. 4.2, 4.3, 4.4, 4.5, and 4.6).

Localized antibiotic therapy plays a crucial role in eradicating biofilm-associated infections. Delivery systems include both non-absorbable polymethyl methacrylate (PMMA)-based carriers and absorbable calcium sulfate-based carriers. However, antibiotic selection is critical, as some antibiotics, such as rifampicin, are incompatible with PMMA due to curing interference, while others, like gentamicin, may degrade due to PMMA's heat during polymerization [31].

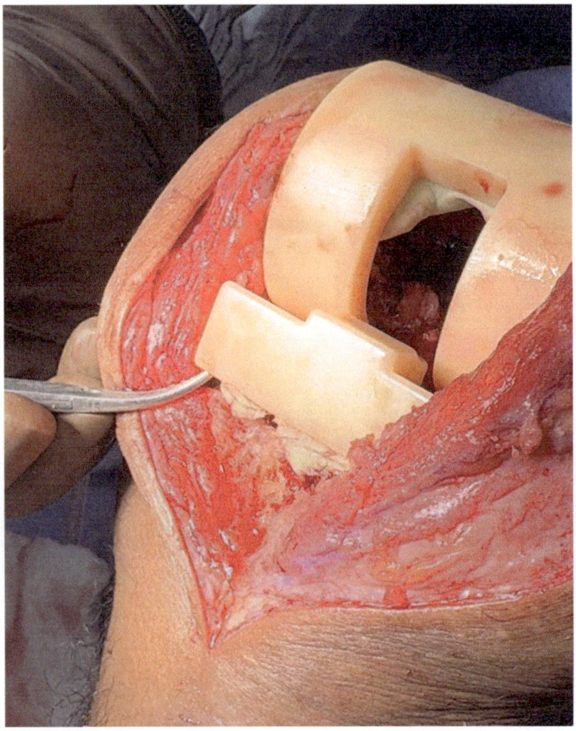

Fig. 4.4 Intraoperative image after inserting antibiotic-coated articulating spacer

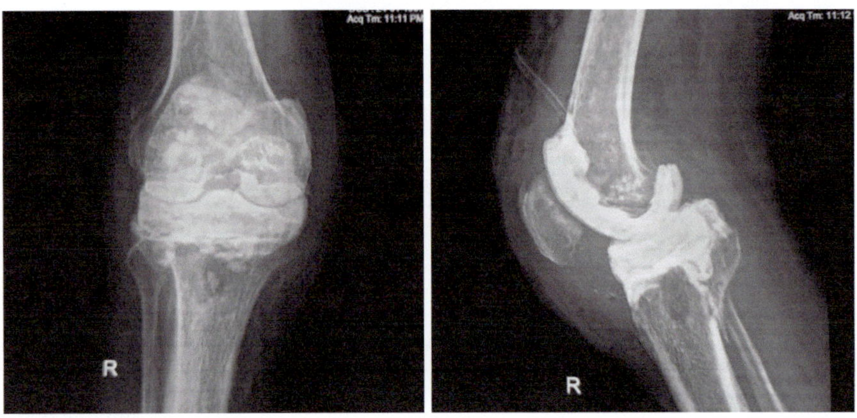

Fig. 4.5 Postoperative radiograph after first stage revision depicting articulating spacer in situ

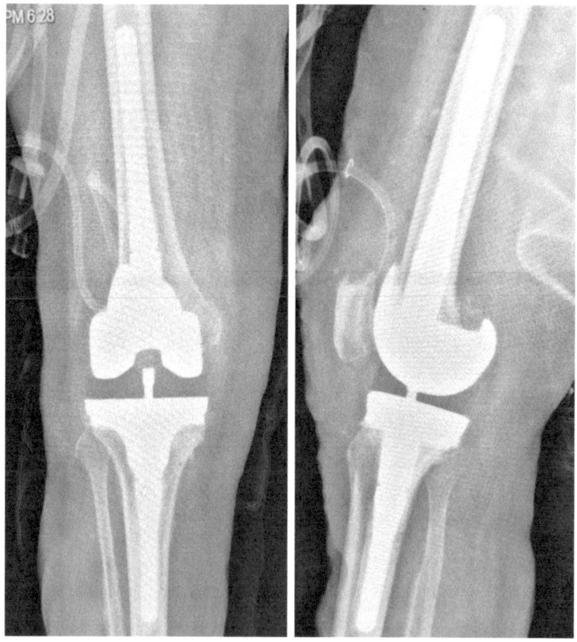

Fig. 4.6 Postoperative radiograph after the second stage definitive reconstruction using a condylar constrained knee system with wedges and stem extenders

A combination of systemic and local antibiotic therapy, along with surgical debridement, is necessary for effective treatment. Monotherapy is generally avoided to prevent resistance development. Antibiotic selection is guided by sensitivity testing, with rifampicin proving effective against *Staphylococcus* biofilms and colistin being beneficial against Gram-negative biofilms. The duration of antibiotic therapy varies based on the severity of infection, typically ranging between 6 and 12 weeks [32].

Case 1 A 68-year-old woman who had previously undergone an uncomplicated right total knee arthroplasty presented 3 years post-surgery with swelling, erythema, and pain while walking. Radiographs revealed osteolysis around the implant, along with the loosening of both components. A diagnosis of periprosthetic joint infection (PJI) was confirmed, and a two-stage revision procedure was planned. In the first stage, thorough debridement was performed, the implant was removed, and an antibiotic-coated articulating spacer was placed to manage the infection. Once infection control was achieved, the second stage involved definitive reconstruction after 6 weeks using a condylar constrained knee system with additional support from wedges and stem extenders.

4.8 Emerging Technologies for Biofilm Treatment

New technologies are being developed to improve the management of biofilm infections. Surface modification techniques, such as implant coatings with antifouling polyurethanes, have shown promise in preventing biofilm formation. Nanotechnology is also being explored to enhance drug delivery, allowing antibiotics or biofilm-degrading enzymes to penetrate biofilms more effectively [33, 34].

Other innovative approaches include photodynamic therapy, which utilizes a photosensitizing agent and specific light wavelengths to destroy bacterial biofilms [35]. Enzymatic treatments such as dispersin B, a beta-N-acetylglucosaminidase, can break down biofilm structures, making bacteria more susceptible to antibiotics [36]. Additionally, the use of predatory bacteria like *Bdellovibrio* has shown potential in depleting resources for biofilm-forming bacteria such as *E. coli* and *Pseudomonas* [37]. While these technologies have demonstrated promise in laboratory studies, further in vivo research is needed before widespread clinical adoption.

4.9 Conclusion

The management of biofilm-related infections requires a multifaceted approach involving surgical debridement, combination of antibiotic therapy, and emerging technologies. While traditional methods such as two-stage revision and local antibiotic delivery remain the mainstay of treatment, novel strategies, including surface modifications, nanotechnology, and enzymatic therapies, hold promise for the future. Continued research and clinical trials will be essential in integrating these advancements into standard practice, ultimately improving patient outcomes.

References

1. Limoli DH, Jones CJ, Wozniak DJ. Bacterial extracellular polysaccharides in biofilm formation and function. Microbiol Spectr. 2015;3(3):10.
2. Zhao A, Sun J, Liu Y. Understanding bacterial biofilms: from definition to treatment strategies. Front Cell Infect Microbiol. 2023;13:1137947.
3. Keely Boyle K, Rachala S, Nodzo SR. Centers for Disease Control and Prevention 2017 guidelines for prevention of surgical site infections: review and relevant recommendations. Curr Rev Musculoskelet Med. 2018;11(3):357–69.
4. He SY, Yu B, Jiang N. Current concepts of fracture-related infection. Int J Clin Pract. 2023;2023:4839701.
5. Mallon C, Gooberman-Hill R, Blom A, Whitehouse M, Moore A. Surgeons are deeply affected when patients are diagnosed with prosthetic joint infection. PLoS One. 2018;13(11):e0207260.
6. Preda VG, Săndulescu O. Communication is the key: biofilms, quorum sensing, formation and prevention. Discoveries (Craiova). 2019;7(3):e100.
7. Michaelis C, Grohmann E. Horizontal gene transfer of antibiotic resistance genes in biofilms. Antibiotics (Basel). 2023;12(2):328.
8. Schilcher K, Horswill AR. Staphylococcal biofilm development: structure, regulation, and treatment strategies. Microbiol Mol Biol Rev. 2020;84(3):e00026–19.

9. Kumar A, Alam A, Rani M, Ehtesham NZ, Hasnain SE. Biofilms: survival and defense strategy for pathogens. Int J Med Microbiol. 2017;307(8):481–9.
10. Kernien JF, Snarr BD, Sheppard DC, Nett JE. The interface between fungal biofilms and innate immunity. Front Immunol. 2017;8:1968.
11. Yin W, Wang Y, Liu L, He J. Biofilms: the microbial "Protective Clothing" in extreme environments. Int J Mol Sci. 2019;20(14):E3423.
12. Colin R, Ni B, Laganenka L, Sourjik V. Multiple functions of flagellar motility and chemotaxis in bacterial physiology. FEMS Microbiol Rev. 2021;45(6):fuab038.
13. Paharik AE, Horswill AR. The staphylococcal biofilm: adhesins, regulation, and host response. Microbiol Spectr. 2016;4(2):10.
14. Zhang X, Bai R, Sun Q, Zhuang Z, Zhang Y, Chen S, Han B. Bio-inspired special wettability in oral antibacterial applications. Front Bioeng Biotechnol. 2022;10:1001616.
15. Sharma S, Mohler J, Mahajan SD, Schwartz SA, Bruggemann L, Aalinkeel R. Microbial biofilm: a review on formation, infection, antibiotic resistance, control measures, and innovative treatment. Microorganisms. 2023;11(6):1614.
16. Guzmán-Soto I, McTiernan C, Gonzalez-Gomez M, Ross A, Gupta K, Suuronen EJ, Mah TF, Griffith M, Alarcon EI. Mimicking biofilm formation and development: recent progress in *in vitro* and *in vivo*biofilm models. iScience. 2021;24(5):102443.
17. Pinto RM, Soares FA, Reis S, Nunes C, Van Dijck P. Innovative strategies toward the disassembly of the EPS matrix in bacterial biofilms. Front Microbiol. 2020;11:952.
18. Khatoon Z, McTiernan CD, Suuronen EJ, Mah TF, Alarcon EI. Bacterial biofilm formation on implantable devices and approaches to its treatment and prevention. Heliyon. 2018;4(12):e01067.
19. Soto SM. Role of efflux pumps in the antibiotic resistance of bacteria embedded in a biofilm. Virulence. 2013;4(3):223–9.
20. Balducci E, Papi F, Capialbi DE, Del Bino L. Polysaccharides' structures and functions in biofilm architecture of antimicrobial-resistant (AMR) pathogens. Int J Mol Sci. 2023;24(4):4030.
21. Redanz S, Enz A, Podbielski A, Warnke P. Targeted swabbing of implant-associated biofilm formation-a staining-guided sampling approach for optimizing routine microbiological diagnostics. Diagnostics (Basel). 2021;11(6):1038.
22. Shoji MM, Chen AF. Biofilms in periprosthetic joint infections: a review of diagnostic modalities, current treatments, and future directions. J Knee Surg. 2020;33(2):119–31.
23. Trampuz A, Piper KE, Jacobson MJ, Hanssen AD, Unni KK, Osmon DR, Mandrekar JN, Cockerill FR, Steckelberg JM, Greenleaf JF, Patel R. Sonication of removed hip and knee prostheses for diagnosis of infection. N Engl J Med. 2007;357(7):654–63.
24. Arciola CR, Montanaro L, Costerton JW. New trends in diagnosis and control strategies for implant infections. Int J Artif Organs. 2011;34(9):727–36.
25. Tzeng A, Tzeng TH, Vasdev S, Korth K, Healey T, Parvizi J, et al. Treating periprosthetic joint infections as biofilms: key diagnosis and management strategies. Diagn Microbiol Infect Dis. 2015;81(3):192–200.
26. Dibartola AC, Swearingen MC, Granger JF, Stoodley P, Dusane DH. Biofilms in orthopedic infections: a review of laboratory methods. APMIS. 2017;125(4):418–28.
27. Moley JP, McGrath MS, Granger JF, Sullivan AC, Stoodley P, Dusane DH. Mapping bacterial biofilms on recovered orthopaedic implants by a novel agar candle dip method. APMIS. 2019;127(3):123–30.
28. Shaw JD, Brodke DS, Williams DL, Ashton NN. Methylene blue is an effective disclosing agent for identifying bacterial biofilms on orthopaedic implants. J Bone Jt Surg Am. 2020;102(20):1784–91.
29. Florio W, Baldeschi L, Rizzato C, Tavanti A, Ghelardi E, Lupetti A. Detection of antibiotic-resistance by MALDI-TOF mass spectrometry: an expanding area. Front Cell Infect Microbiol. 2020;10:572909.
30. Vaz K, Taylor A, Kendrick B, Alvand A. A guide to debridement, antibiotics, and implant retention. Ann Jt. 2022;7:5.

31. Howlin RP, Brayford MJ, Webb JS, Cooper JJ, Aiken SS, Stoodley P. Antibiotic-loaded synthetic calcium sulfate beads for prevention of bacterial colonization and biofilm formation in periprosthetic infections. Antimicrob Agents Chemother. 2015;59(1):111–20.
32. Tuon FF, Suss PH, Telles JP, Dantas LR, Borges NH, Ribeiro VST. Antimicrobial treatment of *Staphylococcus aureus* Biofilms. Antibiotics (Basel). 2023;12(1):87.
33. Tunney MM, Gorman SP. Evaluation of a poly(vinyl pyrollidone)-coated biomaterial for urological use. Biomaterials. 2002;23(23):4601–8.
34. Lin CD, Kou YY, Liao CY, Li CH, Huang SP, Cheng YW, Liao WC, Chen HX, Wu PL, Kang JJ, Lee CC, Lai CH. Zinc oxide nanoparticles impair bacterial clearance by macrophages. Nanomedicine (Lond). 2014;9(9):1327–39.
35. Qi M, Chi M, Sun X, Xie X, Weir MD, Oates TW, Zhou Y, Wang L, Bai Y, Xu HH. Novel nanomaterial-based antibacterial photodynamic therapies to combat oral bacterial biofilms and infectious diseases. Int J Nanomedicine. 2019;14:6937–56.
36. Kaplan JB, Mlynek KD, Hettiarachchi H, Alamneh YA, Biggemann L, Zurawski DV, Black CC, Bane CE, Kim RK, Granick MS. Extracellular polymeric substance (EPS)-degrading enzymes reduce staphylococcal surface attachment and biocide resistance on pig skin in vivo. PLoS One. 2018;13(10):e0205526.
37. Bratanis E, Andersson T, Lood R, Bukowska-Faniband E. Biotechnological potential of *Bdellovibrio* and like organisms and their secreted enzymes. Front Microbiol. 2020;11:662.

Diagnostic Approaches and General Principles of Management of Orthopedic Infections

5

Vivek P. Ksheerasagar and Vijay G. Goni

Abstract

Orthopedic infections, ranging from superficial soft-tissue infections to complex cases of osteomyelitis and septic arthritis, present significant diagnostic and therapeutic challenges. Prompt recognition and effective management are crucial to prevent complications such as chronic pain, functional loss, and systemic spread. This chapter provides a comprehensive overview of the diagnostic strategies and general principles in the management of orthopedic infections. Emphasis is placed on systematic clinical evaluation, utilization of laboratory investigations (such as CRP, ESR, and blood cultures), and advanced imaging modalities including MRI and PET-CT. The role of microbiological testing through culture, sensitivity, and molecular diagnostics is discussed in guiding targeted antibiotic therapy. Surgical interventions, ranging from debridement to staged procedures with antibiotic-loaded cement spacers, are outlined based on the chronicity and severity of infection. Multidisciplinary collaboration involving orthopedic surgeons, infectious disease specialists, microbiologists, and plastic surgeons is highlighted as essential for optimizing patient outcomes. Preventive strategies, including preoperative optimization, prophylactic antibiotics, and sterile techniques, are also emphasized to minimize the risk of infection.

Keywords

Orthopedic infections · Osteomyelitis · Septic arthritis · Antibiotic therapy · Surgical debridement · Biofilm management · Diagnostic imaging · Multidisciplinary approach · Infection prevention · Prosthetic joint infection

V. P. Ksheerasagar (✉) · V. G. Goni
Department of Orthopedics, PGIMER, Chandigarh, India

P. Kumar et al. (eds.), *Textbook of Orthopedic Infections*,
https://doi.org/10.1007/978-981-95-5029-6_5

Learning Objectives

- Conduct a comprehensive clinical assessment and utilize laboratory investigations effectively in diagnosing bone infection
- Employ appropriate imaging techniques
- Administer effective antibiotic therapy
- Implement surgical management strategies
- Address chronic infections and biofilm management
- Promote multidisciplinary care
- Implement prevention strategies and evaluate treatment outcomes

Orthopedic infections present significant challenges in terms of diagnosis, treatment, and long-term management. They range from superficial soft-tissue infections to deep-seated bone infections (osteomyelitis) and septic arthritis. Left untreated, these infections can cause chronic pain, functional impairment, and potentially life-threatening complications such as sepsis. Thus, timely diagnosis and a structured, multidisciplinary approach are essential in ensuring successful management. This chapter explores the diagnostic approaches and general management principles of orthopedic infections, including key clinical, laboratory, and imaging tools, as well as the role of surgery and antibiotics in treatment.

5.1 Diagnostic Approaches

5.1.1 Clinical Assessment

The first and most crucial step in diagnosing orthopedic infections is a comprehensive clinical assessment that includes a detailed patient history and physical examination.

- *Patient history*: Understanding the patient's medical history is essential for recognizing potential risk factors for infection. These include recent trauma, surgery (especially involving hardware or prosthetics), and conditions such as diabetes, immune suppression, peripheral vascular disease, or chronic kidney disease [1]. A history of recurrent or prior infections, particularly in patients with prosthetic joints, significantly raises the suspicion of infection. Patients with a history of intravenous drug use, recent dental procedures, or distant infections (e.g., urinary tract infections) may also develop hematogenous seeding of a joint or bone, leading to infection.
- *Clinical symptoms*: Localized signs of infection include pain, redness, warmth, and swelling, with joint stiffness or restricted movement in cases of septic arthritis. Acute infections typically present with more overt symptoms, such as fever, chills, and acute onset of pain, while chronic infections can manifest with more insidious symptoms, such as mild discomfort and intermittent swelling. Patients

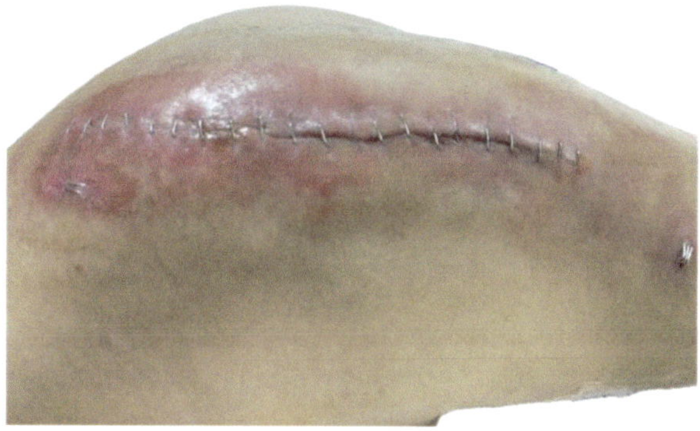

Fig. 5.1 Shows local signs of infection—erythema and swelling (author's original)

with chronic osteomyelitis, for instance, may report recurring episodes of pain and drainage from a sinus tract [2].

- *Physical examination*: Physical signs of orthopedic infections include erythema, swelling, tenderness, and warmth over the affected area [2]. In septic arthritis, joint effusion and severe pain with movement are classic findings. Sinus tract formation with discharge should rise suspicion of infection [3]. Abscesses may cause fluctuation on palpation, indicating a collection of pus. Systemic signs such as fever, tachycardia, and hypotension can point to a more disseminated infection or sepsis [4, 5] (Figs. 5.1 and 5.2).

5.1.2 Laboratory Investigations

Laboratory testing is an important adjunct to the clinical examination and helps to confirm the presence of infection, determine its severity, and monitor treatment response.

- *Complete blood count* (*CBC*): An elevated white blood cell (WBC) count, particularly neutrophilia, is indicative of infection, though this is a nonspecific finding. In chronic infections, the WBC count may be normal or only mildly elevated.
- *Erythrocyte sedimentation rate* (*ESR*) *and C-reactive protein* (*CRP*): Both ESR and CRP are nonspecific markers of inflammation, but they are highly sensitive for infection [4]. CRP typically rises and falls more quickly than ESR, making it a valuable marker for monitoring treatment response. Elevated ESR and CRP levels are common in both acute and chronic infections, and they can be used to track disease progression or response to therapy.
- *Blood cultures*: Blood cultures are particularly useful when bacteremia or systemic infection is suspected, especially in patients with prosthetic joints or in those presenting with fever and other systemic signs of infection [6]. Positive blood cultures may be the only clue to the diagnosis of a hematogenous infection.

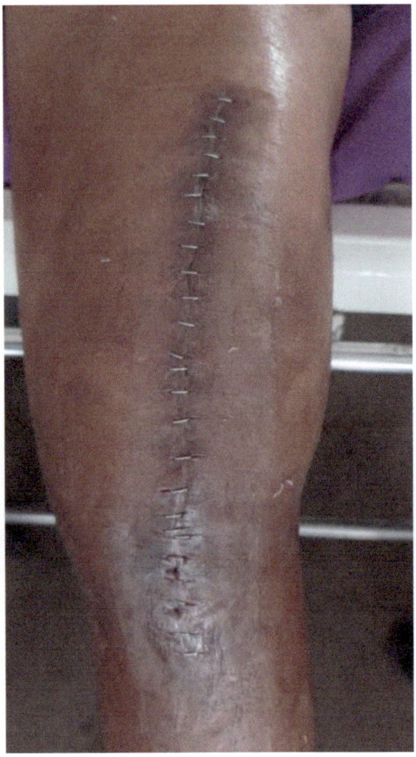

Fig. 5.2 Shows sinus tract formation at the distal end of the surgical wound (author's original)

5.1.3 Imaging Studies

Imaging plays a pivotal role in diagnosing orthopedic infections, particularly when clinical and laboratory findings are inconclusive.

- *X-rays*: Plain radiographs are often the first imaging modality used but may not show changes in the early stages of infection. In cases of osteomyelitis, radiographic signs such as periosteal elevation, bone erosion, and sequestra (dead bone) typically become evident 10–14 days after the onset of infection [1]. X-rays are more useful in detecting chronic infections, where bony destruction is more prominent [7] (Figs. 5.3 and 5.4).
- *Magnetic resonance imaging* (*MRI*): MRI is the gold standard for detecting soft-tissue and bone infections, especially in the early stages when X-rays may be inconclusive. MRI is highly sensitive for detecting bone marrow edema, abscess formation, and soft tissue involvement [7]. It is particularly useful in diagnosing osteomyelitis and septic arthritis [4] (Fig. 5.5).
- *Computed tomography* (*CT*): CT scanning provides better visualization of cortical bone than MRI and is useful for detecting sequestra in chronic osteomyelitis. CT is also helpful in guiding biopsy or drainage procedures in deep infections.

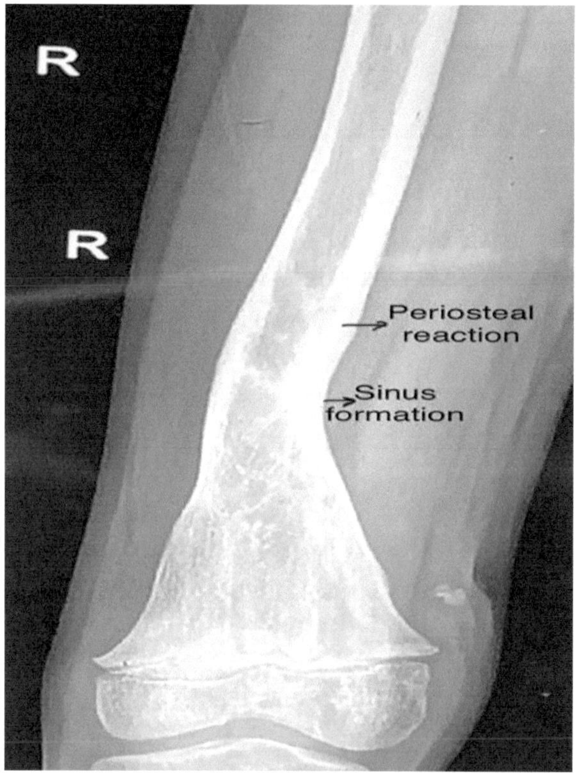

Fig. 5.3 Radiograph of chronic osteomyelitis with sinus and periosteal reaction (author's original)

- *Ultrasound*: Ultrasound is a valuable tool for detecting joint effusions or abscesses, particularly in soft tissue infections. It is often used to guide aspiration of joint fluid or abscesses for diagnostic purposes.
- *Bone scintigraphy and PET scans*: In cases where MRI or CT is contraindicated or when the source of infection is unclear, nuclear medicine techniques like bone scintigraphy or PET-CT are useful. These techniques are sensitive in detecting inflammation and infection in bones and joints, particularly in cases of prosthetic joint infections (Fig. 5.6).

5.1.4 Microbiological Testing

Accurate microbiological diagnosis is essential for selecting the appropriate antibiotic therapy.

- *Aspiration and biopsy*: Joint aspiration and bone biopsy are critical for confirming septic arthritis or osteomyelitis. Synovial fluid or bone samples are sent for gram staining, culture, and sensitivity testing to identify the causative organism and guide antibiotic therapy. In cases of prosthetic joint infection, aspiration or

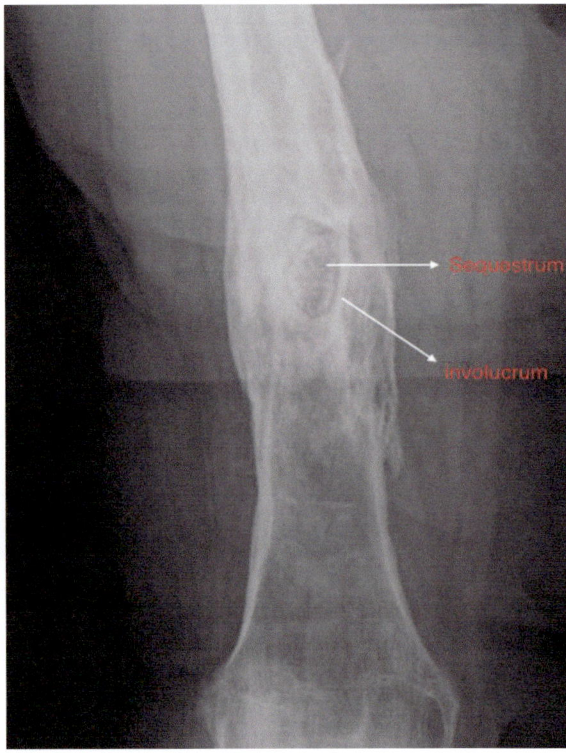

Fig. 5.4 Radiograph of chronic osteomyelitis showing sequestrum and involucrum formation around it (author's original)

tissue samples may be used to detect biofilm-forming bacteria, which are difficult to eradicate and often require prolonged or targeted therapy.

- *Culture and sensitivity*: Identifying the causative organism through culture and sensitivity testing is crucial for guiding antibiotic therapy. The most common pathogens include *Staphylococcus aureus* (including MRSA) [1, 7], *Streptococcus species*, and Gram-negative bacteria. In chronic infections, anaerobes or atypical organisms (e.g., *Mycobacterium tuberculosis*, *Brucella*) should be considered.
- *Molecular techniques*: Polymerase chain reaction (PCR) and next-generation sequencing (NGS) are increasingly being used for rapid identification of organisms in culture-negative infections. These techniques are especially valuable for identifying slow-growing or difficult-to-culture bacteria, such as those that form biofilms (Fig. 5.7).

5.2 General Principles of Management

Early Diagnosis and Intervention

The prognosis for patients with orthopedic infections largely depends on early diagnosis and prompt intervention. Delays in treatment can lead to the spread of infection, permanent damage to bones and joints, and chronic disability. The management

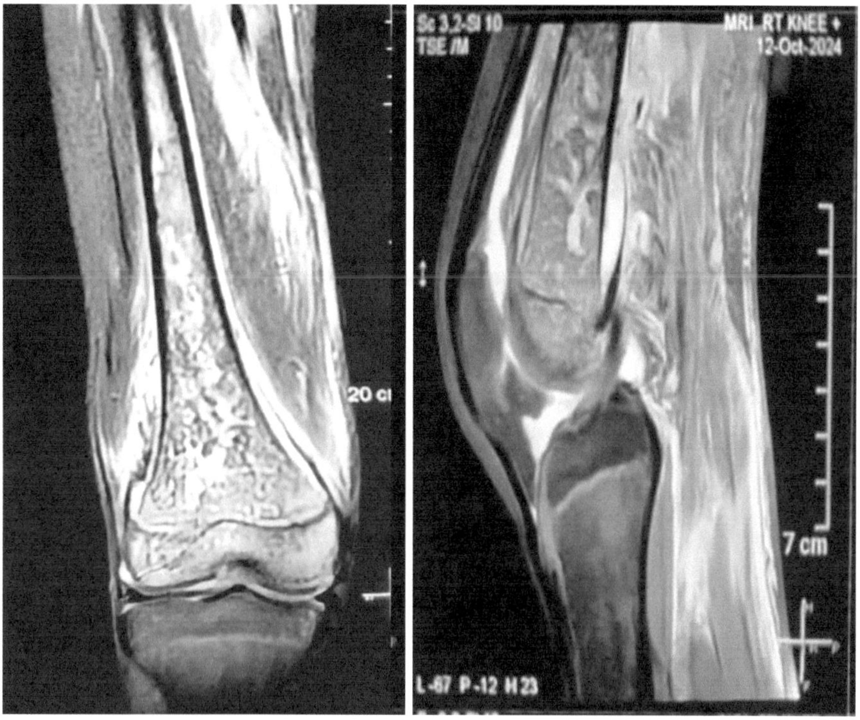

Fig. 5.5 MRI image of distal femur osteomyelitis showing bone marrow edema, cortical destruction, periosteal reaction, and abscess formation (author's original)

of orthopedic infections typically involves a combination of surgical and medical approaches, with the goal of eradicating the infection, preserving function, and preventing recurrence.

5.2.1 Acute Osteomyelitis Management

Empirical antibiotic therapy

- Based on likely pathogens
- Adjust according to culture results

Surgical drainage or debridement (if needed)

- Abscess drainage
- Removal of infected tissue

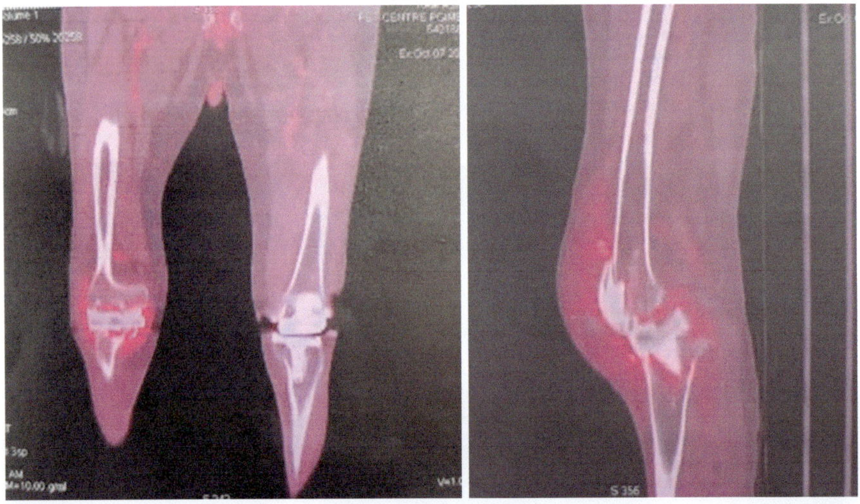

Fig. 5.6 WBC-labelled nuclear scan showing infected cement spacer in knee. Image shows localized bright spot due to tracer uptake by the leukocytes (author's original)

5.2.2 Chronic Osteomyelitis Management

Long-Term Antibiotic Therapy

- Based on culture and sensitivity.
- Oral or IV antibiotics for several weeks/months.

Surgical Management

Surgical intervention plays a key role in the management of most orthopedic infections. The primary goals of surgery are to remove infected tissue, drain abscesses, and optimize conditions for healing.

Debridement

- *Procedure*: Surgical removal of necrotic (dead) bone, infected tissue, or any foreign material that may be contributing to the infection.
- *Goal*: To remove all infected tissue to reduce bacterial load and promote healing.
- *Indications*: Especially important in chronic osteomyelitis, where necrotic bone (sequestrum) is present.
- *Outcome*: It may be followed by filling the void with bone grafts or other materials.

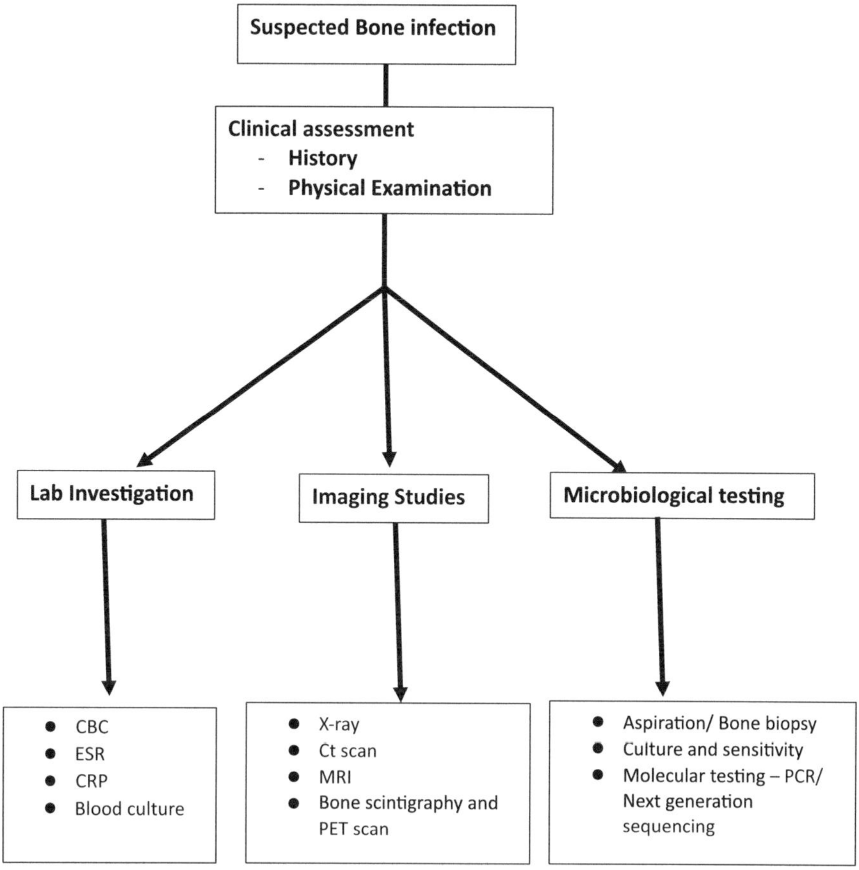

Fig. 5.7 Diagnostic approach in bone and joint infection

Sequestrectomy

- *Procedure*: Specific removal of the sequestrum, which is the dead piece of bone isolated from viable bone.
- *Goal*: To eradicate the source of chronic infection, particularly in cases of long-standing osteomyelitis.
- *Outcome*: Helps stop the persistence of infection, allowing for new bone formation and healing [8].

Curettage

- *Procedure*: Scraping of the infected bone to remove diseased areas.
- *Goal*: To clean out infected areas of bone without extensive removal of healthy bone.

- *Outcome*: It can be combined with debridement to ensure thorough cleaning of the infected site.

Bone Resection (Segmental Resection)

- *Procedure*: Removal of an entire section of infected bone.
- *Goal*: Reserved for more extensive cases where a significant part of the bone is involved, and healing is not possible without removing a larger segment of bone.
- *Outcome*: May require bone grafting or reconstructive surgery afterwards.

Amputation

- *Procedure*: Removal of the infected limb or portion of a limb.
- *Goal*: This is a last-resort treatment when the infection is so severe that limb salvage is not feasible.
- *Outcome*: Used in life-threatening or non-healing infections where other treatments have failed.

Bone Grafting/Bone Graft Substitute

- *Procedure*: After the removal of infected bone, bone grafts or substitutes may be used to fill the defect and encourage healing.
- *Goal*: To restore structural integrity and promote new bone formation.
- *Outcome*: Helps maintain limb function and prevents deformities.

Insertion of Antibiotic-Loaded Cement Spacers

- *Procedure*: Use of antibiotic-impregnated cement spacers (temporary) in the bone cavity after debridement.
- *Goal*: To deliver high local concentrations of antibiotics directly to the infection site.
- *Outcome*: These spacers can help control the infection while maintaining space for later reconstructive surgery [9].

Stabilization and Internal Fixation

- *Procedure*: Use of internal fixation devices (plates, screws, or rods) to stabilize the bone after debridement or resection.
- *Goal*: To allow the bone to heal properly, especially in long bones like the femur or tibia.

- *Outcome*: May be combined with bone grafting for long-term structural support.

Vacuum-Assisted Closure (VAC) Therapy

- *Procedure*: A vacuum dressing (negative pressure wound therapy) is applied after debridement.
- *Goal*: To promote wound healing by reducing infection, increasing blood flow, and drawing fluid out of the wound.
- *Outcome*: Enhances the healing of soft tissue and promotes granulation over exposed bone [10].

Chronic Drainage or Sinus Tract Surgery

- *Procedure*: Surgical closure or removal of draining sinus tracts connected to the infected bone.
- *Goal*: To eliminate any external draining channels that serve as a conduit for bacteria to the bone.
- *Outcome*: Prevents the recurrence of infection and promotes healing.

Staged Procedures
In cases of prosthetic joint infection, a two-stage revision is often required. The first stage involves removal of the infected prosthesis and placement of an antibiotic-impregnated spacer. Once the infection has been eradicated, a new prosthesis is implanted in the second stage [11]. This approach has a high success rate in eradicating infection and restoring function.

5.2.3 Antibiotic Therapy

Antibiotic therapy is a critical component of managing orthopedic infections and is typically initiated as soon as the diagnosis is suspected. Treatment is guided by microbiological results, but empirical therapy is often started while awaiting culture results.

- *Empirical antibiotics*: Initial empiric antibiotic therapy should cover the most likely pathogens, particularly *Staphylococcus aureus* and MRSA. Empiric regimens commonly include vancomycin or daptomycin (for MRSA coverage), combined with a broad-spectrum agent such as piperacillin-tazobactam or cefepime, especially in cases of suspected Gram-negative involvement [2, 12]. The choice of antibiotics should be guided by local resistance patterns and adjusted based on culture and sensitivity results.

- *Definitive antibiotics*: Once culture results are available, antibiotic therapy should be tailored to the specific pathogen. For septic arthritis, antibiotics are typically continued for 4–6 weeks [13], whereas chronic osteomyelitis often requires prolonged therapy (6–12 weeks), particularly when hardware is involved. Intravenous (IV) antibiotics are generally preferred initially, followed by oral antibiotics once clinical improvement is achieved and laboratory markers normalize.
- *Local antibiotic delivery*: Local antibiotic delivery systems, such as antibiotic-impregnated cement or beads, are commonly used in the treatment of osteomyelitis and prosthetic joint infections [14]. These devices allow for high local concentrations of antibiotics while minimizing systemic toxicity. Antibiotic-impregnated spacers are particularly useful in staged procedures for prosthetic joint infections.

5.2.4 Management of Chronic Infections

Chronic infections, particularly those involving biofilm-forming organisms or multi-drug-resistant bacteria, require prolonged and aggressive management strategies.

- *Biofilm management*: Biofilm-producing bacteria, such as *Staphylococcus epidermidis* [15], are difficult to eradicate due to their resistance to antibiotics and host immune responses. Infections involving biofilms typically require prolonged antibiotic therapy and complete removal of infected hardware. Strategies to disrupt biofilms, such as using antibiotics with biofilm activity (e.g., rifampin) or employing local antibiotic delivery systems, may improve outcomes [16].
- *Suppressive therapy*: In patients who are not candidates for curative surgery (e.g., due to advanced age or medical comorbidities), long-term suppressive antibiotic therapy may be used to control chronic infections. This approach is particularly common in cases of chronic prosthetic joint infections, where complete removal of the prosthesis is not feasible [2] (Fig. 5.8).

5.2.5 Multidisciplinary Care

Successful management of orthopedic infections often requires a multidisciplinary approach, involving collaboration between orthopedic surgeons, infectious disease specialists, microbiologists, and plastic surgeons.

- *Infectious disease specialists*: Infectious disease specialists play a key role in guiding antibiotic selection, duration of therapy, and monitoring for adverse effects. They are also essential in managing complex cases of chronic or multi-drug-resistant infections.

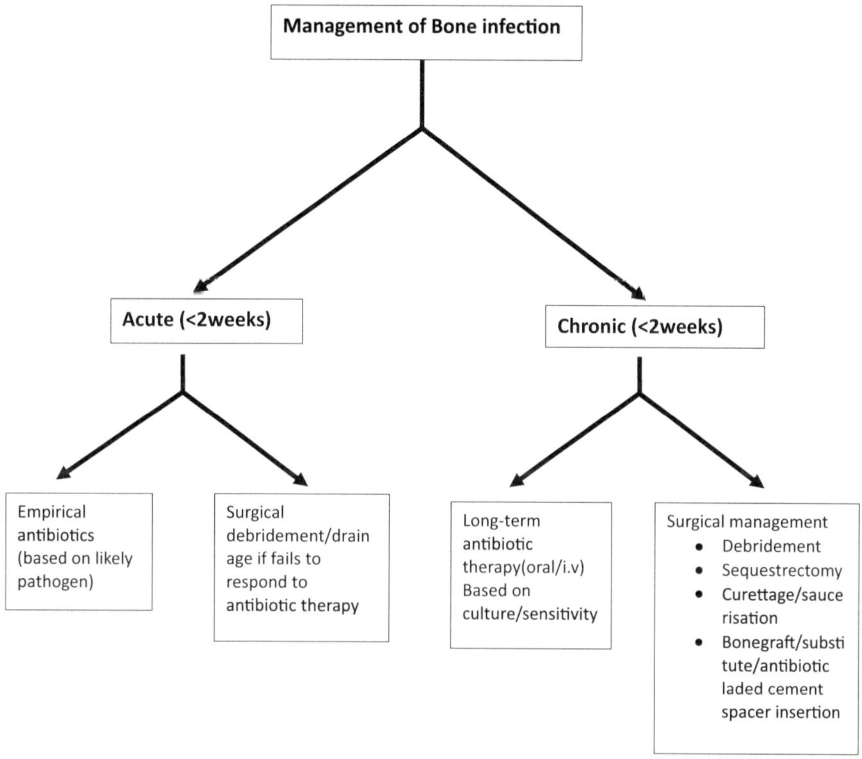

Fig. 5.8 Management of bone infection

- *Microbiologists*: Microbiologists help to identify the causative organisms and guide antibiotic therapy based on culture and sensitivity results. Advanced molecular techniques, such as PCR and NGS, are increasingly being used to detect difficult-to-culture organisms.
- *Plastic surgeons*: In cases of extensive soft tissue loss, particularly following aggressive debridement, plastic surgeons may be needed for flap coverage or reconstructive procedures. Ensuring adequate soft tissue coverage is critical to prevent wound breakdown and recurrence of infection.

5.2.6 Prevention and Risk Reduction

Preventing orthopedic infections is a key goal in both surgical and non-surgical patients. Strategies for reducing the risk of infection include optimizing patient health, adhering to sterile surgical techniques, and using prophylactic antibiotics when appropriate.

- *Preoperative optimization*: Optimizing the patient's health before surgery is essential for reducing the risk of post-operative infections. This includes managing chronic conditions such as diabetes, malnutrition, and immune suppression. Smoking cessation and weight management are also important in reducing the risk of infection and improving wound healing.
- *Prophylactic antibiotics*: The use of prophylactic antibiotics before surgery is standard practice in orthopedics, particularly in procedures involving prosthetic implant [5]. Antibiotics should be administered within 1 h of incision and discontinued within 24 h post-operatively to reduce the risk of surgical site infections without contributing to antibiotic resistance [17].
- *Sterile techniques*: Adhering to strict sterile techniques during surgery is critical for preventing infections. This includes proper hand hygiene, sterile draping, and the use of antimicrobial-impregnated dressings in high-risk patients [18]. Post-operative wound care should also emphasize early detection and treatment of any signs of infection.
- *Follow-up and monitoring*: Close follow-up is essential for detecting early signs of infection, particularly in high-risk patients. Monitoring inflammatory markers (CRP, ESR) can help identify subclinical infections or relapses in patients with prosthetic joints or previous infections.

5.3 Conclusion

Orthopedic infections, whether acute or chronic, require a systematic and multidisciplinary approach to achieve successful outcomes. Early diagnosis is essential, and a combination of clinical assessment, laboratory investigations, and imaging studies is critical for confirming the diagnosis. Surgical management, including debridement and drainage, plays a central role in eradicating infection, particularly when biofilms or prosthetic materials are involved. Antibiotic therapy, both systemic and local, is crucial in controlling the infection and preventing recurrence. Close collaboration between orthopedic surgeons, infectious disease specialists, and microbiologists is key to ensuring optimal patient outcomes.

Take-Home Message

- Effective management of orthopedic infections requires early diagnosis through comprehensive clinical assessment, laboratory tests, and imaging studies.
- Surgical intervention, including debridement and drainage, is often essential alongside tailored antibiotic therapy.
- A multidisciplinary approach enhances patient outcomes, while prevention strategies are critical for reducing infection risk.
- Timely intervention is key to preventing complications and ensuring optimal recovery.

References

1. Schmitt SK. Osteomyelitis. Infect Dis Clin N Am. 2017;31:325–38.
2. Fritz JM, McDonald JR. Osteomyelitis: approach to diagnosis and treatment. Phys Sportsmed. 2008;36:nihpa116823.
3. Klim SM, Amerstorfer F, McNally MA, Trebse R, Slokar U, Sigmund IK, et al. The sinus tract in bone and joint infection: minimally invasive salvation or prolonged suffering? A multicenter study. J Pers Med. 2023;13:737.
4. Zimmerli W. Clinical practice. Vertebral osteomyelitis. N Engl J Med. 2010;362:1022–9. Available from: https://pubmed.ncbi.nlm.nih.gov/20237348/.
5. Berbari EF, Kanj SS, Kowalski TJ, Darouiche RO, Widmer AF, Schmitt SK, et al. 2015 Infectious Diseases Society of America (IDSA) clinical practice guidelines for the diagnosis and treatment of native vertebral osteomyelitis in adults. Clin Infect Dis Off Publ Infect Dis Soc Am. 2015;61:e26–46.
6. Tande AJ, Patel R. Prosthetic joint infection. Clin Microbiol Rev. 2014;27:302–45.
7. Hatzenbuehler J, Pulling TJ. Diagnosis and management of osteomyelitis. Am Fam Physician. 2011;84:1027–33. Available from: https://pubmed.ncbi.nlm.nih.gov/22046943/.
8. Sulaiman A, Mahfoud M, Abdalrahman M. Comparison of sequestrectomy with or without nucleotomy in patients with sequestered fragment and small perforations within the fibrous ring: 2 years' experience. Interdiscip Neurosurg. 2021;24:101098.
9. Bor N, Dujovny E, Rinat B, Rozen N, Rubin G. Treatment of chronic osteomyelitis with antibiotic-impregnated polymethyl methacrylate (PMMA)—the Cierny approach: is the second stage necessary? BMC Musculoskelet Disord. 2022;23:38.
10. Cozza V, Pepe G, Cintoni M, De Maio F, Tropeano G, Magalini S, et al. Vacuum-assisted closure (VAC®) systems and microbiological isolation of infected wounds. World J Emerg Surg WJES. 2018;13:53.
11. Lum ZC, Holland CT, Meehan JP. Systematic review of single stage revision for prosthetic joint infection. World J Orthop. 2020;11:559–72.
12. Gutierrez K. Bone and joint infections in children. Pediatr Clin North Am. 2005;52:779–94, vi.
13. Lew DP, Waldvogel FA. Osteomyelitis. Lancet Lond Engl. 2004;364:369–79.
14. Gogia JS, Meehan JP, Di Cesare PE, Jamali AA. Local antibiotic therapy in osteomyelitis. Semin Plast Surg. 2009;23:100–7.
15. Vestby LK, Grønseth T, Simm R, Nesse LL. Bacterial biofilm and its role in the pathogenesis of disease. Antibiotics. 2020;9:59.
16. Sen CK, Roy S, Mathew-Steiner SS, Gordillo GM. Biofilm management in wound care. Plast Reconstr Surg. 2021;148:275e–88e.
17. Baseel D, Kim J, Mohammed S, Lowe A, Siddiqi J. The ideal time to administer pre-operative antibiotics: current and future practices. Cureus. 2022;14:e24979.
18. da Silva AA, Marques AF, di Biase CB, Zingg W, Dramowski A, Sharland M. Interventions to prevent urinary catheter-associated infections in children and neonates: a systematic review. J Pediatr Urol. 2018;14:556.e1–9. Available from: https://pubmed.ncbi.nlm.nih.gov/30126746/.

Antimicrobial Therapy

6

K. Niveditha, Nusrat Shafiq, and Ankit Dadra

Abstract

Musculoskeletal infections, including osteomyelitis and septic arthritis, pose significant challenges due to poor antibiotic penetration, biofilm formation, and rising antimicrobial resistance. This chapter outlines the burden of surgical site infections, principles of antimicrobial susceptibility testing, and the classification and application of prophylactic, empirical, and definitive therapies. Key antibiotics such as vancomycin, piperacillin-tazobactam, cefuroxime, and carbapenems are reviewed with respect to dosage, indications, and pharmacokinetics. The chapter emphasizes factors affecting treatment efficacy, including tissue penetration and host-specific considerations. It also highlights recent FDA-approved antibiotics targeting multidrug-resistant organisms and underscores the importance of antibiotic stewardship and multidisciplinary care. Emerging strategies focused on local drug delivery, optimized pharmacodynamics, and biofilm disruption are discussed to improve outcomes in managing bone and joint infections.

Keywords

Musculoskeletal infections · Antimicrobial therapy · Biofilm resistance · Osteomyelitis · Septic arthritis

K. Niveditha · N. Shafiq
Department of Pharmacology, PGIMER, Chandigarh, India

A. Dadra (✉)
Department of Orthopedics, PGIMER, Chandigarh, India

P. Kumar et al. (eds.), *Textbook of Orthopedic Infections*,
https://doi.org/10.1007/978-981-95-5029-6_6

Learning Objectives

- *Understand musculoskeletal infections* and their management challenges.
- *Explain antimicrobial therapy principles* in orthopedic infections.
- *Recognize biofilms' role* in infection persistence and resistance.
- *Evaluate emerging antimicrobial therapies* and their limitations.
- *Apply antimicrobial stewardship* to optimize treatment outcomes.
- *Explore future innovations* in infection management.
- *Appreciate a multidisciplinary approach* for effective infection control.

6.1 Background

Bone and joint infections pose significant challenges in orthopedic practice, often requiring a multidisciplinary approach. Osteomyelitis (bone infection) and septic arthritis (joint infection) can result from trauma, surgery, hematogenous spread, or adjacent soft tissue infections. Without timely intervention, these infections can cause permanent damage and chronic disease [1, 2].

Unlike other infections, antimicrobial therapy for bone and joint infections is complicated by poor vascularity, dense bone matrix, and biofilm formation, which hinder antibiotic penetration and efficacy. Biofilm-associated bacteria exhibit increased resistance, making eradication difficult [3].

Successful management requires:

- Early diagnosis through clinical, imaging, and microbiological studies.
- Targeted antimicrobial therapy with prolonged administration.
- Surgical intervention to remove infected tissue and enhance antibiotic effectiveness.
- Adjunctive strategies, such as local antibiotic delivery and biofilm-targeted approaches.

This chapter explores the principles of antimicrobial therapy, systemic and local antibiotic strategies, biofilm challenges, and emerging treatment approaches to optimize outcomes.

6.1.1 Burden and Challenges of Musculoskeletal Infections

The *2024 CDC Healthcare-Associated Infection (HAI) Prevalence Survey* estimated that *110,800 surgical site infections (SSIs)* were associated with inpatient surgeries—a *4% increase* from the previous year. Despite advancements in infection prevention, including improved ventilation, sterilization techniques, and antimicrobial prophylaxis, SSIs continue to contribute significantly to morbidity, prolonged hospital stays, and mortality [4].

SSIs account for *20% of all HAIs*, increasing mortality risk *by 2–11 times*, with *75% of SSI-related deaths* directly attributed to infection. These infections are also the *costliest type of HAI*, with an annual financial burden of *$3.3 billion* in the U.S. and an average *hospital stay extension of 9.7 days*, leading to *an additional $20,000 per patient* in hospitalization costs.

In *India, approximately 300,000 SSIs* occur each year, necessitating an *additional 6.5 days of hospitalization* per patient. This significantly increases surgery costs—by up to *five times*—and imposes a considerable financial strain on healthcare systems. Bone and joint infections further contribute to prolonged hospital stays and patient morbidity, emphasizing the need for improved prevention and management strategies [5, 6].

6.2 Antimicrobial Susceptibility Testing

Clinical microbiology laboratories play a crucial role in diagnosing and guiding the treatment of infectious diseases. The isolation of bacteria from clinical samples allows for the selection of appropriate antibiotics based on known susceptibility profiles.

With the increasing prevalence of *antimicrobial resistance (AMR)* in both community and healthcare settings, empirical antibiotic selection has become increasingly complex. Routine *antimicrobial susceptibility testing (AST)* is now more critical than ever in ensuring effective, targeted therapy [7].

6.2.1 Reporting of Antimicrobial Susceptibility Results

Various methods are used for AST, including conventional, automated, and molecular techniques. A clear understanding of these methods enables clinicians to accurately interpret laboratory-reported results.

Antibiotics selected for susceptibility testing depend on factors such as the *bacterial species, infection site, and hospital formulary*. Following testing, the clinical microbiology laboratory must determine which results should be released into the hospital information system. Typically, an institutional committee comprising *microbiologists, infectious disease specialists, and pharmacologists* oversees the selection of antimicrobial agents to be reported in different clinical scenarios.

Selective reporting plays a key role in antimicrobial stewardship by discouraging the unnecessary use of broad-spectrum antibiotics when narrower-spectrum agents would suffice. For example, while *Streptococcus pyogenes* isolates may be tested for *carbapenem* susceptibility, routinely reporting such results could lead to inappropriate prescribing. Therefore, certain susceptibility data should only be disclosed when specifically required, such as in cases of *unexpected resistance or multidrug resistance (MDR)* [8].

The *Clinical and Laboratory Standards Institute (CLSI)* provides guidelines on appropriate antimicrobial selection for commonly encountered and rare pathogens.

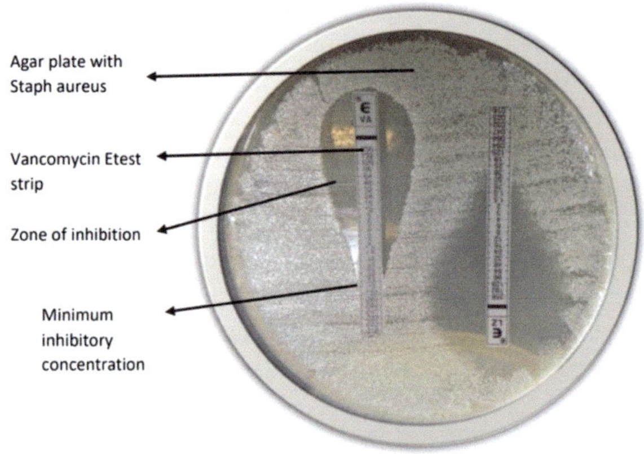

Fig. 6.1 Epsilometer (E-test) of vancomycin susceptibility in methicillin-resistant *Staphylococcus aureus*

Clinical microbiology laboratories should *retain bacterial isolates for at least 1 week* after finalizing culture reports, allowing for further testing if needed [9].

6.2.2 Interpretation of Antimicrobial Susceptibility Results

AST methods, such as *disk diffusion and minimum inhibitory concentration (MIC) testing*, yield measurable results that must be interpreted based on established breakpoints from *CLSI, EUCAST, or the FDA*.

The *CLSI interpretive categories* include:

- *Susceptible* (*S*): The antibiotic achieves sufficient concentrations at the infection site to inhibit bacterial growth, ensuring effective treatment (Fig. 6.1).
- *Intermediate* (*I*): The MIC is near achievable blood/tissue levels, and response rates may be lower than in susceptible isolates. In certain cases, clinical efficacy can still be achieved, particularly when antibiotics are concentrated at the infection site (e.g., *β-lactams, aminoglycosides, and fluoroquinolones in urine*). The intermediate category also acts as a *buffer zone* to account for minor technical variability.
- *Resistant* (*R*): The antibiotic fails to achieve inhibitory concentrations at the infection site, suggesting *the presence of resistance mechanisms* or *insufficient clinical efficacy*.

For commonly encountered bacteria, *breakpoints are determined through a comprehensive review of microbiological, clinical, and pharmacodynamic data* to ensure optimal classification.

6.3 Types and Goals of Antimicrobial Therapy

Antimicrobial therapy is categorized into *prophylactic, empirical, and definitive (targeted) therapy* based on the clinical context.

6.3.1 Prophylactic Therapy

Prophylaxis involves administering antibiotics *before infection develops* to prevent bacterial colonization and subsequent infection. *Primary prophylaxis* aims to prevent initial infection in high-risk patients, whereas *secondary prophylaxis* is used to prevent recurrence in those with a history of infection.

While prophylaxis can significantly reduce infection rates, its indiscriminate use may lead to *microbiome disruption, antibiotic resistance, toxicity, and increased costs*. Therefore, prophylactic antibiotics should be *narrow-spectrum, appropriately timed, and administered for the shortest necessary duration* [10].

The choice of prophylactic antibiotic depends on *the surgical site and most likely contaminating pathogens. Staphylococcus aureus and coagulase-negative staphylococci* are the primary culprits in post-surgical infections following clean procedures [11, 12].

6.3.2 Empirical Therapy

Empirical therapy is initiated *before pathogen identification*, based on *clinical presentation and local antibiograms*. Broad-spectrum antibiotics covering the most probable pathogens are typically selected in line with *institutional and international guidelines*.

6.3.3 Definitive (Targeted) Therapy

Definitive therapy involves *narrowing antibiotic coverage* once pathogen identification and susceptibility results are available. This approach minimizes *unnecessary broad-spectrum antibiotic use*, reducing resistance development and toxicity.

It is crucial to *train residents and clinicians* in institutional antibiotic policies to ensure optimal antimicrobial therapy outcomes. Misuse of antibiotics can lead to *inferior clinical results*, as seen in cases where *vancomycin is inappropriately prescribed for methicillin-susceptible Staphylococcus aureus (MSSA)* when *cloxacillin* is the preferred agent.

6.4 Management of Bone and Joint Infections

The primary antibiotics used in musculoskeletal infections include cephalosporins, carbapenems, vancomycin, and piperacillin-tazobactam, among others. This section highlights essential principles of antibiotic selection, their pharmacological characteristics, spectrum of microbial coverage, and specific clinical applications [13, 14].

Vancomycin

Vancomycin is primarily utilized for empirical or pathogen-specific treatment of *methicillin-resistant Staphylococcus aureus (MRSA) and Enterococcus spp* [15, 16].

Indications, Dosage, and Duration

- *Bloodstream Infections/Sepsis/Septic Shock*: 15–20 mg/kg/dose every 8–12 h, adjusted based on therapeutic drug monitoring. Uncomplicated *S. aureus* infections require a minimum of 14 days from the first negative blood culture.
- *Osteomyelitis*: Typically, treatment extends for ≥6 weeks. If the affected bone is completely resected, shorter courses may be considered.
- *Prosthetic Joint Infections* (*off-label use*): Therapy duration varies from 2 to 6 weeks, depending on prosthesis management.
- *Septic Arthritis*: Treatment spans *3–4 weeks* in the absence of osteomyelitis, with oral step-down therapy as appropriate. A 4-week intravenous (IV) course is recommended for cases with concurrent bacteremia.
- *Skin and Soft Tissue Infections* (*Hospitalized Patients*): Adjust dosing according to therapeutic monitoring of vancomycin trough levels, especially in severe cases.
- *Surgical Site Infections*: For uncomplicated *S. aureus* infections, a 14-day treatment duration is optimal.
- *Surgical Prophylaxis*: Recommended for MRSA or gram-positive coverage in patients who cannot tolerate beta-lactams. Vancomycin should be administered *within 60–120 min prior to the initial incision*, with intraoperative dose adjustments if the procedure is prolonged or there is significant blood loss. If extended prophylaxis is necessary, the total duration should not exceed 24 h.

Monitoring Regular renal function tests, vancomycin trough levels (15–20 μg/mL in severe infections), and vigilance for infusion-related adverse effects such as *Red Man Syndrome* are essential.

Piperacillin-Tazobactam

Piperacillin-tazobactam is a broad-spectrum penicillin derivative active against *Streptococci, Enterococci, Enterobacterales, and Pseudomonas aeruginosa*. It is exclusively administered parenterally and requires renal dosage adjustments.

Indications and Dosage

- *Skin and Soft Tissue Infections* (*Moderate to Severe*): Administered IV at *3.375 g every 6 h* or *4.5 g every 8 h*, particularly in necrotizing infections or cases at risk for *P. aeruginosa*.
- *Bloodstream Infections* (*Gram-negative Bacteremia*): Used as empirical therapy for known or suspected gram-negative pathogens. Extended infusions (30 min or 4 h) enhance efficacy.
- *General Duration*: Treatment typically spans *7–14 days*, with shorter durations (7 days) sufficient for uncomplicated *Enterobacteriaceae* infections demonstrating a favorable response.

Cefuroxime

Cefuroxime is effective against *both gram-positive and gram-negative organisms*, making it a valuable agent in postoperative infections.

Surgical Prophylaxis [17]

- *Adults*: IV *1.5 g* administered within 60 min prior to incision; an additional dose is required intraoperatively if the procedure lasts ≥4 h or if there is significant blood loss. If postoperative prophylaxis is deemed necessary, the total duration should be ≤24 h.
- *Children and Adolescents*: IV *50 mg/kg*, with a maximum dose of *1500 mg/dose*; repeat as needed during prolonged procedures.

Carbapenems (Imipenem, Meropenem, Meropenem/Vaborbactam)

Carbapenems exhibit a *broad spectrum of activity against aerobic and anaerobic microorganisms*, offering resistance to beta-lactamase-mediated hydrolysis.

Microbial Coverage

- Active against *Streptococci, Enterococcus faecalis, staphylococci (excluding MRSA), Enterobacterales*, and many strains of *Pseudomonas* and *Acinetobacter*.
- Carbapenem resistance among these organisms is increasing, necessitating cautious use.

Indications and Dosage

- *Skin and Soft Tissue Infections* (*Moderate to Severe*)
  - *Necrotizing Infections*: IV *1 g every 6–8 h* until further debridement is unnecessary, clinical improvement is evident, and the patient has been afebrile for ≥48 h.

  - *Non-necrotizing Infections*: IV *500 mg every 6 h*, with treatment duration (including oral step-down therapy) ranging from *5 to 14 days*, depending on severity and response.
- *Bloodstream Infections* (*Gram-negative Bacteremia*)
  - Used for empirical or pathogen-directed therapy in infections resistant to other agents.
  - Standard treatment duration is *7–14 days*, with shorter courses (7 days) recommended for uncomplicated *Enterobacteriaceae* infections in responsive patients. Prolonged therapy may be required in immunocompromised individuals.

Dosage Considerations

- *Imipenem*: IV *500 mg every 6 h* (infused over 30 min) or *1 g every 6–8 h* (infused over 40–60 min). Extended infusion (off-label) at *500 mg–1 g over 3 h* may be beneficial, particularly in sepsis.
- *Meropenem*: IV *1–2 g every 8 h* in normal renal function.
- *Meropenem/Vaborbactam*: Reserved for *multidrug-resistant gram-negative* infections, dosed at *2 g meropenem + 2 g vaborbactam every 8 h.*

Clinical Considerations

- Extended infusion strategies optimize pharmacokinetic/pharmacodynamic targets and may improve outcomes in severe infections.
- *Renal dose adjustments* are necessary for patients with impaired kidney function.

The antibiotic selection in musculoskeletal infections should be rational, considering microbial spectrum, patient-specific factors, and pharmacokinetic properties. Adherence to recommended dosages, monitoring for adverse effects, and adjusting therapy based on patient response remain fundamental to optimizing treatment outcomes.

Tissue Penetration of Antibiotics and Infection Severity [18–21]
The effectiveness of antimicrobial therapy depends on the ability of antibiotics to reach the infection site at adequate concentrations. Compared to plasma or serum levels, antibiotic concentrations in infected tissues and bones are often lower. Several factors contribute to this reduced penetration, including local vascularization, tissue permeability, and protein binding of the antibiotic.

Due to limited research in this area, it remains unclear whether these lower concentrations at infection sites lead to therapeutic failure or contribute to bacterial resistance (Fig. 6.2). However, excessive dosing to compensate for low penetration may lead to toxicity, such as nephrotoxicity. Optimizing pharmacokinetic/

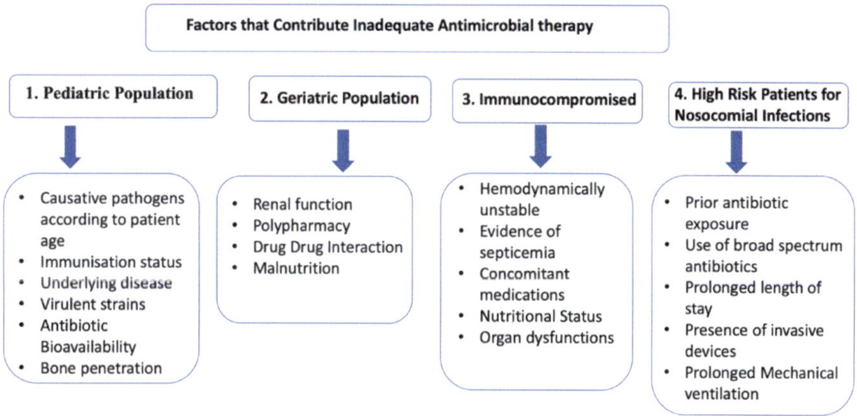

Fig. 6.2 Factors leading to inadequate antimicrobial therapy in special populations [22–25]

pharmacodynamic (PK/PD) parameters is critical to ensuring effective treatment while minimizing adverse effects. An appropriate dosing regimen based on target-site concentrations can improve treatment outcomes and reduce unnecessary side effects.

Lessons from Existing Antimicrobial Agents

Antibiotic dose optimization based on infection site characteristics is essential for improving treatment efficacy while minimizing adverse effects. Choosing the most effective antibiotic with the least toxicity enhances patient outcomes. Additionally, monitoring the use of WHO reserve-category antibiotics in clinical settings is crucial for better infection control and antibiotic stewardship.

A multidisciplinary approach involving an infectious disease team alongside the treating physician can help optimize antibiotic selection and dosing. Rational prescribing that incorporates PK/PD principles ensures effective treatment while reducing toxicity and cost. Adhering to antimicrobial stewardship guidelines enhances overall healthcare performance by promoting evidence-based prescribing practices.

New Antimicrobials Approved for Multidrug-Resistant Infections

With the increasing prevalence of multidrug-resistant (MDR) bacterial infections, the development of novel antibiotics remains a critical priority. Below is an overview of recently approved antibacterial agents by the United States Food and Drug Administration (US FDA) from 2018 to 2024, highlighting their mechanisms of action, indications, and clinical relevance (Table 6.1) [20, 26].

By incorporating these newly approved antibiotics into clinical practice, healthcare providers can enhance treatment strategies for multidrug-resistant infections while ensuring judicious antibiotic use to mitigate resistance (Fig. 6.3).

Table 6.1 Recent FDA-approved antimicrobial agents (2018–2024)

Antimicrobial agent	Indications
Ceftobiprole medocaril sodium (2024)	Staphylococcus aureus bloodstream infections, acute bacterial skin and skin structure infections (ABSSSI), and community-acquired bacterial pneumonia (CABP)
Cefepime-enmetazobactam (2024)	Treatment of complicated urinary tract infections (cUTIs)
Sulopenem etzadroxil/probenecid (2024)	Approved for uncomplicated urinary tract infections (uUTIs)
Cefiderocol (2019)	A siderophore cephalosporin used for the treatment of complicated urinary tract infections (cUTIs). It is administered as an intravenous (IV) infusion, 2 g every 8 h for 7–14 days
Omadacycline (2018)	A tetracycline-class antibiotic approved for community-acquired bacterial pneumonia (CABP) and ABSSSI. *Dosage*: Loading dose on day 1: 200 mg IV over 60 min or 100 mg IV over 30 min twice, followed by 100 mg IV daily. *Oral dosage*: 450 mg once daily on days 1 and 2, then 300 mg once daily for a total duration of 7–14 days
Plazomicin (2018)	Designed for treating infections caused by gram-negative aerobic bacteria in complicated urinary tract infections (cUTIs).

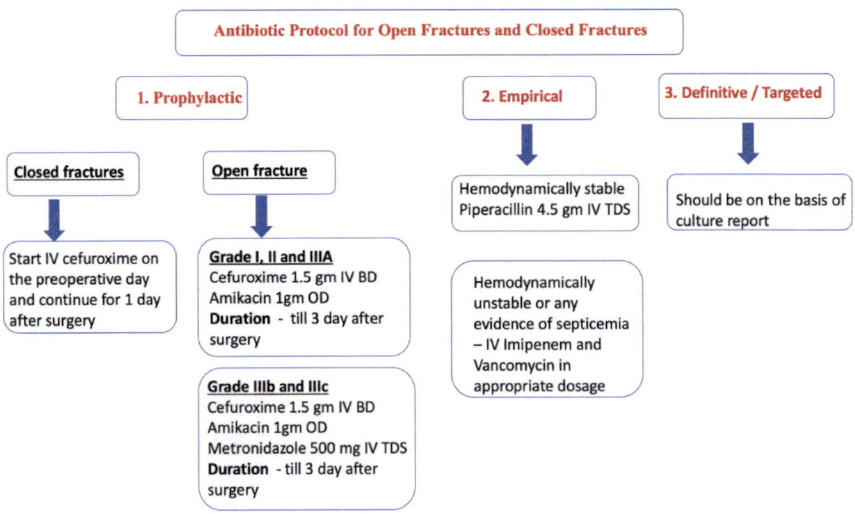

Fig. 6.3 Flowchart: Institutional antibiotic protocol for open fractures and closed fractures

Clinical Implications of New Antimicrobials

1. *Addressing Multidrug Resistance (MDR):*
    - Novel β-lactam/β-lactamase inhibitor combinations (e.g., cefepime-enmetazobactam, sulopenem) enhance treatment options for ESBL-producing bacteria.
    - Cefiderocol, with its unique siderophore-mediated entry, provides a promising solution against carbapenem-resistant infections.
    - Plazomicin expands aminoglycoside therapy for MDR *Enterobacterales.*
2. *Optimizing Pharmacokinetics and Dosing Strategies:*
    - Prolonged β-lactam infusions and combination therapies are being explored to maximize bacterial eradication.
    - Omadacycline offers an oral treatment alternative, improving outpatient therapy options.
    - Sulopenem combined with probenecid improves oral bioavailability and extends its half-life.
3. *Enhancing Antibiotic Stewardship:*
    - The introduction of these agents highlights the need for careful antibiotic selection to prevent the emergence of resistance.
    - Surveillance of WHO reserve-category antibiotics ensures judicious use in healthcare settings.
    - Combining antimicrobial stewardship programs with infectious disease expertise optimizes treatment regimens while minimizing toxicity.

6.5 Conclusion

Managing musculoskeletal infections is complex, requiring an understanding of microbial resistance, antibiotic pharmacokinetics, and biofilms. Effective treatment balances prophylactic, empirical, and definitive therapy while minimizing resistance risks. Emerging antimicrobials offer new options but demand judicious use, guided by antimicrobial stewardship programs. Future advancements should focus on local antibiotic delivery, biofilm disruption, and optimized pharmacokinetics. A multidisciplinary approach combining surgery, targeted antimicrobial therapy, and infection prevention remains essential for successful management.

References

1. Colston J, Atkins B. Bone and joint infection. Clin Med. 2018;18(2):150–4.
2. Matthews PC, Berendt AR, McNally MA, Byren I. Diagnosis and management of prosthetic joint infection. BMJ. 2009;338:b1773.
3. Baldan R, Sendi P. Precision medicine in the diagnosis and management of orthopedic biofilm infections. Front Med (Lausanne). 2020;7:580671.
4. Metsemakers WJ, Moriarty TF, Morgenstern M, Marais L, Onsea J, O'Toole RV, Depypere M, Obremskey WT, Verhofstad MH, McNally M, Morshed S. The global burden of fracture-related infection: can we do better? Lancet Infect Dis. 2024;24(6):e386–93.
5. Vedachalam SK, Siromany VA, VanderEnde D, Malpiedi P, Vasquez A, Dikid T, et al. Implementing a healthcare-associated bloodstream infection surveillance network in India: a mixed-methods study on the best practices, challenges and opportunities, 2022. Antimicrob Resist Infect Control. 2024;13(1):1–4.
6. Skender K, Machowska A, Singh V, Goel V, Marothi Y, Lundborg CS, Sharma M. Antibiotic use, incidence and risk factors for orthopedic surgical site infections in a teaching hospital in Madhya Pradesh, India. Antibiotics. 2022;11(6):748.
7. Tamma PD, Heil EL, Justo JA, Mathers AJ, Satlin MJ, Bonomo RA. Infectious Diseases Society of America 2024 guidance on the treatment of antimicrobial-resistant gram-negative infections. Clin Infect Dis. 2024:ciae403. https://doi.org/10.1093/cid/ciae403. Epub ahead of print.
8. Wang B, Wang Q, Hamushan M, Yu J, Jiang F, Li M, Guo G, Tang J, Han P, Shen H. Trends in microbiological epidemiology of orthopedic infections: a large retrospective study from 2008 to 2021. BMC Infect Dis. 2023;23(1):567.
9. Clinical and Laboratory Standards Institute (CLSI). Performance standards for antimicrobial susceptibility testing. CLSI supplement M100. 31st ed. Wayne: CLSI; 2021.
10. Bratzler DW, Dellinger EP, Olsen KM, Perl TM, Auwaerter PG, Bolon MK, Fish DN, Napolitano LM, Sawyer RG, Slain D, Steinberg JP, Weinstein RA. Clinical practice guidelines for antimicrobial prophylaxis in surgery. Am J Health Syst Pharm. 2013;70(3):195–283.
11. Upadhyyaya GK, Tewari S. Enhancing surgical outcomes: a critical review of antibiotic prophylaxis in orthopedic surgery. Cureus. 2023;15(10):e47828.
12. Dhammi IK, Haq RU, Kumar S. Prophylactic antibiotics in orthopedic surgery: controversial issues in its use. Indian J Orthop. 2015;49(4):373.
13. Subbiah VB. Principles of antibiotic therapy in orthopedic surgery. J Orthop Joint Surg. 2021;3(1):51–3.
14. Oliphant CM. Management of orthopedic infections. J Nurse Pract. 2015;11(10):1036–42.
15. Miller WR, Arias CA. ESKAPE pathogens: antimicrobial resistance, epidemiology, clinical impact and therapeutics. Nat Rev Microbiol. 2024;22(10):598–616.
16. Pinchera B, Buonomo AR, Schiano Moriello N, Scotto R, Villari R, Gentile I. Update on the management of surgical site infections. Antibiotics. 2022;11(11):1608.
17. Leaper DJ, Edmiston CE. World Health Organization: global guidelines for the prevention of surgical site infection. J Hosp Infect. 2017;95(2):135–6.
18. Cancienne JM, Burrus MT, Weiss DB, Yarboro SR. Applications of local antibiotics in orthopedic trauma. Orthop Clin. 2015;46(4):495–510.
19. Koch BC, Zhao Q, Oosterhoff M, van Oldenrijk J, Abdulla A, de Winter BC, Bos K, Muller AE. The mysteries of target site concentrations of antibiotics in bone and joint infections: what is known? A narrative review. Expert Opin Drug Metab Toxicol. 2022;18(9):587–600.
20. Andrei S, Droc G, Stefan G. FDA approved antibacterial drugs: 2018–2019. Discoveries (Craiova). 2019;7(4):e102.
21. Thabit AK, Fatani DF, Bamakhrama MS, Barnawi OA, Basudan LO, Alhejaili SF. Antibiotic penetration into bone and joints: an updated review. Int J Infect Dis. 2019;81:128–36.

22. Falcone M, Paul M, Tiseo G, Yahav D, Prendki V, Friberg LE, Guerri R, Gavazzi G, Mussini C, Tinelli M. Considerations for the optimal management of antibiotic therapy in elderly patients. J Global Antimicrob Resist. 2020;22:325–33.
23. Kollef MH. Inadequate antimicrobial treatment: an important determinant of outcome for hospitalized patients. Clin Infect Dis. 2000;31(Suppl_4):S131–8.
24. Autore G, Bernardi L, Esposito S. Update on acute bone and joint infections in paediatrics: a narrative review on the most recent evidence-based recommendations and appropriate antinfective therapy. Antibiotics (Basel). 2020;9(8):486.
25. Masters EA, Ricciardi BF, Bentley KL, Moriarty TF, Schwarz EM, Muthukrishnan G. Skeletal infections: microbial pathogenesis, immunity and clinical management. Nat Rev Microbiol. 2022;20(7):385–400.
26. https://www.fda.gov/drugs/novel-drug-approvals-fda/novel-drug-approvals-2024.

Surgical Principles of Management of Orthopedic Infections

7

Rakesh John, Tarkik Thami, and Prasoon Kumar

Abstract

Orthopedic infections, including osteomyelitis, septic arthritis, and necrotizing soft tissue infections, remain a significant clinical challenge due to their variable presentations and potential for serious functional impairment. This chapter outlines key surgical strategies required for effective infection control, focusing on early recognition, meticulous surgical debridement, and close coordination with multidisciplinary teams. Management of acute osteomyelitis often involves drainage and removal of necrotic material, while chronic infections require sequestrectomy, dead space management, and stabilization techniques such as external fixation or antibiotic-coated implants. Septic arthritis demands urgent joint lavage to protect cartilage integrity, and severe soft tissue infections may necessitate radical excision or amputation in life-threatening scenarios. Techniques such as negative pressure wound therapy, antibiotic-loaded PMMA beads, and reconstructive plastic surgery are discussed as adjuncts in wound and defect management. The chapter emphasizes that surgical intervention, combined with tailored antibiotic therapy and systemic support, is vital to achieving favourable outcomes in orthopedic infection care.

Keywords

Osteomyelitis · Septic arthritis · Dead space management · Antibiotic loaded PMMA beads

R. John (✉)
Macclesfield District General Hospital, Macclesfield, UK

T. Thami
Department of Orthopedics, AIMS, Mohali, Punjab, India

P. Kumar
Department of Orthopedics, PGIMER, Chandigarh, Punjab, India

P. Kumar et al. (eds.), *Textbook of Orthopedic Infections*,
https://doi.org/10.1007/978-981-95-5029-6_7

7.1 Introduction

Musculoskeletal infections are a complex and multifaceted medical concern, affecting both adults and children across a broad spectrum of conditions. These infections can impact various structures, including bones (osteomyelitis), joints (septic arthritis), muscles, and soft tissues, each posing distinct diagnostic and treatment challenges [1, 2].

These infections can be difficult to tackle due to factors such as delayed detection, antibiotic resistance, prolonged treatment duration, and the risk of severe complications like joint damage, chronic pain, and long-term disability. Treatment often necessitates a combination of medical and surgical approaches, including antibiotic therapy, surgical debridement, and, in severe cases, reconstructive procedures [3].

In addition to clinical complexities, musculoskeletal infections place a significant financial strain on both patients and healthcare providers. Patients may experience high costs due to extended hospital stays, multiple surgeries, rehabilitation, and potential loss of income. For orthopedic specialists and other medical professionals, addressing these infections demands considerable expertise, time, and resources, highlighting the importance of early diagnosis, preventive strategies, and evidence-based management [4, 5]. The musculoskeletal infections generally managed by an orthopedic surgeon can be broadly classified as:

(a) Bone infection (osteomyelitis)
(b) Joint infection (septic arthritis)
(c) Soft tissue infection (STI)

The management of orthopedic infections requires both medical (antimicrobial treatment) and surgical treatment options which go hand in hand [3]. Although surgery is not always necessary, surgical debridement is essential to eradicate infection when there is purulent and necrotic tissue or if there is no response to antimicrobial medications to augment the host response [6].

In this chapter, we will focus on the basic surgical principles of management of musculoskeletal infections—both bone and soft tissue infections. Prosthetic joint infections will be covered separately in a different chapter and is outside the scope of this chapter.

7.2 Osteomyelitis

Acute osteomyelitis is a bacterial infection that may develop through hematogenous spread, direct inoculation, or infection from nearby structures (Fig. 7.1). *Staphylococcus aureus* is the most common causative pathogen, initiating an inflammatory response upon colonization [2]. This response leads to the release of proinflammatory cytokines, resulting in increased vascular permeability, tissue swelling, and infiltration by neutrophils. As the infection advances, pus accumulates within the bone, raising intraosseous pressure and restricting blood flow, which

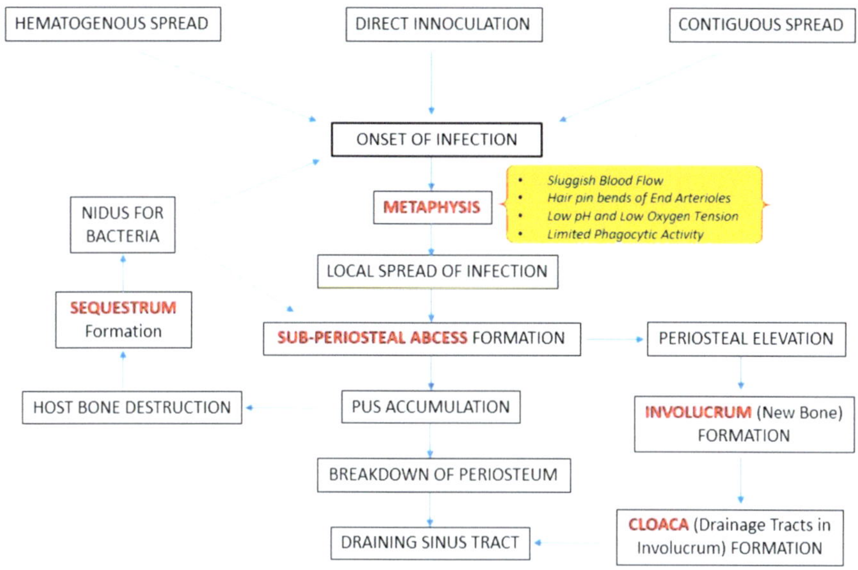

Fig. 7.1 Pathophysiology of osteomyelitis

ultimately causes local ischemia and necrosis of surrounding bone. The formation of sequestra, or dead bone fragments, serves as a reservoir for ongoing infection, while the body may attempt to counteract the damage by generating new bone, known as Involucrum [3]. If not promptly managed, acute osteomyelitis can transition into a chronic state, characterized by persistent infection, progressive bone destruction, and the formation of sinus tracts (Fig. 7.2).

Historically, management of osteomyelitis has been challenging for the orthopedic surgeon. The resultant morbidity and mortality are much lower in the modern era with the advent of antimicrobial therapy and aggressive surgical management [3, 4]. Successful management of osteomyelitis relies on diagnosing the infection early, aggressive and radical surgical debridement, early initiation of antibiotics and continued medical treatment in liaison with microbiologist, and the involvement of multidisciplinary care—especially the involvement of plastic surgeon to cover soft tissue defects.

Osteomyelitis can be broadly classified (based on Temporality) into:

- Acute osteomyelitis
- Subacute osteomyelitis
- Chronic osteomyelitis

In this chapter, we shall focus on the surgical principles in the management of acute and chronic osteomyelitis.

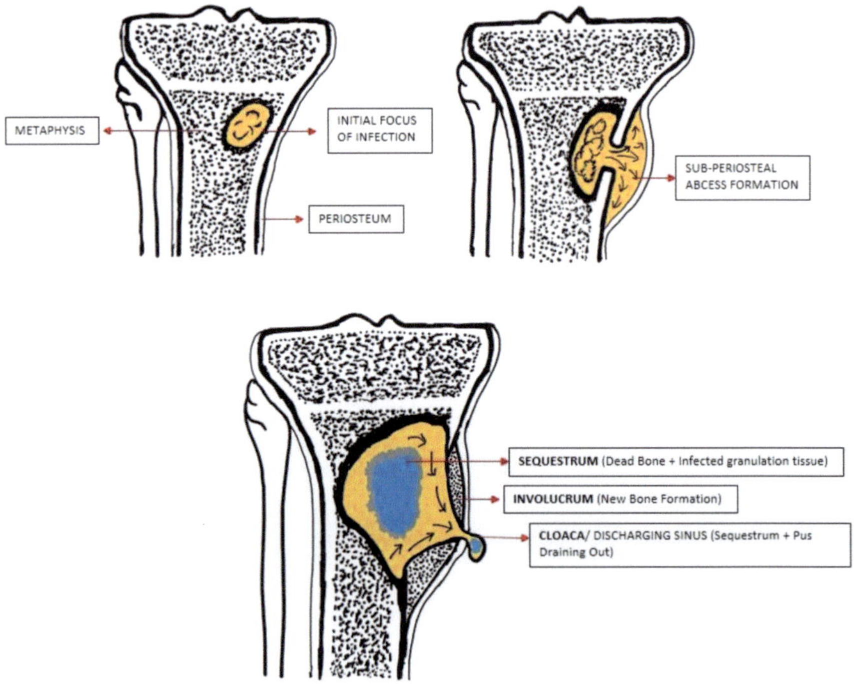

Fig. 7.2 Pathoanatomy of osteomyelitis of tibia

7.2.1 Acute Osteomyelitis

There are two indications for surgery in acute osteomyelitis:

(a) To evacuate an abscess.
(b) Failure of patient to improve clinically despite 24–48 h of initiation of intravenous antibiotics.

The key aims of surgery are to drain any abscess, excise all necrotic tissue, and send plenty of samples for microbiological testing [7].

Surgical Principles of Incision and Drainage of Acute Osteomyelitis

- Tourniquet use is encouraged whenever possible without exsanguinating the limb. The amount of blood loss in these procedures is often underestimated during these procedures.
- Expose the affected part of the bone through the appropriate surgical approach.
- Periosteum is incised longitudinally—subperiosteal abscess should be evacuated at this stage.

- Drill multiple 3.5 mm holes through the bone cortex—if pus escapes out, it confirms the presence of intramedullary abscess.
- Use a drill to outline an oval cortical window and remove the bony window with an osteotome to gain access to the intramedullary canal.
- Evacuate pus and debride all necrotic tissue with a combination of curettage and bony rongeurs.
- Ensure multiple samples are sent for microbiology and pathological examination before commencing the washout.
- Thorough washout of the intramedullary pus is done with at least 3 L of warmed normal saline with or without antibiotics/aqueous betadine.
- Closure of skin should be loose and preferably done with drains. Do not attempt closure if the skin tension is high during closure.
- There will invariably be a high risk of pathological fracture and therefore the limb must be protected for several weeks till there is clinic-radiologic evidence for bone healing and resolution of osteomyelitis. This can be with plaster or with an external fixator based on the location, size of the infection and patient-specific factors.

Surgical and medical management always go hand in hand for management of acute orthopedic infections. It is important to continue broad-spectrum IV antibiotics post-operatively in liaison with the Microbiology team. Although there is no consensus on the optimal duration of antibiotics, it is now commonplace to give a short course of IV antibiotics (2–3 weeks) followed by oral antibiotics (3–4 weeks) with serial monitoring of inflammatory markers and serum antibiotic levels [4, 5].

1. *Chronic osteomyelitis*

   A three-pronged, holistic approach is necessary to treat chronic bone infections:

   (a) *Host immunity*—improve nutrition, smoking cessation, strict glycaemic control in diabetics, optimal management of medical comorbidities to ensure good renal and hepatic function etc.
   (b) *Antibiotic therapy*—ideally initiated after tissue samples have been sent from the surgical debridement for microbiological examination to reduce the probability of false negative results.
   (c) *Surgical debridement*—cornerstone of successful management of chronic osteomyelitis.

As a rule, chronic osteomyelitis cannot be cured without surgery. The reason is bacteria adhere to bone matrix and/or orthopedic implants through a variety of receptors and/or form a slimy layer to evade phagocytes. Therefore, pure antibiotic therapy cannot eradicate a chronic bone infection [6]. The sequestrum (formed as a result of accumulation of infected granulation tissue around dead necrotic bone) also serves as a nidus for further bacterial colonization and multiplication (Fig. 7.3).

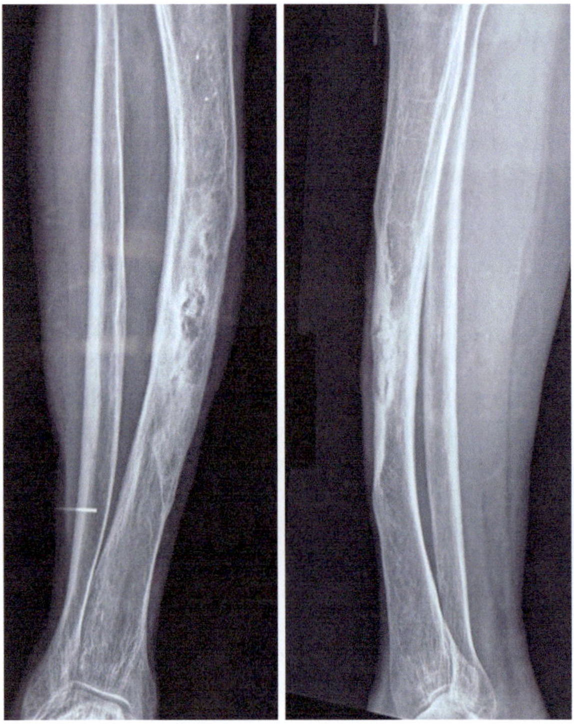

Fig. 7.3 Chronic osteomyelitis of tibia leading to a deformity in sagittal and coronal planes

Surgery consists of sequestrectomy and thorough resection of dead and non-viable soft tissue with a goal of creating a vascular, viable environment for bone regrowth. The thoroughness of debridement of necrotic bone and soft tissue directly correlates with the number of trips to the operation theatre and therefore the resolution of the established infection.

Debridement in chronic osteomyelitis is a double-edged sword. On one hand, inadequate debridement is the most important reason for failure in treating chronic osteomyelitis. On the other hand, adequate debridement often leaves a large dead space and bony instability which needs to be managed [7, 8].

External fixators are generally used after debridement to provide stability, reduce the risk of pathological fractures, and encourage patient mobilization and care [6].

Surgical Principles of Debridement in Chronic Osteomyelitis (Sequestrectomy and Curettage)

- Ensure patient is medically optimized, all relevant investigations have been completed to ensure proper pre-operative planning and make sure that cross-matched blood is available. The amount of blood loss is often under-estimated by an inexperienced orthopedic surgeon.
- Sinus tracts can be injected with methylene blue dye 24 h before surgery to light it up during surgery enabling complete resection.

- Use tourniquet when possible without exsanguinating the limb.
- Expose the infected area of bone with the appropriate surgical approach and excise all sinus tracts completely—send for biopsy and microbiological examination.
- Incise the indurated periosteum and elevate it 1–2.5 cm on each side.
- Outline an oval cortical window with a drill at the site and use an osteotome to remove the bone window (Fig. 7.4).
- Excise the pus, sequestrum, and all dead, necrotic tissue.
- Use a reamer to open both ends of the intramedullary canal to encourage vascularization.
- A combination of high-speed burr, curette and bony rongeur are used to debride necrotic bone until the "paprika sign" is observed (active punctate bleeding bone) (Fig. 7.4a).
- Multiple tissue samples should be sent for culture and pathological examination.
- Excise the overhanging edges of the bone at the mouth of the cavity to reduce the chances of re-collection.
- Thorough washout with at least 3 L of warmed normal saline and aqueous betadine/antibiotic-laden saline.
- The resultant dead space is usually filled with antibiotic-eluting PMMA beads or with bone grafting whichever is appropriate.
- If there is non-union with any bony instability, the bone must be stabilized with:

    (a) External fixator preferably with an Ilizarov-type circular frame.

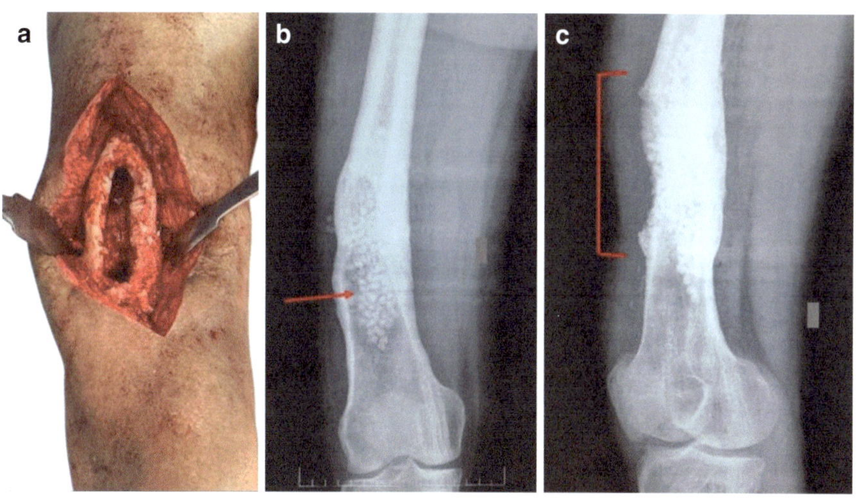

Fig. 7.4 (**a**) Depiction of sequestrectomy, followed by saucerization to open a walled off cavity inside the bone, (**b**) arrow highlights the use of calcium sulphate beads as an antibiotic delivery agent and to reduce dead space, (**c**) saucerization as visible on the lateral view

(b) Antibiotic-eluting cemented intramedullary nail can be used in certain long bone infections and avoids the common complications associated with the bulky circular external fixators.

- If possible, close the skin loosely over drains and ensure that no excessive skin tension is present. If closure is impossible, pack the wound open loosely or apply an antibiotic bead pouch and plan for delayed closure or skin grafting at a later time in liaison with plastic surgeons.
- Appropriate post-operative antibiotic therapy should be initiated in liaison with Microbiology team.

7.2.2 Dead Space Management

Various methods have been described to manage the empty defect left after a radical debridement for chronic osteomyelitis [9–11]. This has to be chosen according to the specific infection factors and patient-specific factors. Generally, the modes of management are:

1. Bone grafting with primary or secondary closure [9].
2. Use of antibiotic loaded poly methyl methacrylate (PMMA) beads as a temporary filler for dead space management before definitive reconstruction of the bone defects (Fig. 7.5) [10].
3. Flap cover by plastic surgical team.
    - Local muscle flaps and skin grafting with or without bone grafting.

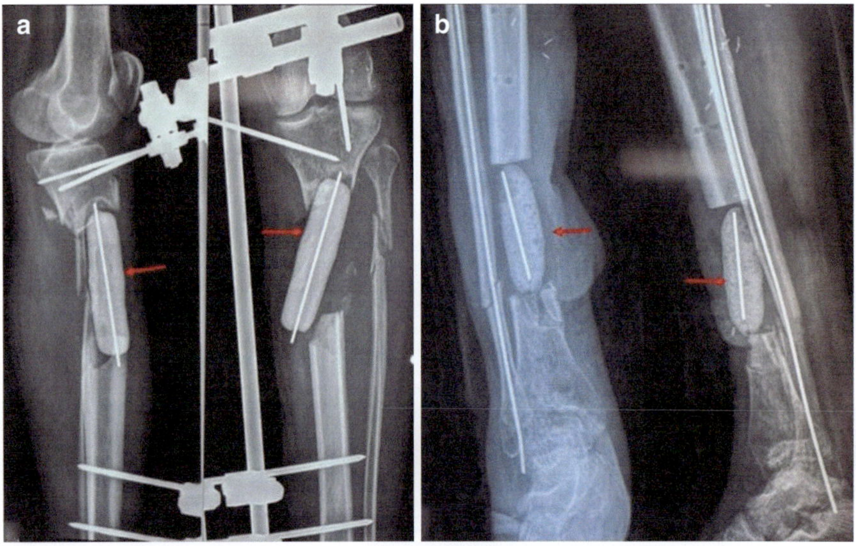

Fig. 7.5 PMMA bead insertion for dead space management (Red Arrows)

- Free flaps: microvascular transfer of muscle, myocutaneous, or fasciocutaneous flaps.

4. Use of bone transport (Ilizarov/Taylor spatial frames).

7.2.3 Antibiotic-Impregnated PMMA Beads and Bead Pouch Technique

Use of antibiotic-impregnated PMMA beads in the treatment of chronic osteomyelitis is now commonplace and provides the advantage of delivering high local dose of antibiotics that exceed the MIC (minimally inhibitory concentration) (Fig. 7.5). These antibiotic-loaded PMMA spacers can achieve local antibiotic concentrations up to 200 times higher than those reached through the systemic route [8]. As the need for systemic antibiotic administration is reduced, the adverse effects of antibiotics are reduced.

Primary wound closure is necessary to achieve high local concentration of antibiotics; however, if this cannot be achieved, the wound can be covered with a water-impermeable dressing to create an artificial pouch. This is called as the bead pouch technique [11, 12].

7.2.4 Negative Pressure Wound Therapy (NPWT)

This is an increasingly popular technique to manage open wounds after debridement procedure. The NPWT or VAC (vacuum-assisted closure) dressing system consists of a pump that generates a vacuum within a sealed wound creating a negative pressure environment, tubing to remove the fluid sucked out of the cavity and a container to collect the biowaste (Fig. 7.6) [13].

7.2.5 Amputation

Amputation is no longer performed commonly for osteomyelitis. However, it may be the preferred option in certain patients [14, 15].

The indications for amputation are:

1. Multiple operations and prolonged antibiotic therapy
2. Secondary malignancy—chronic osteomyelitis can turn malignant in up to 1.6% of the patients. The most common malignancy is a squamous cell carcinoma of the sinus tract. Amputation is the most reliable treatment for this complication.
3. Arterial insufficiency
4. Major nerve paralysis
5. Joint contractures and stiffness with a resultant non-functional limb

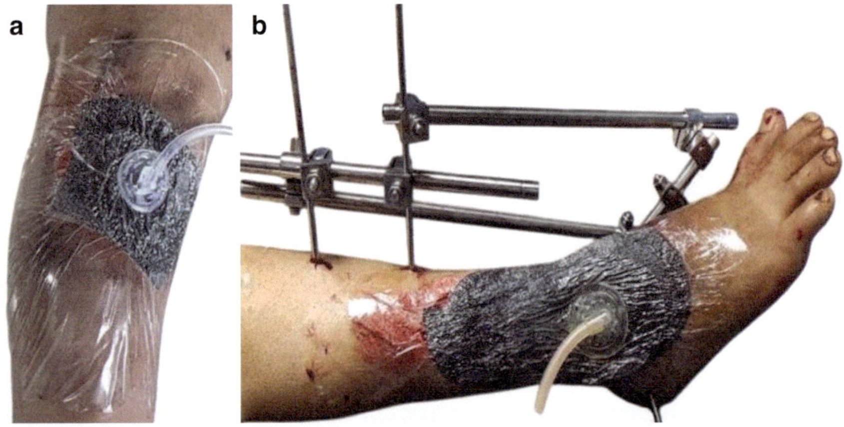

Fig. 7.6 Negative pressure wound therapy (NPWT)/vacuum-assisted closure (VAC) for wound management. (**a**) VAC applied for a soft tissue defect created post debridement and curettage; (**b**) VAC applied over the joint with an ankle spanning external fixator in place

7.3 Septic Arthritis/Infectious Arthritis

Septic arthritis is more common in adults; however, sequelae of septic arthritis are more significant in the younger population. Septic arthritis is secondary to inoculation of the sterile joint fluid by bacteria either through a haematogenous route; by direct inoculation from trauma; or by contiguous spread from adjacent infection foci (e.g. adjacent osteomyelitis, cellulitis).

Prompt identification and early drainage and evaluation of purulent joint fluid is crucial for preservation of articular cartilage and for resolution of the infection. Progression to sepsis and probability of suffering with septic sequelae is directly proportional to the initiation of treatment and timing of surgical drainage [16, 17].

The three core principles in the surgical management of acute septic arthritis include:

1. A thorough washout of the joint and debridement of all infected tissue.
2. Prompt initiation of systemic antibiotics to arrest local spread of infection.
3. Splinting the joint in a stable position to prevent contractures and stiffness.

Initiation of broad-spectrum antibiotics should be ideally done after samples have been obtained through joint aspiration prior to the surgical drainage. This reduces the chances of obtaining false-negative results from the intra-operative samples.

The drainage of the infected joint can be done by:

(a) Open incision and drainage
(b) Arthroscopic drainage
(c) Multiple joint aspirations (preferably image-guided)

All three methods have shown excellent results, and the choice of the drainage method is selected based on patient-specific factors, chronicity and spread of the infection and availability of hospital resources. The incidence of open drainage procedures for septic arthritis of large joints has decreased considerably in the last few decades with emphasis shifting to minimally invasive, arthroscopic joint washouts which have shown equal efficacy in multiple studies. Although, the choice of method of joint drainage can be controversial, there is no question about the importance of early surgical drainage in the management of septic arthritis.

As always, multidisciplinary care and involvement of a microbiologist to tailor the antibiotics for the patient is key to ensure resolution of a joint infection.

7.4 Soft Tissue Infections (STI)

Soft tissue infections can vary from the relatively benign cellulitis to the more malignant and life-threatening Necrotizing Soft Tissue Infections (NSTI), such as gas gangrene and necrotizing fasciitis. We will briefly touch upon the surgical principles of management of NSTI in this chapter as detailed description is outside the scope of this chapter.

1. *Gas gangrene/clostridial myonecrosis*

This is a highly lethal, deep soft tissue infection caused by flesh-eating bacteria belonging to the Clostridium family. This is a gram positive, anaerobic, spore forming bacteria with the most common bacteria being the C perfringens. The infection is characterized by rapidly progressive gangrene with production of foul-smelling gas and relatively rapid descent into sepsis and multi-organ failure [18].

The infection can be post-traumatic (especially in highly contaminated wounds), post-surgery (especially after colon or biliary surgery) or spontaneous in immunosuppressed patients. This is a true surgical emergency and requires concerted multidisciplinary team care, immediate initiation of antibiotic therapy and urgent trip to theatre for limb and life-saving surgery [18].

Treatment is radical surgical debridement and there is no role for non-operative treatment. The debridement is often combined with fasciotomy as there is a high risk of development of compartment syndrome and reperfusion syndrome. If detected relatively late, amputation could be the only option left for the surgeons but potentially a life-saving surgery.

2. *Necrotizing fasciitis*

This is a life-threatening soft tissue infection caused by different bacteria that spread rapidly along soft tissue planes. The most common type (80%–90%) is a polymicrobial infection especially in the immunosuppressed patients. Monomicrobial infection is usually secondary to group A beta haemolytic streptococcal infection often seen in healthy individuals [19–21].

The diagnosis is mainly clinical and suspicions are raised in the presence of skin discoloration, bullae, subcutaneous crepitus, and the classical dishwasher fluid on finger sweep test. The mortality rate can be as high as 30% with direct correlation to time to surgical intervention.

Aggressive radical debridement is the cornerstone to arrest the spread of fasciitis and to reduce mortality along with early initiation of broad-spectrum antibiotics and multidisciplinary care. Wong et al. introduced the zonal approach to make debridement for necrotizing soft tissue infection more systematic and objective [22].

The infected soft tissue is divided into three zones (Fig. 7.7):

- Zone 1 is necrotic tissue,
- Zone 2 is infected but potentially salvageable soft tissue, and
- Zone 3 is non-infected skin.

The junction between zones 2 and 3 frequently indicates the extent of the underlying fasciitis. Blunt probing of the wound defines the extent of infection which is followed by systematic excision. Zone 1 is completely excised. Zone 2 is

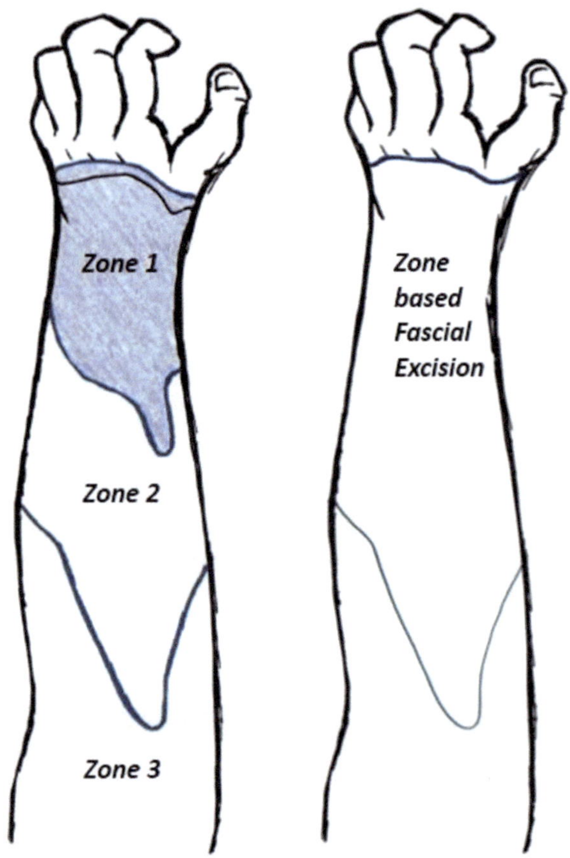

Fig. 7.7 Classification of skin and subcutaneous tissue involvement in necrotizing fasciitis to help in decision-making during debridement of non-viable skin

meticulously assessed and debrided with maximal preservation of salvageable tissue. Zone 3 is left alone. Evaluating skin viability through clinical assessment is crucial in determining the necessary extent of skin excision. The debridement has to be thorough to allow excision of all necrotic tissue and minimize unnecessary returns to the operating room.

References

1. Schmitt SK. Osteomyelitis. Infect Dis Clin N Am. 2017;31(2):325–38.
2. Calhoun JH, Manring MM. Adult osteomyelitis. Infect Dis Clin N Am. 2005;19(4):765–86.
3. Hofstee MI, Muthukrishnan G, Atkins GJ, et al. Current concepts of osteomyelitis: from pathologic mechanisms to advanced research methods. Am J Pathol. 2020;190(6):1151–63.
4. Birt MC, Anderson DW, Bruce Toby E, Wang J. Osteomyelitis: recent advances in pathophysiology and therapeutic strategies. J Orthop. 2016;14(1):45–52.
5. Steer AC, Carapetis JR. Acute hematogenous osteomyelitis in children: recognition and management. Paediatr Drugs. 2004;6(6):333–46.
6. Parsons B, Strauss E. Surgical management of chronic osteomyelitis. Am J Surg. 2004;188:57–66.
7. Daoud A, Saighi-Bouaouina A. Treatment of sequestra, pseudarthroses, and defects in the long bones of children who have chronic hematogenous osteomyelitis. J Bone Joint Surg Am. 1989;71(10):1448–68.
8. Van de Belt H, Neut D, Schenk W, van Horn JR, van der Mei HC, Busscher HJ. Infection of orthopedic implants and the use of antibiotic-loaded bone cements. A review. Acta Orthop Scand. 2001;72(6):557–71.
9. Lalidou F, Kolios G, Drosos GI. Bone infections and bone graft substitutes for local antibiotic therapy. Surg Technol Int. 2014;24:353–62.
10. Van Vugt TA, Geurts J, Arts JJ. Clinical application of antimicrobial bone graft substitute in osteomyelitis treatment: a systematic review of different bone graft substitutes available in clinical treatment of osteomyelitis. Biomed Res Int. 2016;2016:6984656.
11. Van Vugt TAG, Arts JJ, Geurts JAP. Antibiotic-loaded polymethylmethacrylate beads and spacers in treatment of orthopedic infections and the role of biofilm formation. Front Microbiol. 2019;10:1626.
12. Kulkarni GS, Kulkarni S, Babhulkar S. Cement beads and cement spacers: indications, techniques, and clinical results. OTA Int. 2021;4:e118(1–6).
13. Normandin S, Safran T, Winocour S, Chu CK, Vorstenbosch J, Murphy AM, Davison PG. Negative pressure wound therapy: mechanism of action and clinical applications. Semin Plast Surg. 2021;35(3):164–70.
14. Masters EA, Ricciardi BF, Bentley KLM, Moriarty TF, Schwarz EM, Muthukrishnan G. Skeletal infections: microbial pathogenesis, immunity and clinical management. Nat Rev Microbiol. 2022;20(7):385–400.
15. Schmidt BM, Keeney-Bonthrone TP, Hawes AM, Karmakar M, Frydrych LM, Cinti SK, Pop-Busui R, Delano MJ. Comorbid status in patients with osteomyelitis is associated with long-term incidence of extremity amputation. BMJ Open Diabetes Res Care. 2023;11(6):e003611.
16. He M, Arthur Vithran DT, Pan L, Zeng H, Yang G, Lu B, Zhang F. An update on recent progress of the epidemiology, etiology, diagnosis, and treatment of acute septic arthritis: a review. Front Cell Infect Microbiol. 2023;2(13):1193645.
17. Montgomery NI, Epps HR. Pediatric septic arthritis. Orthop Clin North Am. 2017;48(2):209–16.
18. Hussain H, Fadel A, Garcia E, Hernandez RJ, Saadoon ZF, Naseer L, Casmartino E, Hamad M, Schnepp T, Sarfraz R, Angly S, Jayakumar AR. Clostridial myonecrosis: a comprehensive review of toxin pathophysiology and management strategies. Microorganisms. 2024;12(7):1464.

19. Stevens DL, Bryant AE, Goldstein EJ. Necrotizing soft tissue infections. Infect Dis Clin N Am. 2021;35(1):135–55.
20. Tessier JM, Sanders J, Sartelli M, et al. Necrotizing soft tissue infections: a focused review of pathophysiology, diagnosis, operative management, antimicrobial therapy, and pediatrics. Surg Infect. 2020;21(2):81–93.
21. Allaw F, Wehbe S, Kanj SS. Necrotizing fasciitis: an update on epidemiology, diagnostic methods, and treatment. Curr Opin Infect Dis. 2024;37(2):105–11.
22. Wong CH, Yam AK, Tan AB, Song C. Approach to debridement in necrotizing fasciitis. Am J Surg. 2008;196(3):e19–24.

Pediatric Osteomyelitis

8

Ankit Dadra, Karthick Rangasamy, Nirmal Raj Gopinathan, and Jasmine Kaur

Abstract

Acute hematogenous osteomyelitis (AHO) is the most common musculoskeletal infection in children, primarily caused by hematogenous spread of pathogens—most notably *Staphylococcus aureus*—to the metaphyseal regions of long bones. Early diagnosis remains challenging due to nonspecific clinical signs, particularly in neonates and younger children, necessitating a high index of suspicion and thorough evaluation. This chapter provides a detailed overview of the etiopathogenesis, clinical features, diagnostic workup—including imaging and laboratory investigations—and management strategies for AHO. Emphasis is placed on the importance of a multidisciplinary approach combining empirical antibiotic therapy with timely surgical intervention, especially in cases involving abscess formation, persistent infection, or complications such as sequestrum or septic arthritis. Adjunctive therapies like calcium sulfate beads, nutritional support, and immobilization are also discussed. Recognizing early signs, such as pseudoparalysis and localized bone pain, and promptly initiating appropriate treatment are crucial to preventing long-term sequelae such as growth disturbances, chronic osteomyelitis, or limb-length discrepancies.

Keywords

Pediatric osteomyelitis · Acute hematogenous osteomyelitis · MRSA · Sequestrectomy · Infection · *Staphylococcus aureus*

A. Dadra · K. Rangasamy · N. R. Gopinathan
Department of Orthopedics, PGIMER, Chandigarh, India

J. Kaur (✉)
Department of Pediatrics, BRAIMS, Mohali, India

P. Kumar et al. (eds.), *Textbook of Orthopedic Infections*,
https://doi.org/10.1007/978-981-95-5029-6_8

8.1 Introduction

Pediatric Osteomyelitis is a significant musculoskeletal infection affecting children, characterized by inflammation of the bone and bone marrow [1]. The acute hematogenous form (AHO) is the most common, occurring due to bacterial seeding of the bone from the bloodstream [2]. With an incidence of approximately eight cases per 100,000 children/year in high-income countries [2] and a male predominance, AHO presents a significant clinical challenge, particularly in regions where variations in local microbiota and seasonal factors may influence disease occurrence. Early recognition and timely intervention are crucial, as prompt diagnosis and effective treatment significantly improve outcomes. However, more severe forms of the disease—often associated with virulent bacterial strains such as methicillin-resistant *Staphylococcus aureus* (MRSA)—can lead to adverse outcomes, including chronic osteomyelitis, osteonecrosis, joint destruction, limb length discrepancies, and deformities requiring orthopedic intervention [3].

Despite advances in diagnostic techniques and treatment protocols, pediatric musculoskeletal infections remain diagnostically and therapeutically challenging. Children may present with vague, nonspecific symptoms, and the insidious onset of disease can delay diagnosis. Moreover, pediatric patients often struggle to articulate their symptoms, necessitating a thorough history and physical examination to differentiate AHO from other musculoskeletal pathologies. The presence of orthopedic implants or previous surgical interventions further complicates management. Given these complexities, a multidisciplinary approach—integrating pediatricians, orthopedic surgeons, infectious disease specialists, radiologists, and emergency physicians—is essential for optimizing outcomes [4]. Standardized treatment protocols, early transition to oral antibiotics, and careful outpatient follow-up help reduce complications, shorten hospital stays, and minimize long-term morbidity [5].

8.2 Etiopathogenesis

Pediatric osteomyelitis, particularly in its acute hematogenous form (AHO), arises from bacterial seeding of bone through hematogenous spread [6]. Unlike in adults, where direct inoculation or contiguous spread is more common, children typically develop osteomyelitis without an identifiable external wound or penetrating injury [7]. The pathophysiology is driven by transient bacteremia, where circulating pathogens escape the bloodstream and establish infection within bone tissue [8]. The metaphyseal regions of long bones are most commonly affected due to their unique vascular anatomy, which includes slow-flowing, sinusoidal capillaries with hairpin turns that create an environment conducive to bacterial adhesion and proliferation [9]. The proximal femur, tibia, and humerus are frequent sites of involvement, though infections can also occur in the calcaneus, pelvis, and spine.

Among the microbial culprits, *Staphylococcus aureus* remains the predominant pathogen across all pediatric age groups, responsible for over 90% of culture-confirmed cases [10]. Its virulence is largely attributed to its ability to evade host immune responses and persist within the bloodstream. Methicillin-resistant *Staphylococcus aureus* (MRSA) strains, in particular, possess an extensive array of virulence genes, contributing to more severe clinical presentations [11]. Other pathogens vary depending on age and underlying conditions. Neonates are at risk for infections from *Escherichia coli*, *Klebsiella pneumoniae*, and *Group B Streptococcus* (GBS), while *Salmonella* species are a well-recognized cause in children with sickle cell disease [12, 13]. *Pseudomonas aeruginosa* is frequently encountered in nosocomial infections, particularly in immunocompromised patients or those with puncture wounds [14]. Less common but clinically significant organisms include *Kingella kingae*, *Streptococcus pneumoniae*, *Mycobacterium tuberculosis* (in endemic areas), and zoonotic pathogens such as *Bartonella henselae* and *Pasteurella* species [15–18]. Additionally, infections associated with implanted orthopedic hardware often involve *Coagulase-negative Staphylococcus* and atypical mycobacteria [19].

Once bacterial colonization occurs, local inflammatory responses ensue, leading to edema, vascular congestion, and subsequent ischemic necrosis of bone. In approximately 65% of cases, a history of minor trauma precedes the infection, suggesting that increased vascular permeability in response to injury may facilitate bacterial deposition. The host immune response, coupled with bacterial virulence factors, can exacerbate local tissue destruction, leading to subperiosteal abscess formation, cortical bone necrosis, and potential spread into adjacent structures. In about 20% of cases, osteomyelitis extends into the adjacent joint, particularly in bones with intra-articular metaphyses such as the proximal femur, proximal humerus, and distal fibula, leading to concurrent septic arthritis [20]. The presence of contiguous joint infection is an independent risk factor for long-term complications, including growth disturbances and joint destruction.

Persistent bacteremia, especially in MRSA infections, contributes to more severe disease courses, often necessitating prolonged hospital stays, surgical intervention, and intensive antibiotic therapy. The genomic heterogeneity of *Staphylococcus aureus* clinical isolates suggests that specific virulence factors play a critical role in determining the severity of infection. These factors not only influence local tissue destruction but also contribute to systemic complications such as deep venous thrombosis, septic emboli, and multiorgan involvement. The interplay between host susceptibility, bacterial virulence, and treatment delays ultimately dictates disease progression, underscoring the importance of early recognition and targeted intervention to prevent devastating complications.

8.3 Clinical Features

Osteomyelitis should be suspected in any child presenting with an unexplained fever. Based on its duration, osteomyelitis is classified as:

- *Acute*: Less than 2 weeks
- *Subacute*: Between 2 weeks and 3 months

- *Chronic*: More than 3 months

The lower limb long bones are the most commonly affected. Neonates often display nonspecific symptoms such as irritability, lethargy, fever, and poor feeding. They may also exhibit pseudoparalysis of the affected limb, localized swelling, or cellulitis. In acute osteomyelitis, *pseudoparalysis* is a notable early sign, especially in infants and young children [21]. Due to intense pain and inflammation, the child avoids moving the affected limb, holding it in a fixed position. This lack of movement can mimic paralysis, but neurological function remains intact. The limb may appear limp, with refusal to bear weight or use the extremity. Recognizing pseudoparalysis is crucial, as it may be the first clinical clue pointing toward acute osteomyelitis in a non-verbal or febrile child. Multifocal bone involvement is more prevalent in neonates than in older children.

Older children typically present with localized pain, swelling, tenderness, warmth, and redness over the affected bone. Limping, reluctance to bear weight, and avoidance of limb use are common indicators. Infections caused by *methicillin-resistant Staphylococcus aureus* (*MRSA*) tend to result in more severe symptoms and higher fevers than those caused by *methicillin-sensitive Staphylococcus aureus* (*MSSA*) [22].

8.4 Evaluation

8.4.1 Physical Examination

Pain is the most frequent symptom in children with osteomyelitis. Tenderness upon palpation over the affected bone is a key finding. As osteomyelitis can increase pressure beyond the primary site, palpating concentrically from the suspected area can aid diagnosis. It is important to differentiate osteomyelitis from septic arthritis, which typically presents with severe pain during both active and passive joint movement. Osteomyelitis, on the other hand, causes diffuse pain within a specific compartment, away from the joint itself.

Other notable physical findings include fever, reluctance to use the affected limb, swelling, warmth, and an overall unwell appearance. The severity of symptoms may vary depending on the bacterial strain.

Over time, if the infection remains unresolved, the formation of a *discharging sinus* becomes evident (Fig. 8.1a). This sinus serves as a pathway for purulent material to exit from the sequestrated bone to the skin surface, often seen over the tibia or femur (Fig. 8.1b, c) Its presence indicates chronicity and ongoing inflammation. The sinus may intermittently close and reopen, with surrounding skin showing signs of induration or granulation.

MSSA osteomyelitis often presents with more subtle signs, whereas MRSA osteomyelitis tends to cause a more severe illness. Acute osteomyelitis may lead to complications such as physeal arrest, which can result in limb length discrepancies

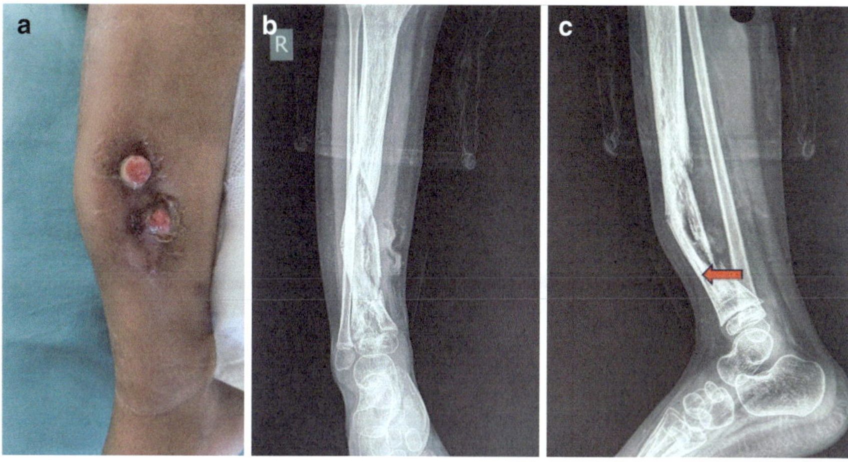

Fig. 8.1 (**a**) Preoperative clinical photographs demonstrate a discharging sinus located on the medial aspect of the leg in a 4-year-old child (**b**, **c**), corresponding AP & Lateral radiographs of the same patient depicting sequestrum (red arrow)

or avascular necrosis. Patients typically require prolonged antibiotic therapy and have a higher risk of recurrence.

8.4.2 Diagnostic Imaging and Testing

For musculoskeletal infections, the first step is typically *plain radiography*. Although initial X-rays may not show early osteomyelitic changes, they are useful in ruling out fractures, neoplasms, or other conditions. Signs of chronic osteomyelitis, such as soft tissue swelling and joint effusions, may be seen. However, bone destruction usually becomes apparent only after 33% of bone mineral density is lost [22].

CT scans can provide additional detail, but *MRI is the preferred imaging modality* due to its ability to differentiate infection from neoplasms and visualize the extent of the disease, including periosteal abscesses, sequestrum formation, and cortical erosion (Fig. 8.2). Young children often require sedation for MRI, and hospital protocols that allow for sedation-assisted MRI transitioning into surgical intervention have shown improved efficiency and outcomes.

An *MRI with and without contrast* should be performed within 24 h of hospital admission for suspected osteomyelitis. Radiologists play a crucial role in the rapid interpretation of these images to facilitate prompt treatment.

In chronic osteomyelitis, a *sinogram* can be a useful imaging tool to delineate the course and extent of a discharging sinus tract (Fig. 8.3) By injecting a water-soluble contrast medium into the sinus opening and taking radiographs, the sinogram helps identify the tract's communication with underlying bone, medullary cavity, or abscess cavities. It aids in surgical planning by mapping the sinus path and locating

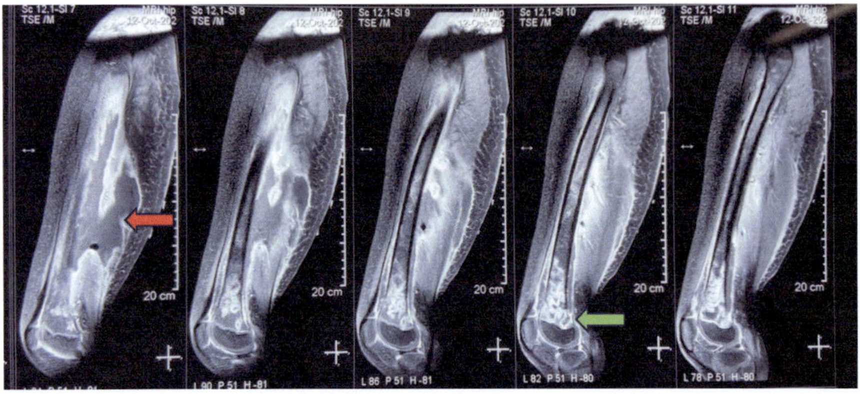

Fig. 8.2 A 7-year-old male with MRI showing intraosseous collection in the distal femoral metaphysis, surrounding marrow edema, and a posterolateral thigh collection (red arrow) in the mid-thigh, confined by the physis (green arrow)

Fig. 8.3 An 8-year-old male with a history of debridement for osteomyelitis 1 year ago now presents with a recurrent discharging sinus visible on the Sinogram

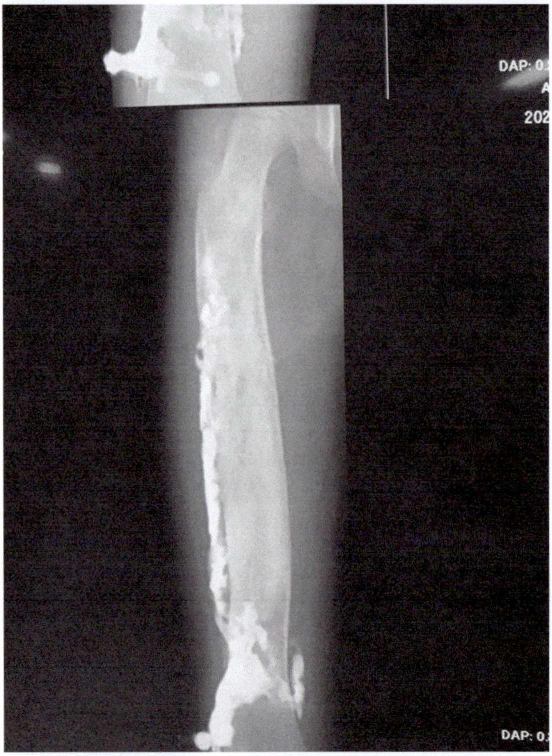

sequestra or areas requiring debridement. Although largely supplanted by MRI, sinography remains valuable in resource-limited settings or when MRI is contraindicated.

8.4.3 Laboratory Investigations

Blood cultures should be collected before administering antibiotics, as they are positive in only 30%–50% of cases. Additionally, *inflammatory markers such as C-reactive protein (CRP), erythrocyte sedimentation rate (ESR), and a complete blood count (CBC)* should be obtained. CRP is the most reliable indicator of treatment response and is closely monitored throughout the course of the illness.

Early assessment of disease severity is critical. A marked elevation in CRP and an increased band percentage in WBCs may indicate a more severe infection, often associated with ICU admission, septic pulmonary emboli (SPE), MRSA bacteremia, and a higher risk of venous thromboembolism (VTE). These patients tend to experience prolonged fever, persistent bacteremia, and require multiple surgical interventions. Additional laboratory findings may include anemia and thrombocytopenia due to rapid blood product consumption.

8.5 Emergency Department Evaluation

Since children with *acute hematogenous osteomyelitis (AHO)* often present with rapid symptom onset, they are frequently evaluated in emergency settings. The initial workup should include a CBC with differential and inflammatory markers (CRP, ESR), alongside aerobic blood cultures obtained before antibiotic administration. *Staphylococcus aureus bacteremia (SAB)* is common in AHO, allowing for pathogen identification without invasive procedures, provided cultures are taken before antibiotics are given. Awareness of antimicrobial stewardship is vital in maintaining high culture yield.

The early evaluation also informs illness severity. *Markedly high CRP values and WBC band counts* correlate with severe illness, increased ICU admissions, SPE on chest X-ray, and MRSA infections. These children have a higher risk of *venous thromboembolism (VTE)* and require early ultrasound assessment to detect deep vein thrombosis (DVT) before surgical intervention.

8.6 Differential Diagnoses

Unlike septic arthritis, which has a broad differential diagnosis, AHO presents with well-defined clinical and laboratory findings. Conditions such as leukemia and *Ewing's sarcoma* should still be considered [2].

- *Leukemia*: Often affects all three blood cell lines (WBC, RBC, platelets) and may present with leukopenia, anemia, or thrombocytopenia. A peripheral smear showing blast cells usually necessitates a hematology consultation and bone marrow biopsy. MRI findings commonly reveal *widespread, patchy bone marrow changes* rather than a localized infection.
- *Ewing's Sarcoma*: Typically affects the *diaphysis* of long bones and appears on X-rays with aggressive periosteal reactions and infiltrative changes suggestive of malignancy. *Biopsy confirmation is essential*, and cultures should be obtained from all biopsied tissues to avoid misdiagnosis.

Advanced imaging, particularly *MRI with extended field of view STIR and T1 sequences*, should be performed bilaterally in cases where leukemia is suspected. Ensuring a multidisciplinary approach, including radiologists, infectious disease specialists, and hematologists, is crucial for accurate diagnosis and management.

8.6.1 Management of Acute Hematogenous Osteomyelitis (AHO)

Early diagnosis and appropriate management are crucial to prevent complications such as chronic osteomyelitis, joint destruction, growth disturbances, and sepsis. The management of AHO involves a multidisciplinary approach, integrating medical therapy with surgical intervention when necessary [23].

8.6.2 Medical Management

8.6.2.1 Empirical Antibiotic Therapy

The primary mode of treatment for AHO is antibiotic therapy, initiated empirically based on the patient's age, local microbiological data, and risk factors (Table 8.1) and later adjusted based on culture and sensitivity results [24].

8.6.2.2 Considerations for Empirical Therapy

- *MSSA infections*: First-generation cephalosporins (cefazolin) or antistaphylococcal penicillin (nafcillin) are preferred.
- *MRSA infections*: Vancomycin is recommended, though it requires renal function monitoring due to nephrotoxicity.
- *Kingella kingae*: Common in children under 4 years, best treated with cefazolin or ceftriaxone.
- *Neonates and immunocompromised patients*: Broader coverage is necessary, including Gram-negative organisms.
- *Septic shock*: Requires immediate broad-spectrum coverage with a combination of vancomycin and ceftriaxone or piperacillin-tazobactam.

Table 8.1 Common pathogens and empirical antibiotic choices

Age group	Common pathogens	Recommended empirical antibiotics
Neonates (<3 months)	*Staphylococcus aureus*, Group B Streptococcus (GBS), gram-negative bacilli (*E. coli*, *Klebsiella*)	Cefotaxime + vancomycin
Infants and children (3 months–4 years)	*Staphylococcus aureus*, *Kingella kingae*, *Streptococcus pneumoniae*, Group A Streptococcus (GAS)	Cefazolin or clindamycin (if MRSA prevalence >10%)
Children (>4 years) and adolescents	*Staphylococcus aureus (MSSA/MRSA), GAS*	Nafcillin or cefazolin (MSSA), vancomycin (MRSA)
Immunocompromised or sickle cell disease	*Salmonella*, *Pseudomonas*	Ceftriaxone + vancomycin (add ciprofloxacin if pseudomonas suspected)
Septic shock or unknown pathogen	Broad-spectrum coverage needed	Vancomycin + ceftriaxone (or piperacillin-tazobactam if polymicrobial infection suspected)

8.6.2.3 Duration of Therapy

- *Intravenous (IV) therapy*: Typically administered for 5–7 days or until clinical and laboratory markers improve.
- *Transition to oral therapy*: Once the patient shows significant clinical improvement, including resolution of fever and declining inflammatory markers (CRP, ESR, WBC).
- *Total duration*: 3–6 weeks, depending on disease severity, response to treatment, and presence of complications.
- *Neonates and severe cases*: Require extended IV therapy up to 6 weeks.

8.6.2.4 Monitoring Response to Treatment

- *Clinical parameters*: Resolution of fever within 48–72 h, reduced pain, improved limb function, and decreased soft tissue swelling.
- *Laboratory markers*:
  - CRP: Peaks early and declines within 10–14 days with effective treatment.
  - ESR: Remains elevated for a longer duration and helps guide therapy.
  - WBC: Less specific but useful in systemic infection monitoring.
- *Imaging*:
  - MRI: Recommended if no clinical response within 48–72 h of initiating therapy.
  - Repeat Ultrasound/X-ray: If there is concern for abscess formation or worsening symptoms.

8.6.3 Surgical Management

Surgical intervention is warranted in approximately 20%–30% of cases and is indicated when:

- *Abscess formation*: Subperiosteal or intramedullary abscess requiring drainage.
- *Failure of medical therapy*: No improvement after 48–72 h of appropriate antibiotics.
- *Septic arthritis*: Contiguous joint involvement requiring urgent drainage.
- *Necrotic bone (sequestrum) formation*: Chronic osteomyelitis development.
- *Hemodynamic instability*: Requires immediate source control.

8.6.3.1 Surgical Techniques

1. *Incision and drainage (I&D)/debridement*
   - Performed under general anesthesia.
   - Used to drain pus, irrigate infected bone, and remove necrotic tissue.
2. *Bone window (corticotomy) for medullary debridement*
   - Creates cortical openings to facilitate drainage and irrigation of the intramedullary canal.
3. *Sequestrectomy* (Fig. 8.4)
   - Sequestrectomy involves the surgical removal of necrotic (sequestrated) bone, which is essential in managing chronic osteomyelitis.
   - It helps eliminate the persistent source of infection and promotes revascularization and bone healing.

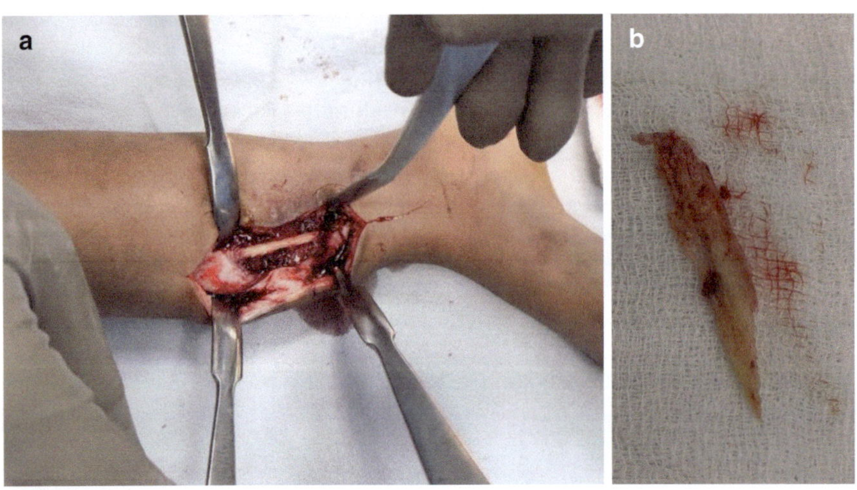

Fig. 8.4 Intraoperative images show a dense, ivory-like sequestrum removed from the posterior aspect of the tibia after *Sequestrectomy*

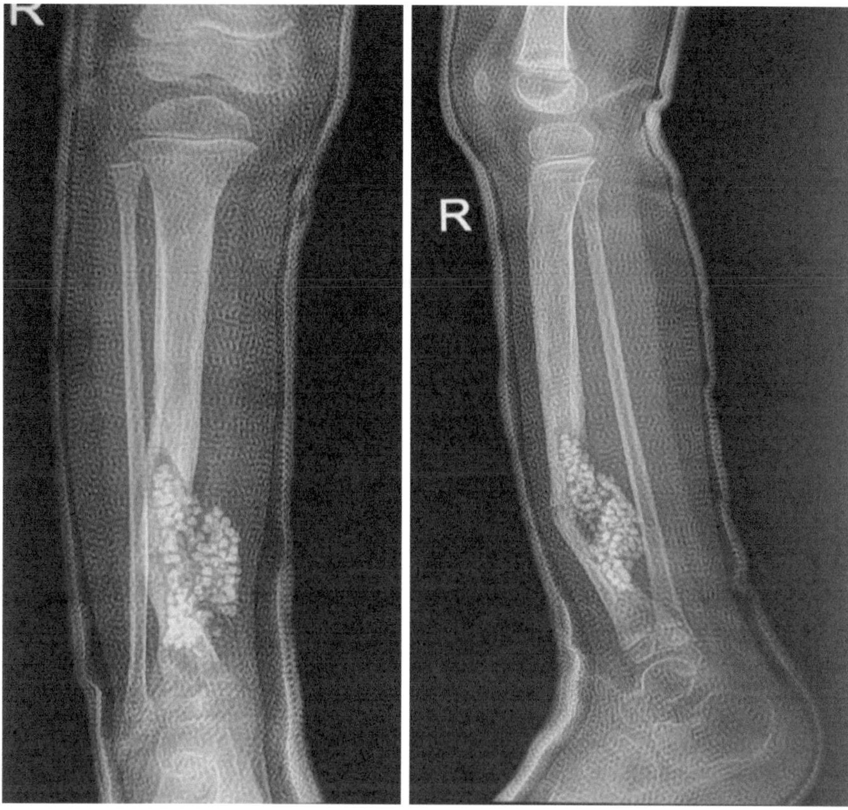

Fig. 8.5 Postoperative X-ray following debridement, sequestrectomy, and placement of STIMULAN® bioabsorbable antibiotic beads

- After debridement, *antibiotic-impregnated calcium sulfate beads* (*e.g., Stimulan*) are inserted into the bone cavity (Fig. 8.5).
- These beads provide high local concentrations of antibiotics directly at the infection site.
- They are *biodegradable*, eliminating the need for a second procedure for removal.

4. *Fluoroscopy-guided biopsy and aspiration*
    - Useful in deep infections and culture-directed therapy.

8.6.3.2 Supportive Care and Adjunct Therapies

Immobilization

- Temporary use of splints or casts to reduce pain and facilitate healing.
- It should be discontinued as soon as the pain subsides to prevent joint stiffness.

Pain Management

- NSAIDs (e.g., ibuprofen) or acetaminophen for pain relief.
- Opioids are reserved for severe pain and used with caution.

Nutritional Support

- High-protein, high-calorie diet to support immune function and bone healing.
- Consider vitamin D and calcium supplementation in patients who are deficient.

8.7 Complications and Follow-Up

8.7.1 Potential Complications

- Chronic osteomyelitis if infection that persists beyond 6 weeks.
- Pathologic fractures due to weakened bone structure.
- Growth disturbances occur if the epiphyseal plate is involved.
- Septic arthritis from contiguous spread.
- Limb-length discrepancies, particularly in young children.

8.7.2 Follow-Up Schedule

- *Weekly follow-ups during the first month* to monitor clinical and laboratory improvements.
- *MRI/X-ray at 3 months* for slow-healing cases or suspected complications.
- *Long-term monitoring* (*up to 1 year*) is required if growth plate involvement is detected.

8.8 Conclusion

AHO is a potentially serious condition that requires a systematic approach for optimal outcomes. Early initiation of empirical antibiotics, close monitoring of treatment response, and timely surgical intervention when necessary are key components of effective management. A multidisciplinary approach, involving infectious disease specialists, orthopedic surgeons, and rehabilitation teams, ensures comprehensive patient care and minimizes long-term morbidity.

References

1. Riise ØR, Kirkhus E, Handeland KS, Flatø B, Reiseter T, Cvancarova M, Nakstad B, Wathne KO. Childhood osteomyelitis-incidence and differentiation from other acute onset musculoskeletal features in a population-based study. BMC Pediatr. 2008;8:45.
2. Thakolkaran N, Shetty AK. Acute hematogenous osteomyelitis in children. Ochsner J. 2019;19(2):116–22.
3. Kaushik A, Kest H. Pediatric methicillin-resistant *Staphylococcus aureus* osteoarticular infections. Microorganisms. 2018;6(2):40.
4. Iliadis AD, Ramachandran M. Paediatric bone and joint infection. EFORT Open Rev. 2017;2(1):7–12.
5. Batchelder N, So TY. Transitioning antimicrobials from intravenous to oral in pediatric acute uncomplicated osteomyelitis. World J Clin Pediatr. 2016;5(3):244–50.
6. McNeil JC. Acute hematogenous osteomyelitis in children: clinical presentation and management. Infect Drug Resist. 2020;13:4459–73.
7. Calhoun JH, Manring MM, Shirtliff M. Osteomyelitis of the long bones. Semin Plast Surg. 2009;23(2):59–72.
8. Christaki E, Giamarellos-Bourboulis EJ. The complex pathogenesis of bacteremia: from antimicrobial clearance mechanisms to the genetic background of the host. Virulence. 2014;5(1):57–65.
9. Ramasamy SK. Structure and functions of blood vessels and vascular niches in bone. Stem Cells Int. 2017;2017:5046953.
10. Kavanagh N, Ryan EJ, Widaa A, Sexton G, Fennell J, O'Rourke S, Cahill KC, Kearney CJ, O'Brien FJ, Kerrigan SW. Staphylococcal osteomyelitis: disease progression, treatment challenges, and future directions. Clin Microbiol Rev. 2018;31(2):e00084–17.
11. Urish KL, Cassat JE. *Staphylococcus aureus* osteomyelitis: bone, bugs, and surgery. Infect Immun. 2020;88(7):e00932–19.
12. Vazquez M. Osteomyelitis in children. Curr Opin Pediatr. 2002;14:112–5.
13. AlFawaz T, Alzumar O, AlShahrani D, Alshehri M. Severity of salmonella infection among sickle cell diseases pediatric patients: description of the infection pattern. Int J Pediatr Adolesc Med. 2019;6(3):115–7.
14. Laughlin TJ, Armstrong DG, Caporusso J, Lavery LA. Soft tissue and bone infections from puncture wounds in children. West J Med. 1997;166:126–8.
15. Yagupsky P. *Kingella kingae*: carriage, transmission, and disease. Clin Microbiol Rev. 2015;28(1):54–79.
16. Agarwal A. Paediatric osteoarticular tuberculosis: a review. J Clin Orthop Trauma. 2020;11(2):202–7.
17. DeMarco G, Chargui M, Coulin B, Borner B, Steiger C, Dayer R, Ceroni D. *Kingella kingae* osteoarticular infections approached through the prism of the pediatric orthopedist. Microorganisms. 2021;10(1):25.
18. Kodama Y, Maeno N, Nishi J, Imuta N, Oda H, Tanaka S, Kono Y, Kawano Y. Multifocal osteomyelitis due to *Bartonella henselae* in a child without focal pain. J Infect Chemother. 2007;13(5):350–2.
19. Ribeiro M, Monteiro FJ, Ferraz MP. Infection of orthopedic implants with emphasis on bacterial adhesion process and techniques used in studying bacterial-material interactions. Biomatter. 2012;2(4):176–94.
20. Oji NM, Sabatini CS. Osteomyelitis and septic arthritis of the upper extremity in pediatric patients. Curr Rev Musculoskelet Med. 2025;18(3):61–72.
21. Stohr K, Xu GX. A case of upper limb osteomyelitis and septic arthritis presenting as pseudoparalysis in a two-week-old. Case Rep Pediatr. 2018;2018:1796831.

22. Levine MA. Assessing bone health in children and adolescents. Indian J Endocrinol Metab. 2012;16(Suppl 2):S205–12.
23. Harik NS, Smeltzer MS. Management of acute hematogenous osteomyelitis in children. Expert Rev Anti-Infect Ther. 2010;8(2):175–81.
24. Peltola H, Pääkkönen M. Acute osteomyelitis in children. N Engl J Med. 2014;370(4):352–60.

Paediatric Septic Arthritis

9

J. P. Khatri, Akash Kumar Ghosh, and Pebam Sudesh

Abstract

Septic arthritis in children remains one of the true orthopedic emergencies—where time truly is joint. This chapter aims to equip practicing orthopedic surgeons with a clear, practical roadmap for recognizing and managing this condition effectively. Most commonly affecting young children, especially toddlers aged 2 to 3, septic arthritis often targets the hip and knee joints and can escalate quickly if not addressed.

The challenge often begins with subtle or nonspecific signs: an infant refusing feeds, a toddler with a limp, or a febrile child who won't bear weight. Early recognition is critical, as cartilage damage can begin within hours of infection onset. This chapter emphasizes the importance of a thorough clinical assessment, supported by lab tests like CRP, ESR, and synovial fluid analysis. Newer tools such as PCR and next-generation sequencing are also discussed for improving diagnosis when cultures fail.

Management begins with timely, empiric antibiotics tailored to age and local resistance patterns. For most cases, a short course of IV antibiotics followed by oral therapy is effective, minimizing hospital stay and complications. When surgery is needed—whether aspiration, arthroscopy, or open arthrotomy—the choice depends on the joint involved, disease severity, and available expertise. The chapter also reviews newer techniques, including image-guided double-lumen catheter drainage.

J. P. Khatri
Department of Orthopedics, Military Hospital Khadki, Range Hills, Pune, India

A. K. Ghosh (✉)
Narayana Hrudayalaya, Bengaluru, India

P. Sudesh
Department of Paediatric Orthopedics, Post-Graduate institute of Medical Education and Research, Chandigarh, India

P. Kumar et al. (eds.), *Textbook of Orthopedic Infections*,
https://doi.org/10.1007/978-981-95-5029-6_9

Beyond acute care, it highlights the need for structured follow-up to detect late complications like avascular necrosis or growth disturbances. With a coordinated, timely, and evidence-informed approach, most children recover fully—often returning to full function with little or no sequelae.

This chapter serves as both a clinical guide and a call to action: to stay vigilant, act early, and always aim for joint preservation.

Keywords

Infectious Arthritis · Synovial Fluid Analysis · Antibacterial Agents Therapeutic Use · Paediatric Population · Bone and Joint Infections Diagnosis and Therapy

Learning Objectives

- Describe the pathophysiological mechanisms and recognize clinical signs of septic arthritis in paediatric patients.
- Outline the diagnostic steps, including laboratory tests, imaging studies, and joint aspiration, for accurate diagnosis.
- Formulate a comprehensive treatment plan, including antibiotic therapy, surgical intervention, and follow-up care.

9.1 Introduction

Septic arthritis in children is a critical orthopedic emergency characterized by bacterial infection within a joint, leading to rapid joint destruction and potential chronic disability. Immediate identification and intervention are crucial to prevent irreversible damage [1]. The condition predominantly affects the lower extremities, with the knees, hips, and ankles involved in approximately 80% of cases. Complaints like refusal of feeds, paradoxical cry, and pseudo-paralysis can be the presenting features.

Despite long-standing principles of management, recent studies have highlighted advancements in the epidemiology, diagnosis, and treatment outcomes of septic arthritis. Early diagnosis is challenging, especially in infants and neonates who may exhibit nonspecific symptoms. Delayed presentation is not uncommon. However, cartilage damage in case of septic arthritis has been documented to start within 8 h of onset of infection in experimental studies. This damage can be compounded by misdiagnosis and inappropriate treatment [2].

This chapter will review the latest evidence-based strategies for diagnosing and managing paediatric septic arthritis, focusing on timely and effective treatment to optimize patient outcomes.

9.2 Epidemiology

The incidence of septic arthritis in paediatric population varies widely in literature ranging from 4 to 10 cases per 100,000 population in developed part of the world and 5–20 in low-income countries [3]. This variation owes to different diagnostic criteria, variability of healthcare access, under-recognition, under-reporting, and epidemiological factors. Sub-clinical presentation and resolving spontaneously as transient bacteraemia with synovitis is also not uncommon that resolves without any intervention [4]. Various studies have failed to document any particular seasonal variation in the incidence rate. It typically leads to mono articular involvement. Hip joint is the most commonly affected joint with septic arthritis in children. Along with knee it comprises up to 80% of the total number of cases. The peak incidence has been reported in the age 2–3 years of age with some male preponderance [5].

9.3 Bacteriology

Paediatric septic arthritis is predominantly caused by *Staphylococcus aureus*, including methicillin-resistant strains (MRSA), complicating treatment due to antibiotic resistance. This pathogen is most common in children over 2 years of age and in nosocomial infections of neonates [3]. *Streptococcus* species, especially *Streptococcus pyogenes*, are significant pathogens, with Group A beta-haemolytic streptococcus being most common following varicella infection and notable for toxin production leading to tissue necrosis.

Kingella kingae, a fastidious, aerobic, gram-negative coccobacillus, is recognized for causing osteoarticular infections in children under five and should be considered in the diagnostic workup of young patients. Other gram-negative bacteria like *Escherichia coli* and *Pseudomonas aeruginosa* are associated with septic arthritis in specific scenarios, such as immunocompromised states or following penetrating joint injuries [6].

Group B streptococcus is a common cause in infants, especially in neonates with community-acquired infections or those exposed during vaginal delivery. Identifying the causative organism is critical for guiding appropriate antibiotic therapy. Empiric treatment typically includes coverage for *Staphylococcus aureus* and *Streptococcus* species, with broader coverage considered based on clinical presentation and patient risk factors.

Neisseria gonorrhoeae remains a common organism in sexually active adolescents or newborns getting exposed to the organism via infected mothers birth canal, characterized by migratory polyarthralgia, multiple joint involvement, and small red papules. This gram-negative pathogen may be treated with large doses of penicillin without requiring surgical debridement. *Haemophilus influenzae* incidence has markedly decreased due to vaccination but remains a consideration in not fully immunized children [7].

Patient history plays a crucial role in identifying potential pathogens. Children with sickle cell disease are more susceptible to *Salmonella* spp. Recent pharyngitis can lead to septic arthritis caused by *Streptococcus pyogenes* or *Fusobacterium necrophorum* (Lemierre disease), while recent diarrheal illness is associated with post-gastrointestinal infection arthritis caused by *Salmonella* spp.

In addition to these primary pathogens, the following findings in patient history are associated with specific diagnoses:

- Not fully immunized: At risk for *Haemophilus influenzae* and *Streptococcus pneumoniae* infections.
- Sickle cell disease: Increased susceptibility to *Salmonella* spp.
- Recent pharyngitis: Risk of septic arthritis caused by *Streptococcus pyogenes* or *Fusobacterium necrophorum*.
- Recent diarrheal illness: Associated with post-gastrointestinal infection arthritis caused by *Salmonella* spp.

Recognizing the spectrum of bacterial pathogens, understanding their typical patient populations and clinical scenarios, and tailoring antibiotic therapy appropriately are crucial for effective diagnosis, treatment, and prevention of long-term complications in paediatric septic arthritis.

9.4 Pathogenesis

The pathogenesis and pathophysiology of septic arthritis involve a complex interplay of factors leading to joint infection and subsequent inflammatory responses. Septic arthritis typically occurs due to the hematogenous spread of pathogens from a distant site of infection to the joint. Less commonly, direct inoculation of the joint following trauma or surgery can also lead to infection. The pathogens adhere to the synovial membrane and articular cartilage, invading the synovial lining and proliferating within the joint space. This invasion triggers the release of inflammatory mediators, initiating an acute inflammatory response [8].

Upon infection, the synovial lining cells become activated, resulting in increased production of proinflammatory cytokines such as interleukin-1 (IL-1) and tumour necrosis factor-alpha (TNF-alpha). Neutrophils are rapidly recruited to the joint in response to chemotactic signals released by the infected synovium. These neutrophils phagocytose bacteria but also release enzymes and reactive oxygen species that contribute to tissue damage. The inflammatory cascade, along with the direct effects of bacterial toxins and enzymes, can lead to cartilage degradation, bone erosion, and potential joint destruction if not promptly treated.

Synovial fluid too displays distinct changes in septic arthritis. There is increased white blood cell count with significant levels of neutrophils and the presence of bacteria identified through staining and culture. In severe cases, systemic manifestations such as fever, leucocytosis, and elevated acute-phase reactants like C-reactive protein (CRP) and erythrocyte sedimentation rate (ESR) may be present, reflecting the systemic inflammatory response to infection. The main determinant of raised ESR is the elevated serum levels of fibrinogen released from liver in response to inflammation (Fig. 9.1).

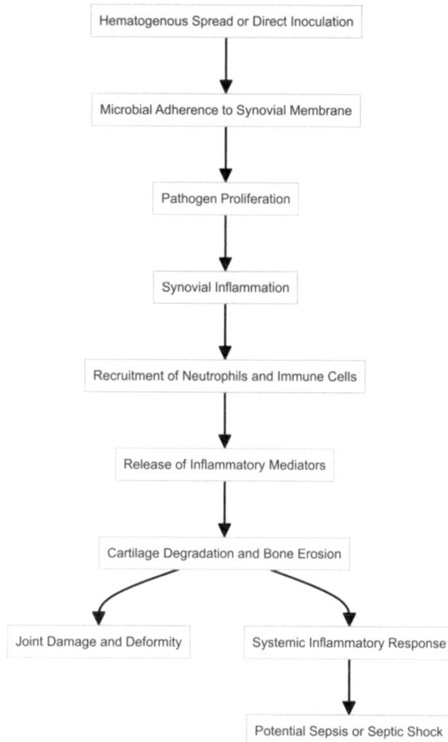

Fig. 9.1 Pathogenesis of septic arthritis

9.5 Clinical Features

Septic arthritis (SA) in children presents a diagnostic challenge due to its varied clinical manifestations and the overlap with other conditions such as transient synovitis and Lyme disease [9]. When evaluating a paediatric patient suspected of having septic arthritis, it is essential to consider a detailed clinical history. Symptoms can develop rapidly, ranging from a few hours to several days, and parents may report a recent history of an upper respiratory tract infection or other minor infections. Risk factors such as recent trauma, surgery, or invasive procedures involving the joint area, as well as underlying medical conditions like immunodeficiency, chronic joint diseases, or recent systemic infections, should also be considered. The child may refuse to ambulate or present with a limp, which is particularly concerning in nonverbal or very young children. Infants may show nonspecific symptoms such as irritability, decreased appetite, or generalized malaise. Additional considerations include travel history, exposure to animals (e.g., cats for *Bartonella henselae*), and ingestion of unpasteurized dairy products to rule out uncommon infections. Verification of immunization status is crucial, especially for pathogens like

Haemophilus influenzae and Pneumococcus, and a family history of conditions such as sickle cell anaemia or immunodeficiency may influence diagnostic and therapeutic decisions.

Local symptoms of SA in children include sudden onset of severe pain, often localized to a single joint, visible joint swelling due to inflammation, increased synovial fluid production, and the affected joint appearing warm and erythematous. The range of motion in the affected joint is typically decreased, and the child may adopt a position that maximizes joint volume to minimize pain, such as hip flexion, abduction, and external rotation. Systemic symptoms may include fever, present in approximately 40–60% of cases, general malaise, chills, lethargy, irritability, decreased appetite, and tachycardia, which often accompanies systemic symptoms and indicates a more severe infection [10].

During physical examination, joint tenderness is commonly observed, with palpation of the joint revealing tenderness and significant discomfort. Joint effusion is a frequent finding, which can be confirmed through palpation or imaging studies, and the joint is often red and warm to the touch. Children may exhibit guarding behaviours, limiting joint movement to avoid pain, and might hold the joint in a position that alleviates pain. The pain arising from septic arthritis of hip and pain arising from pyomyositis around hip can be differentiated by gentle rotatory movement of the hip where septic arthritis would still cause pain but pyomyositis of anterior or posterior muscle group will cause little discomfort comparatively. Systemic signs such as fever and tachycardia indicate a systemic inflammatory response, and the child may appear unwell, with symptoms ranging from mild irritability to signs of sepsis or septic shock in severe cases.

Transient synovitis of the hip presents itself as a very close differential diagnosis and poses a significant diagnostic challenge due to their overlapping symptoms. Correct identification is crucial to prevent poor long-term outcomes associated with untreated septic arthritis. Transient synovitis is common in children, causing up to 0.9% of paediatric emergency visits, and early diagnosis can prevent unnecessary procedures. Kocher et al. identified four predictors to distinguish the two conditions: fever >38.5 °C, non-weight bearing history, ESR > 40 mm/h, and WBC count >12,000 cells/mL. Their method showed predictive probabilities for septic arthritis ranging from 0.2% to 99.6% based on the number of predictors present. However, subsequent studies demonstrated variability in predictive accuracy, suggesting that adjunctive diagnostic tools like ultrasonography and arthrocentesis are beneficial. Clinical judgement remains essential, with a low threshold for admitting children with suspected septic arthritis and close outpatient follow-up recommended for ambiguous cases [11].

Although geographically limited, Lyme disease should also be considered as a differential, especially in endemic areas. Rapid Lyme tests and synovial fluid analysis can help differentiate Lyme disease from SA.

High-risk scenarios include neonates with fever and irritability, who should be evaluated for both bacterial joint infections and CNS infections. Children with recent bacteraemia, especially with pathogens like *Staphylococcus aureus*, require careful joint evaluation. Early recognition of these clinical features, combined with prompt diagnostic evaluation (e.g., joint aspiration for synovial fluid analysis) and initiation of appropriate antibiotic therapy is essential for managing septic arthritis in children and preventing long-term joint damage.

9.6 Laboratory Work-up

Septic arthritis in paediatric patients presents diagnostic challenges that necessitate a combination of clinical evaluation and laboratory investigations. The initial lab investigations for a case of suspected septic arthritis should include a complete blood count (CBC) with a differential leukocyte count, erythrocyte sedimentation rate (ESR), C-reactive protein (CRP), and blood cultures. An elevated white blood cell (WBC) count, although varies in definition across studies, does not substantially alter the odds of septic arthritis. The WBC thresholds ranged from ≥11.0 × 10^9/L to ≥15.0 × 10^9/L.

ESR and CRP are pivotal biomarkers. Elevated ESR, defined variably from >20 mm/hour to >75 mm/hour, demonstrated positive likelihood ratios (LRs) ranging from 1.2 to 12 and negative LRs from 0.1 to 0.9. Similarly, CRP levels, with thresholds from >7 mg/L to >105 mg/L, showed positive LRs of 1.2 to 12.3 and negative LRs of 0.1 to 0.7. A prospective study highlighted a procalcitonin level >0.5 ng/mL to be highly specific (0.97) for septic arthritis. However, it lacks sensitivity (0.13).

Synovial fluid analysis is indispensable for diagnosis. A synovial leucocytes count ≥100,000 cells/μL strongly suggests septic arthritis, while counts ≤25,000 cells/μL generally exclude it. However, values between 25,000 and 100,000 cells/μL lack a clinically useful positive or negative LR. Gram stains are positive in 40–70% of cases, and synovial fluid cultures, although less sensitive in pre-treated patients, remain a cornerstone of diagnosis [12]. Inoculating synovial fluid into blood culture bottles enhances the detection of fastidious organisms [13].

Blood cultures, obtained before initiating antibiotics, are crucial due to bacteraemia in up to 59% of cases [14]. Serologic tests for pathogens like *Bartonella*, *Histoplasma*, or *Brucella*, and tests for tuberculosis (tuberculin skin test or interferon-gamma release assay) may be indicated based on clinical context where clinical possibility of immunocompromised host is high and not recommended routinely.

Molecular diagnostics, including polymerase chain reaction (PCR) and next-generation sequencing (NGS), are emerging as important tools. PCR, targeting specific pathogens or broad bacterial DNA, provides rapid and accurate identification, particularly in culture-negative cases [15]. Next-generation sequencing (NGS) has revolutionized the diagnosis of paediatric septic arthritis by providing a culture-independent method for pathogen detection. Traditional culture methods often fail to identify pathogens in osteoarticular infections, particularly when patients have received prior antibiotic treatment. NGS overcomes these limitations by identifying bacterial DNA directly from clinical samples, resulting in higher sensitivity and specificity. Studies have demonstrated that NGS can detect pathogens in a significant number of cases where traditional cultures remain negative, thereby aiding in accurate and timely diagnosis. For instance, in a study comparing NGS to standard cultures, NGS identified pathogens in 63.4% of cases compared to 43.9% by culture [16]. Furthermore, NGS is particularly valuable in detecting fastidious organisms such as *Kingella kingae*, which are often missed by conventional methods. This advanced diagnostic tool enhances clinical decision-making and treatment strategies, improving outcomes in paediatric patients with septic arthritis [17].

Clinical prediction tools, such as those developed by Kocher et al., which include criteria like fever, guarded weight-bearing, elevated WBC count ($\geq$12 × 10^9/L), and high ESR ($\geq$40 mm/hour), help stratify the probability of septic arthritis. Caird et al. added CRP $\geq$ 20 mg/L to this model, enhancing its predictive value. However, external validation studies show lower performance compared to original derivation studies, with predicted probabilities of septic arthritis ranging from 58.1% to 93%.

9.7 Imaging

Imaging plays a crucial role in the diagnosis and management of septic arthritis, particularly in differentiating it from other conditions and evaluating the extent of infection. The choice of imaging modality often depends on the clinical presentation, the suspected stage of the disease, and the available resources.

9.7.1 Plain Radiographs

Plain radiographs are typically the first imaging study performed in cases of suspected septic arthritis. However, their utility in the acute phase of infection is limited, as significant bony changes usually develop only after 7–10 days from the onset of symptoms. Early radiographs might only reveal soft tissue swelling, joint space widening, and possibly joint effusion (Fig. 9.2). These changes are nonspecific but can help rule out other conditions such as acute fractures or tumours. In the subacute or chronic stages of septic arthritis, radiographs might show joint space

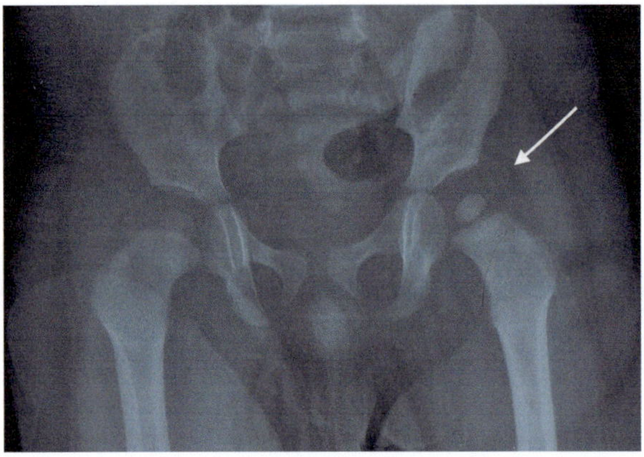

Fig. 9.2 Subtle changes of septic arthritis on plain radiograph pelvis showing increased joint space secondary to capsular distention due to collection on the marked side

narrowing, subchondral bone erosion, and periosteal reaction if osteomyelitis has developed.

9.7.2 Ultrasound

Ultrasound is a rapid, non-invasive, and cost-effective imaging technique that is particularly useful for detecting joint effusions and guiding aspiration or drainage. It has high sensitivity for identifying joint effusion in septic arthritis and can be performed without sedation, making it suitable for young children [18]. However, ultrasound cannot differentiate between purulent, sterile, or haemorrhagic effusions and is less effective at detecting adjacent conditions such as osteomyelitis or pyomyositis. Despite these limitations, a negative ultrasound in the context of a high clinical suspicion for septic arthritis generally rules out the condition, whereas a positive ultrasound indicates the need for further diagnostic or therapeutic interventions [19].

9.7.3 Magnetic Resonance Imaging (MRI)

MRI is the gold standard for evaluating septic arthritis, particularly when there is a high suspicion of adjacent infections or complex involvement. It provides detailed images of both bone and soft tissues, revealing features such as bone marrow oedema, articular cartilage destruction, and subperiosteal abscesses (Fig. 9.3). MRI is highly effective in differentiating septic arthritis from other conditions such as osteomyelitis, psoas abscesses, or pyogenic myositis. It can also help identify complications and guide surgical planning by visualizing the full extent of the infection and any associated abscesses [20]. However, MRI's high cost, requirement for sedation, and limited availability can be significant drawbacks, especially in emergency settings.

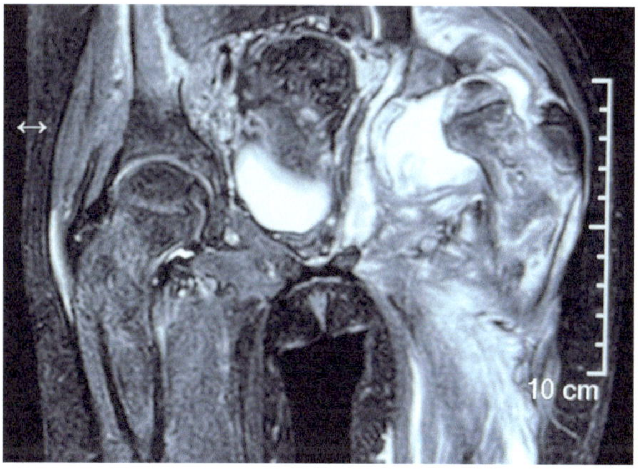

Fig. 9.3 MRI image of a patient with septic arthritis of hip with associated proximal femur osteomyelitis and pyomyositis. One can note the joint subluxation

9.7.4 Bone Scintigraphy

Bone scintigraphy, or bone scanning, uses a radiotracer to identify areas of increased bone metabolism associated with infection. While it is sensitive for detecting multifocal infections, it is less specific and can be challenging to interpret in children due to normal tracer uptake in growth plates. It is generally reserved for cases where MRI is unavailable or when multifocal disease is suspected.

9.7.5 Computerized Tomography (CT)

CT is less commonly used for diagnosing septic arthritis due to its higher radiation dose and lower sensitivity compared to MRI. It may be employed in specific scenarios where MRI is not feasible and can provide additional information on bony structures and potential abscess formation.

Imaging approach for septic arthritis involves an initial plain radiograph to rule out other conditions, followed by ultrasound to assess for joint effusion. MRI is the preferred modality for detailed assessment of infection and its complications, while bone scintigraphy and CT serve as adjuncts in particular clinical situations. The choice of imaging should be guided by the clinical context, the stage of the disease, and resource availability, with a focus on balancing diagnostic accuracy and practicality.

9.8 Treatment

Septic arthritis in children necessitates an urgent and comprehensive approach to prevent joint destruction and systemic complications. This section delineates the medical and surgical management strategies for septic arthritis in children, aiming to provide a thorough overview (Fig. 9.6).

9.9 Medical Management

9.9.1 Empiric Antibiotic Therapy

Empiric antibiotic therapy should be initiated immediately after obtaining blood cultures and synovial fluid samples. The choice of antibiotics is guided by the patient's age, local resistance patterns, and the most likely pathogens. For children with age ranging from 3 months to 5 years, intravenous cefazolin or cefuroxime is recommended [21]. This age group is commonly affected by pathogens such as *Staphylococcus aureus*, *Streptococcus pneumoniae*, *Haemophilus influenzae*, and *Kingella kingae*, and cefazolin and cefuroxime provide effective coverage against these organisms. In children older than 5 years, IV cefazolin or cloxacillin is preferred. *Staphylococcus aureus* (including MRSA) and *Streptococcus* species are common pathogens in this age group, and cloxacillin is effective against MSSA, while cefazolin covers a broader spectrum.

In areas with a high prevalence of methicillin-resistant *Staphylococcus aureus* (MRSA), it is crucial to add vancomycin or teicoplanin to the initial therapy [22]. Vancomycin and teicoplanin are essential to ensure effective initial treatment. For neonates and critically ill children, a combination of IV meropenem and vancomycin is recommended to provide broad-spectrum coverage, including gram-positive, gram-negative, and resistant organisms. This combination is effective in critically ill patients who may be at risk of infections with resistant organisms.

9.9.2 Duration of Intravenous Therapy and Conversion to Oral Antibiotics

The duration of intravenous antibiotic therapy is typically guided by clinical response, resolution of symptoms, and improvement in inflammatory markers such as C-reactive protein (CRP). In uncomplicated septic arthritis, intravenous (IV) antibiotic therapy typically lasts around 4 days, followed by a transition to oral antibiotics for an additional 2–4 weeks once clinical and laboratory improvements are observed. This approach is supported by recent studies that have shown the efficacy and safety of early transition to oral therapy after a short course of IV antibiotics. For instance, a study demonstrated that children could be safely transitioned to oral antibiotics after a median of 5 days of IV therapy, with excellent outcomes observed in the majority of cases. Another study highlighted similar findings, showing that early conversion from IV to oral therapy did not compromise treatment efficacy and resulted in satisfactory clinical outcomes. This early transition helps to reduce hospital stays and minimize the risk of complications associated with prolonged IV therapy [3].

For severe or complicated cases of septic arthritis in children, intravenous (IV) therapy may be extended beyond the typical 4 days, potentially up to 2–3 weeks, before transitioning to oral antibiotics. Criteria for transitioning to oral antibiotics include the patient being afebrile, experiencing decreased joint pain and swelling, and showing improved C-reactive protein (CRP) levels, typically below 2–3 mg/dL. Preferred oral antibiotics for Methicillin-sensitive *Staphylococcus aureus* (MSSA) include cephalexin or clindamycin, for Methicillin-resistant *Staphylococcus aureus* (MRSA), clindamycin or linezolid, and for *Kingella kingae* or other gram-negative organisms, cefuroxime or cefixime. These oral antibiotics must have good bioavailability and penetrate well into the joint spaces.

9.9.3 Culture-Negative Cases

In instances where cultures fail to identify the causative organism, empiric therapy should continue based on the initial clinical suspicion and local epidemiology. If the patient shows clinical improvement, the initial broad-spectrum empiric antibiotics can be continued. However, if there is no clinical response, it is important to reassess the choice of antibiotics. Advanced diagnostic techniques, including polymerase chain reaction (PCR) and extended culture times, may be necessary to identify fastidious organisms such as *Kingella kingae* or *Mycobacterium* species. The duration of therapy for culture-negative cases is based on clinical and laboratory response, typically 2–3 weeks in case of septic arthritis and 3–4 weeks for cases with concomitant osteomyelitis [23].

9.9.4 Controversies in Antibiotic Management

One of the main controversies in antibiotic management is the timing of the transition from intravenous to oral therapy. Recent evidence supports early transition to oral antibiotics given satisfactory clinical and laboratory improvement. This approach reduces hospital stay and the risk of complications associated with prolonged IV access. However, traditional approaches favour prolonged IV therapy to prevent relapse. The decision should be individualized based on the patient's response and the treating physician's judgement. Studies have demonstrated that children could be safely transitioned to oral antibiotics after a median of 5 days of IV therapy, with excellent outcomes observed in the majority of cases [23].

Another area of controversy is whether pre-culture antibiotic administration results in non-diagnostic bone and joint culture results. Studies have shown that antibiotics less than a week's duration does not alter the diagnostic yields of the culture and antibiotics administration should not be withheld unnecessarily waiting for intervention [24]. Also, there is ongoing research for the use of corticosteroids in the treatment of septic arthritis. Some studies suggest that a short course of dexamethasone can lead to earlier resolution of fever and serological improvement, although more research is needed to establish definitive guidelines. The role of corticosteroids remains controversial due to concerns about potential side effects and long-term outcomes. Evidence from clinical trials indicates that corticosteroids can reduce inflammation and accelerate recovery when used adjunctively with antibiotics, but caution is advised due to the variability in patient response.

The optimal duration of antibiotic therapy remains undetermined, with some reports suggesting that shorter courses (10–14 days) can be as effective as longer courses (4–6 weeks) in uncomplicated cases. This discrepancy highlights the need for more research to define the ideal duration of therapy and minimize the risks of both undertreatment and over-treatment. Prospective studies have shown that short-course antibiotic therapy is effective in uncomplicated septic arthritis, supporting a move towards more conservative treatment durations to reduce adverse effects and healthcare costs.

9.9.5 Surgical Management

Surgical intervention is critical for definitive diagnosis, source control, and preservation of joint function. The choice of procedure depends on the severity of infection, the joint involved, and the patient's overall condition.

9.9.6 Joint Aspiration

Joint aspiration, or arthrocentesis, is often the first-line procedure for initial diagnosis and therapeutic relief of joint effusion. This minimally invasive technique is performed under ultrasound guidance to ensure accuracy. Arthrocentesis has the advantage of being minimally invasive with a lower risk of complications compared to more invasive procedures [25]. It is particularly useful for obtaining synovial fluid for culture and sensitivity (Fig. 9.4). However, repeated aspirations may be required, especially in young children where sedation or anaesthesia is needed. The ability to repeat the procedure makes it a valuable diagnostic and therapeutic tool, but the need for repeated procedures can be stressful for patients and families. Recently, preliminary results of treating septic hip arthritis in children with repeated joint aspiration with minimal invasive technique using double luminal catheter under image guidance have been published reporting insignificant complications [26].

9.9.7 Arthroscopic Lavage

Arthroscopic lavage and debridement are less invasive alternatives to open arthrotomy, allowing for thorough irrigation and removal of infected material. This allows for thorough visualization, irrigation, and removal of necrotic tissue with minimal morbidity. It is particularly effective for larger joints such as the knee, hip, ankle, and shoulder. Studies have shown that patients undergoing arthroscopic debridement of the knee recover faster, with earlier return to joint mobility and reduced hospital stay compared to open surgery [27]. The minimally invasive nature of the

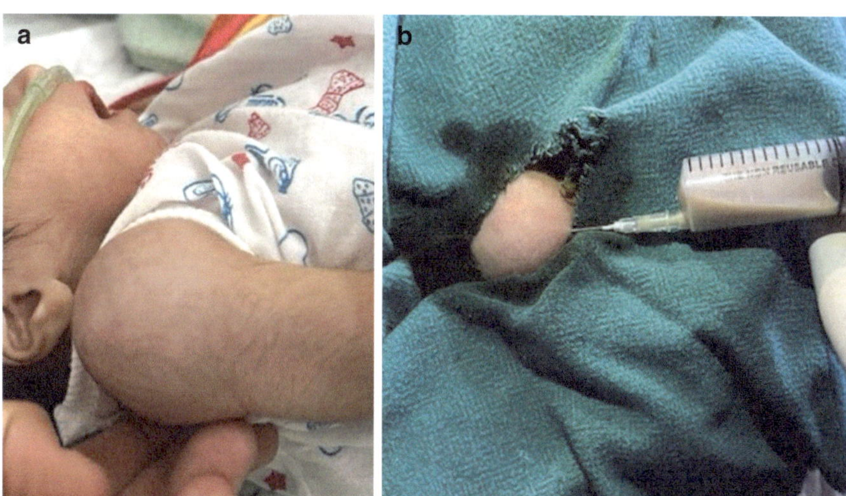

Fig. 9.4 Neonatal septic arthritis of shoulder (**a**), Arthrocentesis of the same yielding frank pus (**b**)

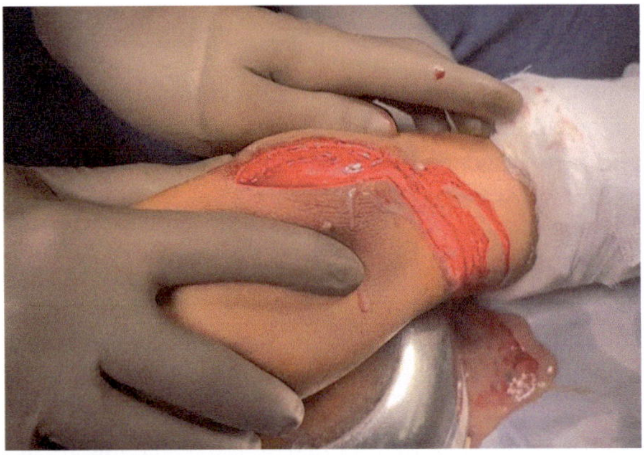

Fig. 9.5 Arthrotomy of knee joint yielding frank pus

procedure reduces postoperative pain and scarring, promoting faster recovery and better patient outcomes [26].

9.9.8 Open Arthrotomy

Open arthrotomy remains the traditional and often definitive surgical procedure for severe septic arthritis, particularly in joints at high risk for complications. This procedure involves a larger incision to provide direct access to the joint, allowing for extensive debridement, irrigation, and placement of drains if necessary (Fig. 9.5). It is indicated for severe septic arthritis with extensive purulent material and involvement of joints at high risk for complications, such as the hip. Open arthrotomy provides thorough debridement and irrigation, which is critical for severe cases, but it is associated with a larger incision, increased postoperative pain, longer recovery, and potential for more significant scarring. The decision to perform an open arthrotomy is often based on the severity of the infection and the need for extensive debridement.

9.10 Postoperative Management

Postoperative care includes the placement of drains, which are typically removed after 2–3 days. If drainage persists or there is no clinical improvement, repeat irrigation and debridement should be considered. Serial operations may be necessary until clinical improvement is achieved [28]. Monitoring of inflammatory markers, such as CRP, helps guide the need for additional interventions. The management of postoperative care is crucial for ensuring the resolution of infection and preventing recurrence.

9.11 Outcome and Follow-up

Prompt diagnosis and timely treatment of septic arthritis can result in excellent outcomes, enabling patients to gain pre-illness function at a faster pace with no or minimal long-standing complications. However, delayed diagnosis or the presence of more virulent organisms can lead to severe outcomes, including growth disturbances, joint destruction, thromboembolism, septicaemia, and even fatality [29]. Previously, complication rates were as high as 50%, but recent advancements have reduced these rates manyfolds. Growth monitoring over time is essential, especially for infections involving physis [30]. In uncomplicated cases, weight-bearing may be allowed as per the tolerance with short period of hospital stay of 3–4 days. This period allows the culture report to be available and conversion of parenteral antibiotic to oral antibiotics once clinical and laboratory improvements are observed. Relapses are rare with appropriate short-course, high-dose antibiotic treatment, though complications such as avascular necrosis of the femoral head necessitate long-term follow-up to detect any sequelae.

Complications of septic arthritis in children can range from minimal lurch in adulthood to devastating joint destruction. Persistent joint subluxation, infection, and pathological fractures are not uncommon occurrences. Early evaluation and swift management including antibiotics and debridement help minimize the acute damage as well as long-term sequalae. Post-treatment follow-up is vital to monitor clinical and laboratory outcomes. It is preferable to keep the child hospitalized in the presence of acute symptoms of pain and fever or initial 3–4 days of IV antibiotics. Patient's white blood cell count, erythrocyte sedimentation rate (ESR), and C-reactive protein (CRP) levels are assessed to look for settling trend indicating the recovery. Occasionally, in view of persistent symptoms and poor recovery, joint aspiration may need to be repeated [31]. Postoperative rehabilitation includes isotonic exercises to gain range of motion and muscle strength expediently. More frequent follow-up visits are scheduled initially for close watch for complications and assessment of function. Long-term follow-up includes repeat laboratory parameters and imaging to look for residual infection, avascular necrosis, or other sequelae [32]. Continuous monitoring for growth aberration, arthrosis, or reactivation of infection is necessary, with patient education on recognizing symptoms of potential complications (Fig. 9.6).

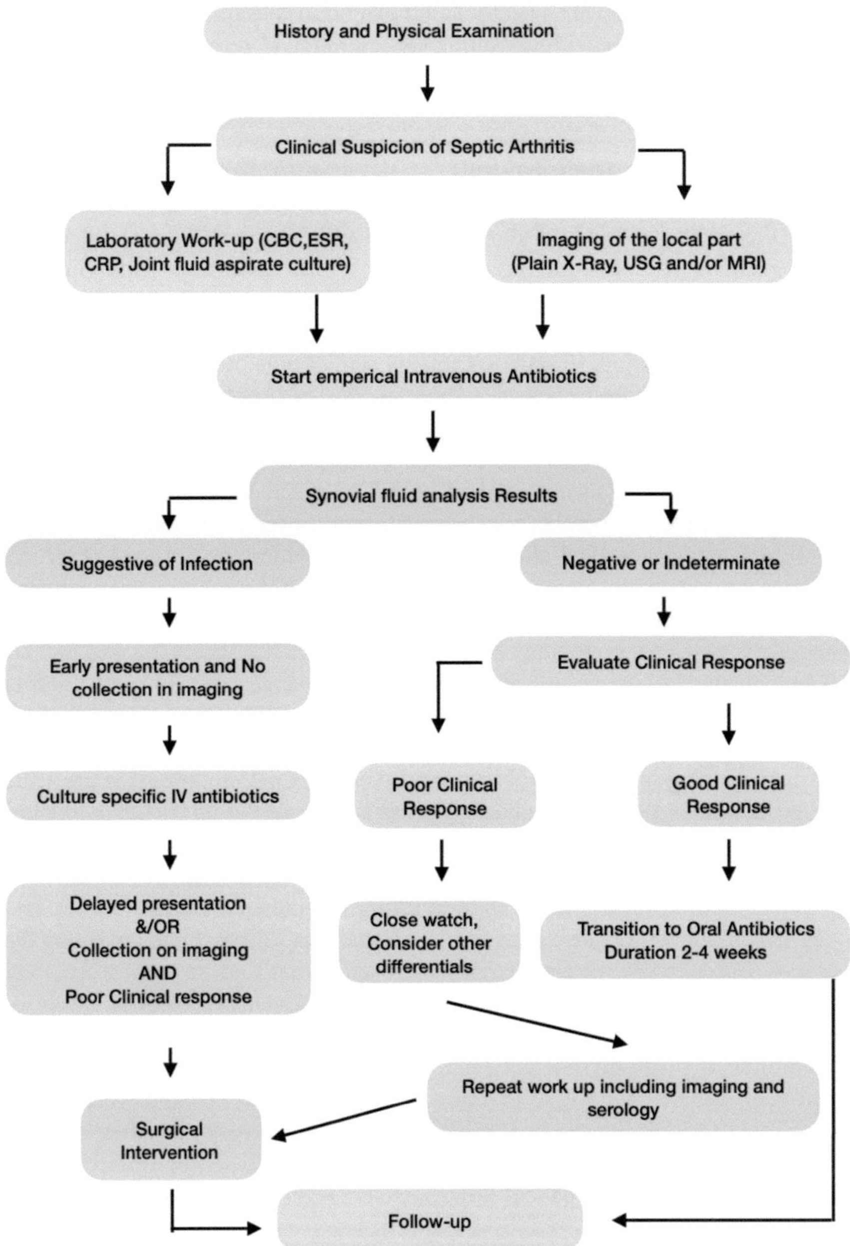

Fig. 9.6 Treatment Algorithm of septic arthritis in paediatric age group

9.12 Take-Home Message

- The treatment of septic arthritis in children requires a well-coordinated multidisciplinary approach to ensure prompt diagnosis, effective antibiotic therapy, and timely surgical intervention.
- The choice of treatment is guided by the patient's age, clinical presentation, and local resistance patterns. Empiric antibiotic therapy should be initiated immediately, with a transition to targeted therapy once culture results are available.
- Surgical intervention, including joint aspiration, arthroscopic lavage, and open arthrotomy, is crucial for source control and preservation of joint function.
- With appropriate management, most children with septic arthritis can achieve good outcomes with minimal long-term sequelae.

References

1. Goldenberg DL, Sexton D. Septic arthritis in children: critical review of the literature. UpToDate [Internet]. 2019; Available from: https://www.uptodate.com.
2. Brown DW, Sheffer BW. Pediatric septic arthritis: an update. Orthop Clin North Am. 2019;50:461–70.
3. Pääkkönen M, Peltola H. Treatment of acute septic arthritis. Pediatr Infect J. 2013;32:684–5.
4. Foster H, Pugmire J, Bache C. Acute septic arthritis: diagnosis and treatment. Lancet. 2021;32:123–8.
5. Donders CM, Spaans AJ, van Wering H, van Bergen CJ. Developments in diagnosis and treatment of paediatric septic arthritis. World J Orthop. 2022;13:122–30.
6. Howard-Jones A, Isaacs D, Gibbons P. Twelve-month outcome following septic arthritis in children. J Pediatr Orthop B. 2013;22:486–90.
7. Kocher M, et al. Clinical prediction rule for differentiating septic arthritis from transient synovitis of the hip in children. J Bone Jt Surg Am. 1999;81:1662–70.
8. Darraj H, Hakami KM, Zogel B, Maghrabi R, Khired Z. Septic arthritis of the knee in children. Cureus [Internet]. 2023 [cited 2024 Jun 17]; Available from: https://www.cureus.com/articles/190733-septic-arthritis-of-the-knee-in-children.
9. Mooney JF, Murphy RF. Septic arthritis of the pediatric hip: update on diagnosis and treatment. Curr Opin Pediatr. 2019;31:79–85.
10. Thompson RM, Gourineni P. Arthroscopic treatment of septic arthritis in very young children. J Pediatr Orthop. 2017;37:e53–7.
11. Kennedy N, Chambers S, Nolan I, Gallagher K, Werno A, Browne M, et al. Native joint septic arthritis: epidemiology, clinical features, and microbiological causes in a New Zealand population. J Rheumatol. 2015;42:2392–7.
12. Pääkkönen M. Septic arthritis in children: diagnosis and treatment. Pediatr Health Med Ther. 2017;8:65–8.
13. Dubost J, et al. Value of gram staining of synovial fluid in the diagnosis of septic arthritis. Joint Bone Spine. 2018;75:627–31.
14. Mathews C, et al. Utility of blood cultures in patients with septic arthritis. Ann Rheum Dis. 2021;78:632–8.
15. Pinsky B, et al. Molecular diagnostics for infectious diseases. Clin Microbiol Rev. 2021;34:e00035–19.
16. Ramchandar N, Burns J, Pennock A, Cannavino C, Farnaes L. Performance of next generation sequencing in isolating a pathogen in pediatric osteoarticular infections. Open Forum Infect Dis. 2020;7:S236–7.

17. He M, Arthur Vithran DT, Pan L, Zeng H, Yang G, Lu B, et al. An update on recent progress of the epidemiology, etiology, diagnosis, and treatment of acute septic arthritis: a review. Front Cell Infect Microbiol. 2023;13:1193645.
18. Monsalve J, Kan JH, Schallert EK, Bisset GS, Zhang W, Rosenfeld SB. Septic arthritis in children: frequency of coexisting unsuspected osteomyelitis and implications on imaging work-up and management. AJR Am J Roentgenol. 2015;204:1289–95.
19. Welling BD, Haruno LS, Rosenfeld SB. Validating an algorithm to predict adjacent musculoskeletal infections in pediatric patients with septic arthritis. Clin Orthop. 2018;476:153–9.
20. Karchevsky M, Schweitzer ME, Morrison WB, Parellada JA. MRI findings of septic arthritis and associated osteomyelitis in adults. AJR Am J Roentgenol. 2004;182:119–22.
21. Ballock RT, Newton PO, Evans SJ, Estabrook M, Farnsworth CL, Bradley JS. A comparison of early versus late conversion from intravenous to oral therapy in the treatment of septic arthritis. J Pediatr Orthop. 2009;29:636–42.
22. Castellazzi L, Mantero M, Esposito S. Update on the management of pediatric acute osteomyelitis and septic arthritiS. Int J Mol Sci. 2016;17:855.
23. Shenoy B, Singhal T, Yewale V, Choudhury J, Kumar AP, Agashe MV, et al. Indian Academy of Pediatrics Consensus statement on diagnosis and management of bone and joint infections in children. Indian Pediatr. 2024;61:209–18.
24. Section J, Gibbons SD, Barton T, Greenberg DE, Jo CH, Copley LAB. Microbiological culture methods for pediatric musculoskeletal infection: a guideline for optimal use. J Bone Jt Surg. 2015;97:441–9.
25. Montgomery NI, Epps HR. Pediatric septic arthritis. Orthop Clin North Am. 2017;48:209–16.
26. Essa A, Asa'af M, Shtarker H. Preliminary results: continuous double luminal catheter drainage for the management of septic hip arthritis in children. J Pediatr Orthop Part B. 2022;31:e11–6.
27. Jaffe J, et al. MRSA: risk factor for unplanned return to the operating room after arthroscopic treatment. J Pediatr Orthop. 2017;37:165–70.
28. Abram S, Nicol F, Hullin D, Spencer S. Clinical outcomes following knee arthroscopy for septic arthritis in England: a data linkage study. Knee. 2020;27:1078–85.
29. Gramlich Y, Winthrop K, von Knoch M. Treatment of septic arthritis of the shoulder. J Bone Jt Surg Am. 2020;102:1179–85.
30. Jung H, Song J, Kekatpure A, Adikrishna A, Hong H, Lee W, et al. The use of continuous negative pressure after open debridement for septic arthritis of the shoulder. Bone Jt J. 2016;98:660–5.
31. Maneiro J, Souto A, Cervantes M, Vázquez-Trinanes C, Carmona L, Gómez-Reino J. Predictors of treatment failure and mortality in native septic arthritis. Clin Rheumatol. 2015;34:1961–7.
32. Hunter J, Bierma-Zeinstra S, Koehler R, Springer B. Diagnostic and therapeutic strategies in septic arthritis: an international survey. Rheumatol Int. 2020;40:243–51.

Adult Osteomyelitis

10

Shahnawaz Khan and Sujit Kumar Tripathy

Abstract

Osteomyelitis, or infection of the bone and marrow, is associated with significant morbidity. The incidence of osteomyelitis is increasing, particularly relating to complications from diabetic foot infections. *Staphylococcus aureus* is the most frequent pathogen, but other organisms may be involved. The primary route of infection is through hematogenous spread. The pathogenesis involves several factors, including pathogenic factors (bacterial virulence, biofilm formation, antibiotic resistance), host factors (local issues including vascular compromise or systemic conditions related to diabetes or immunosuppression), and environmental factors (variations in vascular structures or the presence of an implant). The transition from acute osteomyelitis to chronic osteomyelitis is characterized by the formation of intraosseous abscesses, the development of necrosis of the cortical bone leading to sequestrum formation, and the formation of new bone (involucrum) in the presence of draining sinus tract. Diagnosis consists of clinical history (localized pain, presence of fever, presence of sinus tract), along with imaging studies. Plain X-ray films may show changes at a later stage, whereas CT scans can often present the sequestrum and involucrum, and MRI has the greatest sensitivity and specificity for detecting infection. Further, radiolabeled imaging (radionuclide scans) or PET-CT can be acquired if suggested studies are not conclusive. Across the spectrum of care, management is multidisciplinary. Management typically involves aggressive surgical intervention (debridement or removal of infected and/or necrotic tissues) and directed antibiotic therapy. Surgical techniques address soft tissue and bone loss, ranging from skin grafting and muscle flaps to complex reconstruction of bone, including bone transport, the Masquelet technique, and antibiotic-impregnated cement spacers or mega-

S. Khan (✉) · S. K. Tripathy
Department of Orthopedics, All India Institute of Medical Sciences, Bhubaneswar, India

P. Kumar et al. (eds.), *Textbook of Orthopedic Infections*,
https://doi.org/10.1007/978-981-95-5029-6_10

prostheses. In the most severe cases where surgical options leave a limb unmanageable, amputation may be considered. General management of osteomyelitis involves pain control, nutritional support, and wound care. Advances in recent years have also focused on an understanding of osteoclastic activity, anti-biofilm mechanisms, and drug delivery systems.

Learning Objectives

- To describe the microbiology and pathophysiology of osteomyelitis in adults.
- To study the various clinical features and outline the various investigation modalities
- To formulate a comprehensive management plan for osteomyelitis in adults

10.1 Introduction

Osteomyelitis is an inflammatory condition of the bone primarily caused by infection [1, 2]. This condition is particularly concerning in orthopedics due to the significant morbidity it can cause. Osteomyelitis is one of the oldest known diseases, with evidence dating back to ancient fossils [1, 3]. Various ancient texts have documented this condition in different forms, but it wasn't until 1844, that Nelaton officially coined the term "osteomyelitis" [3]. The advent of penicillin revolutionized the treatment of osteomyelitis; before its introduction, surgery was the only available treatment option. Despite advances in medicine, the exact incidence of osteomyelitis remains unclear, though it is known to affect males more frequently than females [4]. Current evidence shows that the incidence of osteomyelitis is on the rise, and this trend is mostly due to the rise in prevalence of diabetic foot infections [4]. In this chapter, we will discuss various aspects of osteomyelitis from microbiology to treatment.

10.2 Microbiology

Nearly 40% cases are caused by *Staphylococcus aureus*, though the specific pathogen can vary depending on underlying conditions [4, 5]. For instance, *Salmonella typhi* is frequently associated with osteomyelitis in individuals with sickle cell disease, while *Pseudomonas* is common among intravenous drug users, often affecting the clavicle [6–8]. Tubercular osteomyelitis is very common in low- and middle-income countries where tuberculosis is very common. Immunocompromised patients, including those with chronic indwelling catheters, are at risk for fungal osteomyelitis, particularly from *Candida* species [9]. *Bartonella* osteomyelitis has been reported in AIDS patients following cat scratch disease [10]. In individuals with diabetes and chronic ulcers, osteomyelitis is typically polymicrobial.

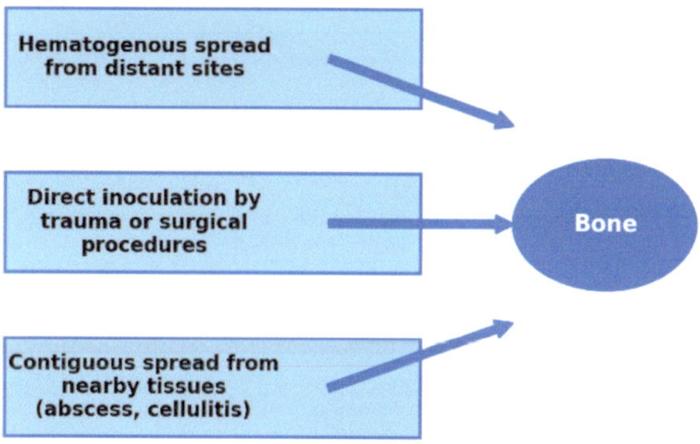

Fig. 10.1 Sources of infection in osteomyelitis

Additionally, *Brucella* and *Salmonella* are known to affect the spine, and infections from Actinomyces and Sporothrix are generally acquired through direct inoculation [9, 11]. *Enterobacter* and *Streptococcus* have also been implicated in adult osteomyelitis cases.

10.3 Sources of Infection

Osteomyelitis can occur when infectious organisms reach the bone through various routes. As suggested in the article by Lew et al. [3], osteomyelitis can be caused by three mechanisms (Fig. 10.1). In adults, direct inoculation of bacteria is often due to trauma or iatrogenic injuries during surgery. Hematogenous spread from a distant infection site is the leading cause of osteomyelitis in children and adult vertebral osteomyelitis. In the presence of implants, infection can spread from surrounding tissues to the bone. Diabetic patients, who are at increased risk due to poor vascular supply and neuropathy, are more susceptible to injuries that can lead to osteomyelitis. Contiguous spread of infection is also a concern in patients with pressure sores located near bones. Open fractures are also an important cause of osteomyelitis with infection rates ranging from 4% to 64% depending upon the contamination [12, 13]. The incidence of osteomyelitis following a joint replacement can vary from 1.5% to 2.5% and can be as high as 20% following a revision surgery [12].

10.4 Pathogenesis

The development of osteomyelitis is a complex process influenced by three main factors: the pathogen, the host, and the local environment (Fig. 10.2).

A. *Pathogen Factors*

The virulence of the infecting organism plays a crucial role in the progression of osteomyelitis. Highly virulent bacteria, especially during their planktonic stage,

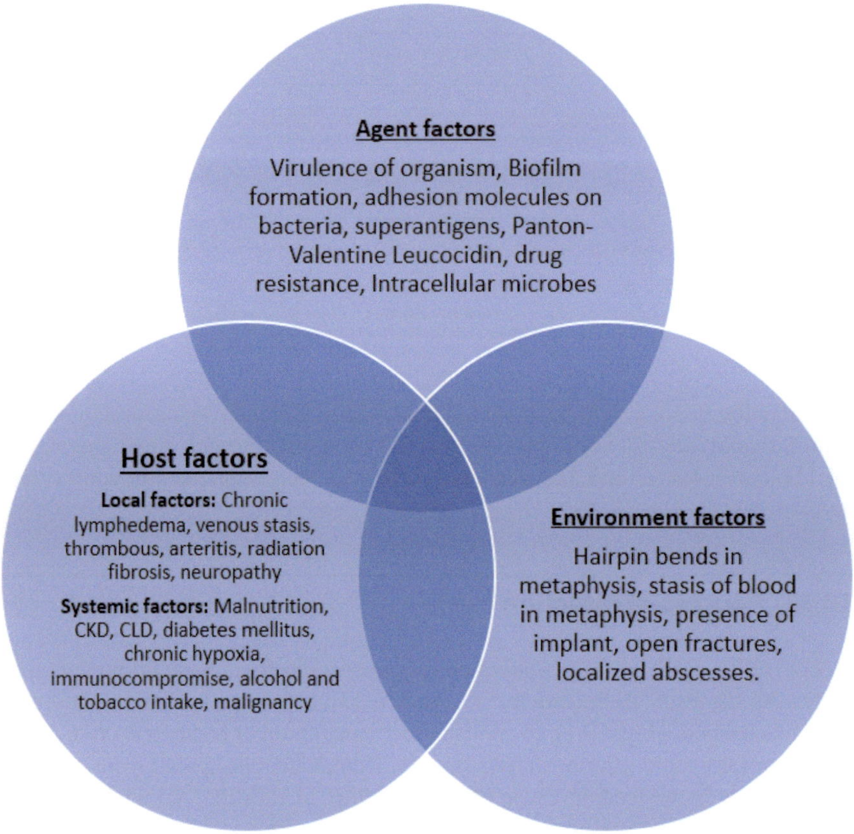

Fig. 10.2 Pathogenesis of osteomyelitis

multiply rapidly and spread the infection quickly [14]. These organisms possess various adhesion molecules that allow them to attach to host cells and evade immune detection. Additionally, some bacteria produce superantigens, which can excessively activate the immune system, leading to a heightened inflammatory response. *Staphylococcus aureus*, for example, secretes staphylococcal protein A (spA), which alters B cell function and survival, thereby modulating the immune response and evading detection [14, 15]. Invasion of *Staphylococcus aureus* into submicron channels called osteocyte lacuna-canalicular networks in the mineral matrix of the bone has led to its persistence in human foot osteomyelitis [16]. Furthermore, certain bacteria have the ability to undergo intracellular colonization within osteoblasts, allowing them to escape the host's immune defenses [15]. Additionally, some bacteria carry plasmids that enable them to alter their surface antigens, making them resistant to antibiotics [17].

Role of Biofilm: Certain bacteria can organize into protective groups known as biofilms, which are covered with a layer of exopolysaccharide [18]. This is particularly common during the sessile stage of the bacterial life cycle. The biofilm acts as a barrier, preventing antibiotics from penetrating and eradicating the infection effectively leading to persistence of infection.

B. *Host Factors*

Host factors significantly influence susceptibility to osteomyelitis. These factors can be divided into local and systemic categories:

Local Factors: Conditions that reduce blood supply to the affected bone increase the risk of infection. For instance, the altered blood flow and lymphedema reduce the phagocytic actions of inflammatory cells. A localized thrombous creates an inflammatory milieu along with stasis of circulation leading to lodgment of bacteria on the bones. Additionally, the presence of an implant or any foreign body can facilitate infection by enhancing bacterial adhesion and biofilm formation [19, 20].

Systemic Factors: Conditions that reduce overall immunity of the host, such as diabetes, chronic illness, or intravenous drug abuse, increase the risk of developing osteomyelitis. Immunocompromised individuals are particularly vulnerable to infections that can progress to osteomyelitis. The recent rise in incidences of osteomyelitis among diabetes is also alarming [4].

C. *Environmental Factors*

The local environment, or milieu, surrounding the bone also plays a crucial role in the pathogenesis of osteomyelitis. The unique vascular structure, particularly the hairpin bends in blood vessels, reduces blood flow and facilitates bacterial adhesion [21]. The presence of implants or foreign bodies further encourages bacterial colonization and biofilm formation. In cases where a localized abscess forms, it can prevent antibiotics from penetrating deep into the tissue, complicating treatment.

10.5 Progression from Acute to Chronic Osteomyelitis

The pathogenesis of osteomyelitis often begins with the formation of septic emboli, which lodge in the metaphysis due to the hairpin arrangement of blood vessels that slow blood flow [22]. The relative lack of phagocytes in this region allows for the development of an intraosseous abscess. This abscess can extend into the medullary cavity through the Haversian canals and spread horizontally via the Volkmann's canals. As the pus accumulates in the medullary cavity of a tubular bone, it seeks the path of least resistance, often piercing the cortex at the metaphyseal area and accumulating beneath the periosteum, forming a subperiosteal abscess.

The subperiosteal abscess elevates the periosteum, cutting off the blood supply to the underlying cortex, which leads to cortical bone necrosis. The combination of high intraosseous pressure from the abscess and the interruption of both periosteal and medullary blood supplies results in the formation of a sequestrum, a piece of dead bone surrounded by living granulation tissue.

Meanwhile, the inner cambium layer of the periosteum, stimulated by the subperiosteal pus, begins to form new bone in a tubular fashion around the sequestrum, creating an involucrum. The pus from the medullary cavity attempts to escape through channels in the sequestrum, known as cloacae, which is a characteristic feature of chronic osteomyelitis.

As the infection progresses, the abscess may break through the periosteum and spread into the muscle plane, sometimes leading to skin breakdown and the formation of a sinus tract. Through this draining sinus, dead pieces of cortical bone, or bony spicules, may be expelled, which is a hallmark sign of chronic osteomyelitis.

10.6 Classification

Numerous classification systems have been used in the past. However, we discuss the most commonly used classification systems in this chapter.

A temporal classification of osteomyelitis is classified into three types:

1. Acute osteomyelitis: Duration of symptoms less than 2 weeks
2. Subacute osteomyelitis: Duration of symptoms is between 2 weeks to 6 months
3. Chronic osteomyelitis: Symptoms are more than 6 months

The chronic osteomyelitis has been further classified according to Cierny-Mader classification summarized in Table 10.1 [23]. It has two components: anatomical location of bone involvement and the physiological class which depicts host's immunity.

The factors affecting the immunity are:

1. Local (B_L): Chronic lymphedema, venous stasis, thrombous, arteritis, radiation fibrosis, neuropathy

Table 10.1 Cierny-Mader classification of chronic osteomyelitis

Anatomical type	
Type	*Characteristics*
I	Medullary osteomyelitis
II	Superficial osteomyelitis
III	Localized osteomyelitis
IV	Diffuse osteomyelitis
Physiological class	
Class	*Characteristics*
A	Good immunity
B	Immunity compromised locally (B_L) or systemically (B_S)
C	Requires suppressive or no treatment as treatment is worse than disease

2. Systemic (B_S): Malnutrition, chronic kidney disease or chronic liver disease, diabetes mellitus, chronic hypoxia, immunocompromise, alcohol and tobacco intake, malignancy

10.7 Clinical Features of Osteomyelitis

The clinical presentation of osteomyelitis differs significantly depending on the duration of the infection, which can manifest as either acute or chronic osteomyelitis.

10.7.1 Acute Osteomyelitis

Acute osteomyelitis is characterized by localized pain and fever. Patients may also present with erythema, swelling, and tenderness over the affected area. In pediatric patients, acute osteomyelitis may present as septic arthritis, particularly when the infection involves intraarticular physes. In cases involving the spine, a sudden onset or worsening of back pain should prompt the clinician to consider vertebral osteomyelitis.

10.7.2 Chronic Osteomyelitis

Chronic osteomyelitis typically presents with a sinus tract that discharges pus, often containing bony spicules. While pain and erythema may be present, fever and other constitutional symptoms are less common in chronic cases. The affected skin may exhibit discoloration, puckering, and adhesions. The underlying bone is often thickened and irregular, with the potential for pathological fractures or gap nonunion. When assessing a patient with suspected chronic osteomyelitis, it is essential to evaluate for signs of immunosuppression, including systemic diseases and the use of immunosuppressive drugs, as well as peripheral vascular disease.

10.8 Investigations for Osteomyelitis

10.8.1 Radiographs

Plain radiographs are typically the first investigation modality employed in suspected cases of osteomyelitis, and it is crucial to obtain orthogonal views of the affected limb to accurately assess the condition. In cases of acute osteomyelitis, radiographic findings often lag behind clinical symptoms by approximately 2 weeks [1]. Significant bone loss—usually at least 50%—is required before radiographic changes become apparent [24, 25]. This delay underscores the importance of correlating clinical findings with imaging results in the early stages of osteomyelitis.

In contrast, chronic osteomyelitis presents with more pronounced radiographic changes. The hallmark feature is the presence of a sequestrum, a segment of dead bone that appears more radio-opaque due to its avascularity. Surrounding the sequestrum is a rim of radiolucency, indicating the presence of pus. Additionally, new bone formation, known as involucrum, can often be observed encasing the sequestrum. This involucrum, lined with granulation tissue and bacterial glycocalyx, appears as irregular cortical thickening resembling a periosteal reaction. In patients with orthopedic hardware, the presence of radiolucency, a sclerotic rim, osteopenia, periosteal reaction, or lysis around the hardware should raise suspicion of infection. It is essential to differentiate chronic osteomyelitis from other conditions with similar radiographic features, such as healing Charcot's disease, Ewing's sarcoma, giant cell tumor, and Langerhans cell histiocytosis.

Brodie's abscess (Fig. 10.3), an intraosseous abscess commonly seen in individuals with good immunity, is another notable radiographic finding. It typically manifests as a radiolucent area within the bone, indicative of the body's attempt to contain the infection in subacute or chronic osteomyelitis.

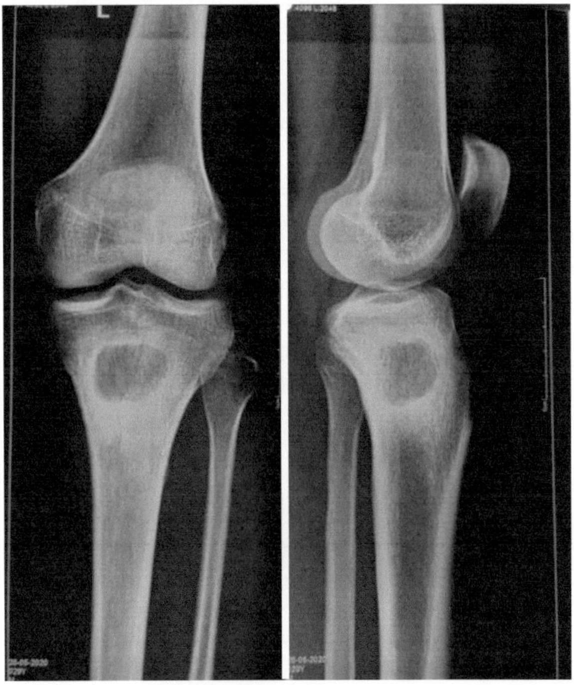

Fig. 10.3 Brodie's abscess

10.8.2 Sinogram

A sinogram is a minimally invasive procedure that involves the injection of a radio-opaque contrast dye into a sinus tract, followed by radiographic imaging to visualize the extent and course of the sinus. Though performed rarely nowadays after the advent of MRI, this test depicts the anatomy and extent of sinus in patients who are not eligible for MRI scan.

10.8.3 Computed Tomography (CT)

Computed Tomography (CT) plays a valuable role in diagnosing osteomyelitis by providing enhanced detail and confirming radiographic findings with greater clarity. CT scans are particularly effective in identifying sequestrum, involucrum, and the presence of intramedullary gas, which are key indicators of the disease. Both CT and the radiographs have a sensitivity and specificity of 50–75% in diagnosis of osteomyelitis [26]. However, the utility of CT scans is limited in the presence of metallic implants, as artifacts can interfere with the accuracy of the acquired images.

10.8.4 Magnetic Resonance Imaging (MRI)

Magnetic Resonance Imaging (MRI) is a critical diagnostic tool for osteomyelitis, providing superior spatial resolution and the highest sensitivity (78–90%) and specificity (60–100%) among imaging modalities [27]. It effectively detects osteomyelitis as a localized abscess that appears hypointense on T1-weighted images and hyperintense on T2-weighted images, with granulation tissue also appearing hyperintense. Contrast-enhanced MRI and STIR sequences are recommended for a more detailed assessment of bone pathology. Enhancement of rim of abscess called "penumbra sign" on T1 weighted MRI is diagnostic of osteomyelitis. Additionally, MRI is invaluable in septic arthritis, as it can precisely detect joint effusion and adjacent bone involvement, such as osteomyelitis, offering a comprehensive evaluation of the infection.

10.8.5 Ultrasound (USG)

Ultrasonography has limited utility in diagnosing osteomyelitis, particularly for bone infections. However, it can be beneficial in detecting associated soft tissue infections. In cases where the metaphyseal region is intracapsular, such as in the hip, ankle, shoulder, and elbow, osteomyelitis may be associated with septic arthritis. In these scenarios, ultrasonography plays a vital role in diagnosing septic arthritis and guiding joint aspiration.

10.8.6 Radionuclide Scanning

Radionuclide scanning, including Technetium (Tc99m), Gallium, and Indium scans, was traditionally used for diagnosing osteomyelitis, though it has largely been supplanted by MRI. However, these scans remain valuable in certain situations, particularly in cases of multifocal osteomyelitis or when MRI is contraindicated. Triple phase bone scan is an improved version of radionuclide scanning which helps in distinguishing bone infection from a soft tissue infection. In case of osteomyelitis, there is uptake in all three phases, namely, flow phase, blood pool phase, and delayed phase. They are highly sensitive and capable of detecting infection-related changes as early as 2 days after the onset of infection.

10.8.7 Positron Emission Tomography-Computed Tomography (PET-CT)

PET-CT is an emerging diagnostic tool that offers precise identification of infected regions and assists in determining the extent of surgical debridement needed. FDG PET has demonstrated superiority over MRI in detecting sequestrum, particularly due to its ability to identify areas with low proton content. With a sensitivity and specificity of more than 90%, this scan is the most advanced form of diagnostics [28]. However, the widespread use of PET-CT is limited by its high cost, limited availability, and the risk of false positives, especially if conducted within 1 month of surgery.

10.8.8 Laboratory Tests

Laboratory tests play a crucial role in diagnosing osteomyelitis and monitoring the response to treatment. A complete blood count (CBC) typically reveals an elevated leucocyte count with a predominance of neutrophils in acute osteomyelitis, while chronic cases may not show significant changes in blood counts. Inflammatory markers such as erythrocyte sedimentation rate (ESR) and C-reactive protein (CRP) are also elevated in osteomyelitis and are useful indicators for tracking the effectiveness of treatment. Although Interleukin-6 and Interleukin-12 levels, along with Alpha-1-acid glycoprotein, may also be elevated, they are not as reliable for diagnostic purposes [29]. Blood cultures are generally positive in cases where the infection has spread hematogenously, providing valuable information for identifying the causative organism.

10.8.9 Biopsy

Bone biopsy is considered the gold standard for confirming the histopathological diagnosis of osteomyelitis and identifying the causative organism. Biopsies can be obtained either percutaneously or through open surgical methods. Current evidence suggests giving antibiotics do not affect the yield of pathogenic cultures [30, 31]. Histopathological examination of acute osteomyelitis typically reveals neutrophilic infiltration, whereas chronic osteomyelitis is characterized by a predominance of mononuclear cells, macrophages, spongy osteogenesis, and fibrotic tissue [32]. Massive necrosis is commonly observed in acute cases, while chronic cases may present with sinuses and fibrosis. For accurate identification, biopsy specimens should be sent for gram staining, as well as aerobic, anaerobic, mycobacterial, and fungal cultures. However, it is important to note that cultures from sinus tracts and superficial wounds are generally unreliable.

10.9 Differential Diagnosis of Osteomyelitis

- *Ewing's sarcoma:* Ewing's sarcoma is the most common differential diagnosis in young adults. Typically, this disease presents with fever and evening rise of temperature with localized pain. MRI and radiographic findings also mimic osteomyelitis. A biopsy is necessary to differentiate the two.
- *Vaso-occlusive crisis:* This disease can mimic osteomyelitis due to frequent bone pains. However, a history of sickle cell disease, absence of infective agent and multiple bone involvement will differentiate this from osteomyelitis.
- *Soft tissue infections:* Soft tissue infections like necrotizing fasciitis and cellulitis also present with localized pain. MRI or bone scans are necessary to differentiate this from osteomyelitis.
- *Osteoid osteoma:* A history of nocturnal bone pain responding to anti-inflammatory drugs is typical of Osteoid osteoma. CT scans are needed to identify the nidus in a osteoïd osteoma.
- *Stress fractures:* Repeated stress on a normal bone leads to stress fractures. This can be differentiated from osteomyelitis based on the history of repeated stressful activities like marching. T1-weighted MRI will show a fracture line leading to its differentiation from osteomyelitis.
- *Bony metastasis:* These are common in old age and present with bone pains. Identification of "penumbra sign" on T1-weighted MRI and a rise in inflammatory blood markers favor the diagnosis osteomyelitis.
- *Charcot arthropathy:* This condition is very common among diabetics and is difficult to differentiate from osteomyelitis. A prior history of ulcer will be present in cases of osteomyelitis. A "dependent rubor" test is positive in Charcot's where the erythema disappears on elevating the affected limb and reappears on lowering the limb. Surrounding joint fragmentations and subluxations with absence of sequestrum is seen in Charcot's arthropathy imaging.

10.10 Treatment of Osteomyelitis

The main goal of treatment is to eliminate the infective foci and promote healing of tissues. This can be achieved effectively by combination of medical and surgical modalities. Treatment can be divided into two categories: general management and treatment of the disease proper.

10.10.1 General Management

The initial management of osteomyelitis focuses on pain control and overall patient stabilization. In cases of acute osteomyelitis, there is severe pain in the affected limb due to accumulation of pus and edema fluid inside the bone. This necessitates the use of analgesics. Most commonly used analgesics are Non-Steroidal Anti-Inflammatory Drugs (NSAIDS) and opioids. Limb elevation and cryotherapy can aid in reduction of the limb edema. In cases of severe pain, splintage of the limb for a short period of time may be done. This can be done by the means of slabs and splints. However, splinting the limb for more than 3 weeks is not recommended as it can lead to joint stiffness. Hence, one must explore other treatment modalities also.

Nutritional support forms a vital cog of treatment. This part is often overlooked by the physicians and surgeons which in turn leads to poor chances of recovery. Infections often increase the basal metabolic rate of the body. A high protein diet (at least 2 g protein/kg body weight daily) along with a high carbohydrate diet is necessary to support immune function [33, 34]. Furthermore, adequate fluid intake must be ensured to cope up with the third space losses and pus discharges and also prevent dyselectrolytemia.

Patients with comorbid conditions, such as diabetes or immunosuppression, require special attention, particularly in maintaining optimal blood glucose levels.

10.10.2 Wound Care

The management of the wounds and sinuses is of paramount importance in cases of chronic osteomyelitis. Dressing of the wound at least twice daily is necessary if there is enough soakage to wet the dressing material. Dressing with normal saline is recommended to reduce the pathogen load at the wound site. Use of povidone iodine and antibiotic solution has not shown any clinical benefit. Vacuum-assisted closure (VAC) dressings are beneficial for reducing edema, enhancing neovascularization, and promoting granulation tissue formation, especially after surgical debridement.

10.10.3 Treatment of Disease Proper

The treatment of the disease varies according to the severity of the disease. This encompasses the use of antibiotic therapy and the surgical treatment.

Role of Antibiotics Antibiotic therapy is initiated after the samples are taken for culture. The choice of antibiotics varies from one hospital to another, depending on the local culture isolates. The antibiotic therapy can be divided into following categories:

- *Empirical Therapy:* Initially, broad-spectrum antibiotics should be initiated immediately after cultures are obtained. The commonly prescribed broad spectrum antibiotics include Flucloxacillin, and 3rd generation Cephalosporins or benzyl-penicillin while Vancomycin, Clindamycin and Fluoroquinolones are used to treat difficult infections.
- *Targeted Therapy:* Once the culture reports are available, the antibiotic regimens need to be tailored accordingly. While there is debate over the optimal duration and route of administration, common regimens include 2 weeks of intravenous antibiotics followed by 4 weeks of oral therapy or vice versa. American Association of Orthopedics recommendations suggest shortening the duration of antibiotics to 4 weeks if the response is adequate [35]. The antibiotic penetration into the infection site increases with neovascularization following the debridement.
- *Local Antibiotic Delivery Systems:* Calcium sulfate or hydroxyapatite beads provide high local antibiotic concentrations with minimal systemic toxicity. In contrast to PolyMethylMethacrylate (PMMA) beads, these beads provide rapid release of antibiotics at local sites. The antibiotic release peaks at 24 h after the surgery and continues up to 4 months [36, 37].
- *Suppressive Antibiotics:* The role of chronic suppressive antibiotics is controversial but may be beneficial in immunocompromised patients who are not candidates for surgery. High recurrence rates are observed when antibiotics are discontinued.

Surgical Management Aggressive surgical debridement is the cornerstone of treatment, aiming to remove sequestra and biofilm-associated pathogens.

Debridement must be done by the senior surgeons. If a hardware is present, it should be removed, as it is often a nidus for biofilm formation. The intraosseous abscess and the necrotic material are removed. The bone ends must be debrided till fresh bleeding spots are observed on the bone surface. This is called the "paprika sign".

The medullary canal also needs to be debrided. This can be done by reaming of the canal till the inner slimy layer is removed from the endosteum. The Reamer Irrigator

Aspirator (RIA) technique, which combines reaming with irrigation, is particularly effective in reducing pathogen load from the medullary canal. Reaming should be done with utmost care as there is a chance of iatrogenic fracture in such weak bones.

Soft tissue debridement is also critical as these surrounding soft tissues often provide a nidus for lodgement of bacteria. The sinus tract should be excised and sent for biopsy to look for malignant changes along with other soft tissue and bony specimen. The surgical wound needs to be irrigated with adequate amounts of normal saline. A high volume and low-pressure system of irrigation is recommended.

In cases where extensive debridement is performed, there is a resultant bone and soft tissue defect. The bone ends need to be stabilized by the means of an external fixator or an antibiotic coated intramedullary nail. We do not recommend the use of slabs as frequent dressing becomes a problem and the soft tissue reconstruction fails in absence of rigid immobilization.

Management of Soft Tissue Loss The soft tissue cover also gets compromised due to extensive debridements. A healthy soft tissue cover is necessary before any bony procedure is attempted. In the earlier phases when the wound condition is not healthy, VAC dressing are applied over the wound. Minor loss of skin can be closed by mobilization of the surrounding skin. Massive skin defects warrant a split thickness skin grafting. Massive defects involving loss of muscle cover and exposed bone need a muscle flap cover. This can be accomplished by rotation flaps. Muscle flaps not only provide coverage but also create a vascular bed conducive to bone healing. Certain regions like distal leg and ankle joint, where the soft tissue cover is not great and muscle bulk is lacking, a free flap or a cross-leg flap is necessary.

Management of Bone Loss The major challenge in management of osteomyelitis is in tackling the bone loss. Reconstruction of debrided bone gaps is crucial to restore limb length and function. The dead spaces can be managed in a single setting or in multiple settings in a staged manner. The bone loss can range from a minor defect in cortex to massive segment loss. Numerous techniques have been described to manage the bone loss.

- *Bone Transport:* Large bone gaps are managed using bone transport, typically with an Ilizarov fixator or Limb Reconstruction System. The principle of distraction histiogenesis not only fills the bone gap but also improves local vascularity enhancing the chances of bone healing. This technique can be used to manage large bone defects with minimal complications. However, the prolonged course of treatment and pin site infections may not be accepted by all patients.
- *Transfer of Adjacent Bone:* This technique is used in forearm and leg where there are two bones. One such procedure is Huntington's procedure which involves tibialization of fibula in a staged manner. Similarly, single bone forearm is an accepted surgery in case of massive defects.

- *Vascularized Bone Grafts:* These grafts have their own blood supply, enhancing survival and integration. It is crucial to ensure that the infection is fully eradicated before proceeding with this technique. Vascularized fibula graft is the most commonly used vascularized graft.
- *Antibiotic-Impregnated Cement Spacers:* These spacers, mixed with heat-stable antibiotics like vancomycin, gentamicin, and tobramycin, can fill the defect and provide local antibiotic delivery [38]. The spacer is typically removed after 6 weeks, followed by bone grafting. After 6 weeks, the spacer acts as a substrate for bacterial growth.
- *Bioactive Glass:* This synthetic osteoconductive and angiogenic material can be used to manage dead space effectively, promoting integration of bone and soft tissues. It has shown to be also effective against the multidrug-resistant organisms and hence has been used as a substitute for bone grafts [39].
- *Papineau Technique:* Introduced in 1973, this technique involves serial debridements and dressings until granulation tissue forms, followed by filling the gap with cancellous bone grafts [40]. This old technique is successful in managing the large bone gaps but the need of large amounts of bone grafts and elimination of local infection is crucial to success of this technique.
- *Primary Bone Grafting:* This method involves filling the defect with cancellous bone graft during the primary debridement. However, the success rate is low, with a high risk of reinfection due to the avascularity of the graft. The graft uptake is also unreliable with donor site morbidities.
- *Masquelet Technique:* This two-stage procedure begins with radical debridement and placement of a PolyMethylMethacrylate (PMMA) spacer in the defect [41]. After approximately 4 weeks, a bio-membrane forms around the spacer, and in the second stage, the spacer is removed and the defect is filled with bone graft. The success of Masquelet technique lies in the quality of the biomembrane. Recently, the use of bone morphogenic proteins, platelet-rich plasma to enhance the quality and vascularity of the membrane is gaining importance.
- *Megaprosthesis:* In recent times, many surgeons have used megaprosthesis to replace the bone defects. This technique is mostly successful in management of bone defects close to the joints. This also prevents the donor site morbidity experienced in bone grafts. But these prostheses may dislocate if the soft tissue reconstruction of soft tissue is not proper. The risk of infection and the chances of implant loosening limit the use of megaprosthesis. Further, high costs of prosthesis and the chances of recurrence of infection in presence of a metal limit the use of megaprosthesis in large bone defects.
- *Allograft Prosthesis Composite (APC):* To overcome the shortcomings of the megaprosthesis, APCs were designed. APC consists of a revision-type prosthesis cemented into an allograft which is then integrated into the host bone. These are also prone to loosening and the integration into host bone is also not predictable. High costs and limited availability of APCs is a big disadvantage.

10.10.4 Amputation

In some cases, despite aggressive treatment, amputation may be necessary to eradicate infection. This option is often considered for patients who are not fit for repeated surgical interventions and in those individuals, where reconstruction of limb is not possible after repeated debridements. With advancements in prosthetics, many patients can achieve a high quality of life post-amputation, returning to normal activities more quickly.

This comprehensive approach to osteomyelitis treatment integrates surgical and medical therapies to achieve optimal patient outcomes, addressing both the infection and the resultant anatomical and functional deficits (Fig. 10.4).

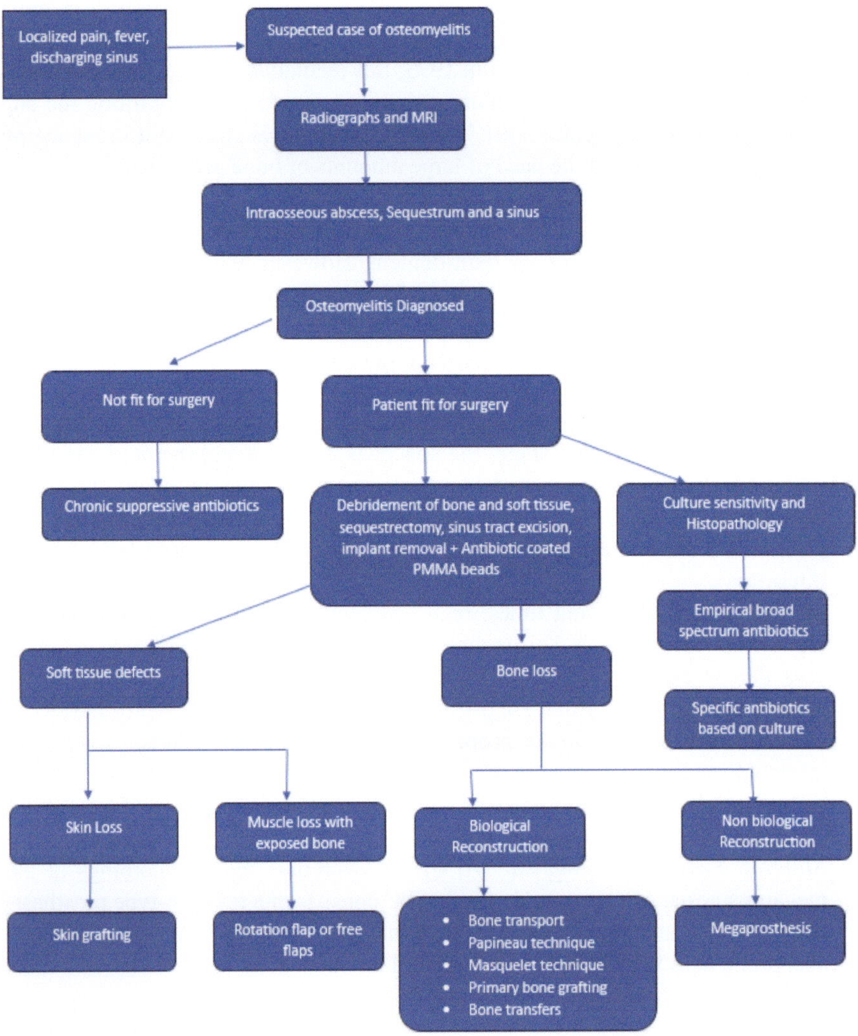

Fig. 10.4 Management algorithm of osteomyelitis

Role of Physical Therapy

Gradual mobilization of the joints by physical therapy is necessary to prevent stiffness and complications like Complex Regional Pain Syndrome. Once the pain subsides, the surrounding joints need to be mobilized. Active and passive exercises are encouraged along with cryotherapy is necessary. Patient should be mobilized at the earliest to prevent venous thrombosis and bed sores. Isometric exercises need to be initiated to maintain the muscle strength. Patients with amputated limbs should be fitted with prosthesis and mobilized immediately.

Psychotherapy

Treatment of osteomyelitis is often prolonged owing to the nature of persistence of infection. Repeated surgeries followed by months of reconstruction often have a psychological bearing on the patient. Recent studies show a whopping 19 patients of osteomyelitis out of 1 lakh have mental during the course of treatment and this may be underestimated [42]. Proper psychotherapy and cognitive behavior therapy should be initiated in all patients of osteomyelitis. Patients undergoing amputation also need special counselling to overcome the grief and post-traumatic stress disorder.

10.11 Complications

The most common complication of osteomyelitis is the persistence of infection, as bony infections can be notoriously difficult to eradicate. Despite the best possible combination of medical and surgical treatment, 20% cases fail to show any response [43]. In rare cases, patients may develop sepsis, a life-threatening condition that requires prompt medical attention. This risk is particularly heightened in immunocompromised individuals, who may not present with typical signs such as fever, necessitating regular evaluation. A serious long-term complication of chronic osteomyelitis is malignant transformation, with 1–23% of cases progressing to squamous cell carcinoma, also known as Marjolin's ulcer (Fig. 10.5) [44]. This transformation typically occurs after the infection has persisted for over 20 years. Treatment for such malignant cases involves wide local excision to remove the cancerous tissue.

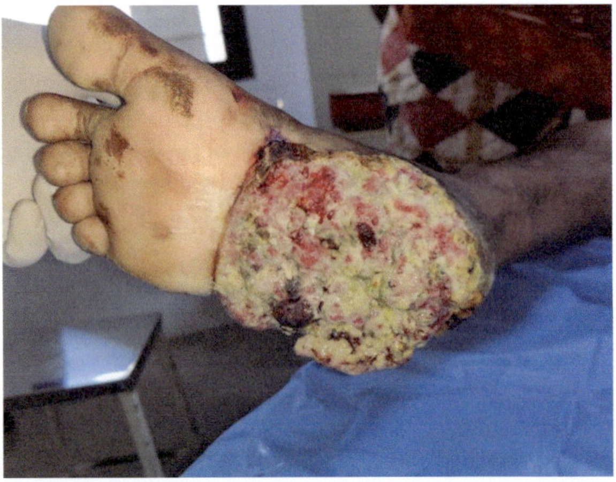

Fig. 10.5 Marjolin's ulcer following osteomyelitis of calcaneum

10.12 Recent Advancements

Though osteomyelitis is a very old disease affecting mankind, numerous advancements have taken place in recent years. The current literature is focusing more on pathogenesis and latest treatment options. Very recently, the role of osteoclasts has been studied in the pathogenesis of osteomyelitis. An upregulation in osteoclastic activity by the Staphylococcal proteins and the neutrophils has been noted at the infection site which manifests as a lytic lesion on radiograph. This fact has been utilized by authors who tried using bisphosphonates in treatment of osteomyelitis [14, 45]. A layer of fibrin is formed over the implants which increases the bacterial adherence to them. A coating of plasminogen activator over the implants impedes the formation of fibrin layer and inhibits the bacterial adhesion [14]. The use of hydrogel coating over the implants prolongs the drug action at the infection site. Recently, the role of lysostaphin is being studied to reduce the severity of osteomyelitis. Lysostaphin is a substance released by *Staphylococcus simulans* and has an inhibitory action on *Staphylococcus aureus* [46]. The use of viruses like bacteriophage to alter plasmids and reduce biofilms is also under consideration [47]. The use of hyperbaric oxygen hastens the wound healing and has shown to reduce the infection rates. Finally, the use of 3D printing in making bone scaffolds will improve the management of dead spaces in osteomyelitis.

10.13 Take-Home Messages

- The incidence of osteomyelitis is rising due to rise in number of diabetics.
- Most of the cases of osteomyelitis are caused by bacteria followed by fungi.
- The management of osteomyelitis requires a multi-disciplinary approach.
- Surgical treatment is the mainstay of the treatment and is combined with the antimicrobial chemotherapy.
- Psychotherapy and physical rehabilitation of the patients is important.

10.14 Clinical Cases

Case Example 1 A 23-year-old male developed chronic osteomyelitis of the mid-diaphyseal part of the humerus 2 years after surgical fixation of an open humerus shaft fracture. The patient presented with an actively discharging sinus, along with pain, tenderness, and abnormal mobility at the fracture site (Fig. 10.6). Surgical intervention was performed using the anterolateral approach, during which the wound was thoroughly debrided. All necrotic skin, muscle, fascia, and bone were excised, and the wound was irrigated with six liters of normal saline mixed with an antiseptic solution (betadine). Following the debridement, vancomycin-mixed absorbable calcium sulfate antibiotic beads were applied (Fig. 10.7a, b), and the fracture was stabilized using an external fixator (Fig. 10.7a, b). After 3 months, the wound healed completely, and the fracture achieved union (Fig. 10.7c). This case clearly demonstrates that a local antibiotic delivery system is highly effective in the treatment of chronic osteomyelitis when combined with thorough debridement.

Case Example 2
An 18-year-old female presented with diaphyseal osteomyelitis of the femur, accompanied by pain, fever, and swelling. Radiographic evaluation revealed mixed lytic and sclerotic features with mild cortical thickening (Fig. 10.8). MRI showed a

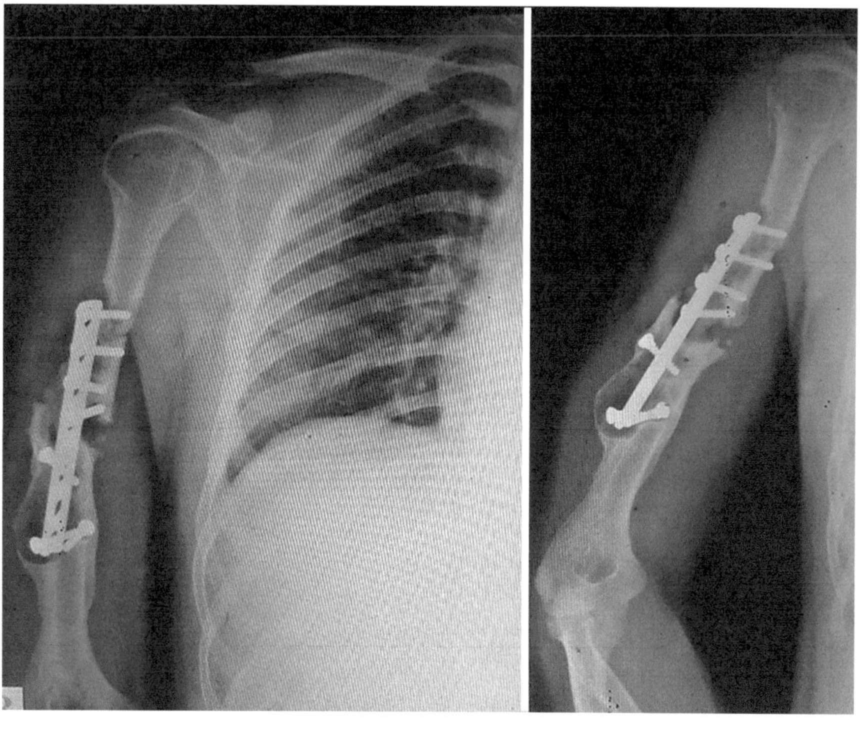

Fig. 10.6 Chronic osteomyelitis of mid-diaphyseal humerus in a 23-year-old male

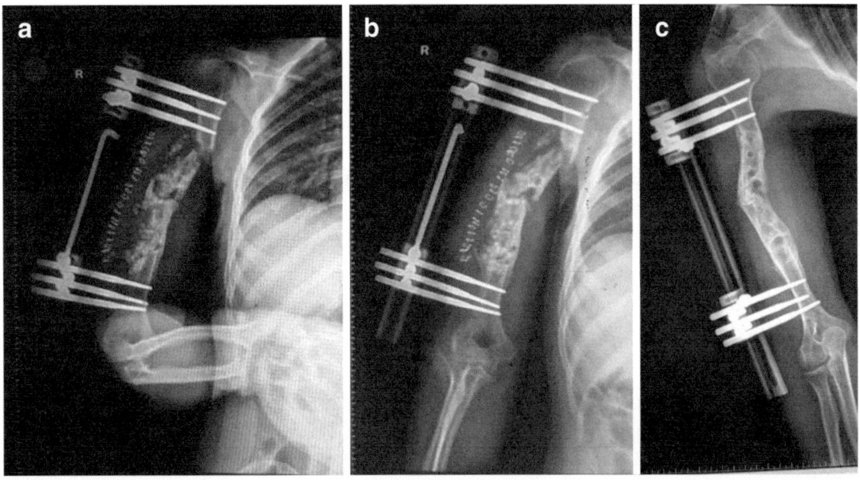

Fig. 10.7 (**a**, **b**) After thorough debridement and the application of antibiotic beads, the fracture was stabilized with an external fixator. (**c**) The infection resolved, and the fracture successfully united within 3 months

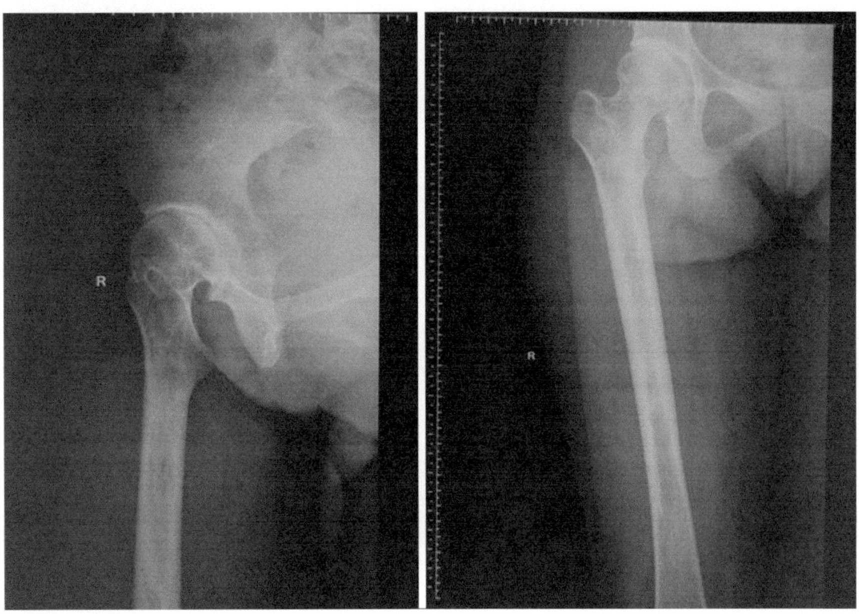

Fig. 10.8 Chronic osteomyelitis of femur

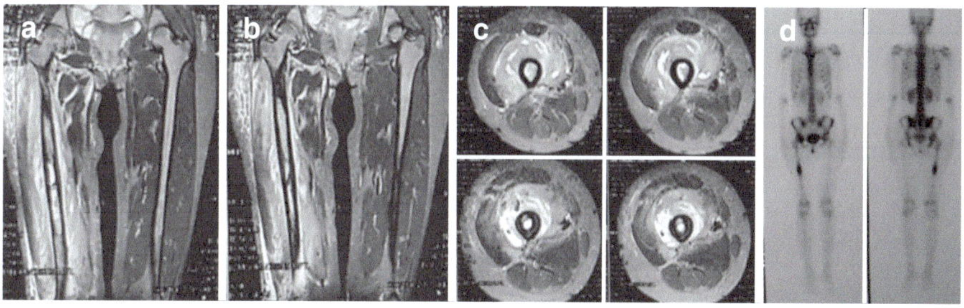

Fig. 10.9 MRI shows T2W hyperintense signal within the medulla and surrounding soft tissues. ^{99m}Tc-diphosphonate scan shows increased tracer uptakes in all three phases

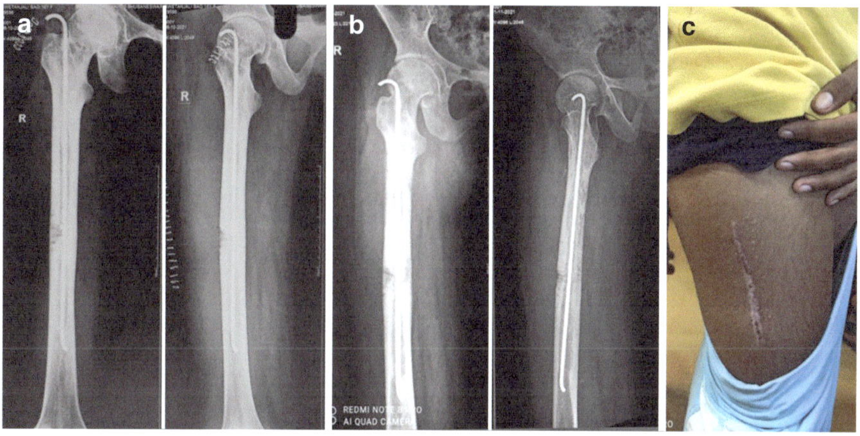

Fig. 10.10 Debridement and antibiotic nail insertion led to complete healing

hyperintense T2-weighted signal in the medulla and surrounding soft tissues (Fig. 10.9). A bone scan demonstrated increased tracer uptake across all phases—venous, arterial, and bone uptake phases. The lesion was accessed through a lateral approach, where a bony window was created to evacuate the pus. Additionally, a hole was made in the piriform fossa, and the medulla was reamed to aspirate the infective contents. Surrounding soft tissues were also debrided. After thorough lavage, an antibiotic cement nail was inserted for stabilization (Fig. 10.10). The infection was successfully controlled, and the lesion healed. Remarkably, even after 4 years of follow-up, there has been no recurrence of the infection.

References

1. Schmitt SK. Osteomyelitis. Infect Dis Clin N Am. 2017;31:325–38. https://doi.org/10.1016/j.idc.2017.01.010.
2. Momodu II, Savaliya V. Osteomyelitis. In: StatPearls. Treasure Island: StatPearls Publishing; 2024.
3. Lew DP, Waldvogel FA. Osteomyelitis. Lancet. 2004;364:369–79. https://doi.org/10.1016/S0140-6736(04)16727-5.
4. Kremers HM, Nwojo ME, Ransom JE, Wood-Wentz CM, Melton LJ, Huddleston PM. Trends in the epidemiology of osteomyelitis. J Bone Joint Surg Am. 2015;97:837–45. https://doi.org/10.2106/JBJS.N.01350.
5. Banerjee B, Shaw T, Mukhopadhyay C, Bhat N S, Singh BMK Epidemiology, resistance characteristics, virulence determinants, and treatment outcomes of Staphylococcus aureus bone and joint infections: a one-year prospective study at a tertiary care hospital in India. Pathog Glob Health. 114:482–6. https://doi.org/10.1080/20477724.2020.1823108.
6. Boroujeni BM, Ghandali MV, Saki N, Ekrami A, Dezfuli AAZ, Yousefi-Avarvand A. Mini review Salmonella: a problem in patients with sickle cell anemia. Gene Rep. 2021;23:101118. https://doi.org/10.1016/j.genrep.2021.101118.
7. Hook EW, Campbell CG, Weens HS, Cooper GR. Salmonella osteomyelitis in patients with sickle-cell anemia. N Engl J Med. 1957;257:403–7. https://doi.org/10.1056/NEJM195708292570904.
8. Saglam F, Saglam S, Gulabi D, Eceviz E, Elmali N, Yilmaz M. Bilateral clavicle osteomyelitis: a case report. Int J Surg Case Rep. 2014;5:932–5. https://doi.org/10.1016/j.ijscr.2014.10.056.
9. Bariteau JT, Waryasz GR, McDonnell M, Fischer SA, Hayda RA, Born CT. Fungal osteomyelitis and septic arthritis. J Am Acad Orthop Surg. 2014;22:390–401. https://doi.org/10.5435/JAAOS-22-06-390.
10. Keret D, Giladi M, Kletter Y, Wientroub S. Cat-scratch disease osteomyelitis from a dog scratch. J Bone Joint Surg Br. 1998;80:766–7.
11. Blinkhorn RJ, Strimbu V, Effron D, Spagnuolo PJ. "Punch" actinomycosis causing osteomyelitis of the hand. Arch Intern Med. 1988;148:2668–70.
12. Panteli M, Giannoudis PV. Chronic osteomyelitis: what the surgeon needs to know. EFORT Open Rev. 2016;1:128–35. https://doi.org/10.1302/2058-5241.1.000017.
13. Mathews JA, Ward J, Chapman TW, Khan UM, Kelly MB. Single-stage orthoplastic reconstruction of Gustilo-Anderson Grade III open tibial fractures greatly reduces infection rates. Injury. 2015;46:2263–6. https://doi.org/10.1016/j.injury.2015.08.027.
14. Hofstee MI, Muthukrishnan G, Atkins GJ, Riool M, Thompson K, Morgenstern M, Stoddart MJ, Richards RG, Zaat SAJ, Moriarty TF. Current concepts of osteomyelitis: from pathologic mechanisms to advanced research methods. Am J Pathol. 2020;190:1151–63. https://doi.org/10.1016/j.ajpath.2020.02.007.
15. Muthukrishnan G, Masters EA, Daiss JL, Schwarz EM. Mechanisms of immune evasion and bone tissue colonization that make Staphylococcus aureus the primary pathogen in osteomyelitis. Curr Osteoporos Rep. 2019;17:395–404. https://doi.org/10.1007/s11914-019-00548-4.
16. de Mesy Bentley KL, Trombetta R, Nishitani K, Bello-Irizarry SN, Ninomiya M, Zhang L, Chung HL, McGrath JL, Daiss JL, Awad HA, Kates SL, Schwarz EM. Evidence of Staphylococcus Aureus deformation, Proliferation, and migration in Canaliculi of live cortical bone in murine models of osteomyelitis. J Bone Miner Res. 2017;32:985–90. https://doi.org/10.1002/jbmr.3055.
17. Ramirez MS, Traglia GM, Lin DL, Tran T, Tolmasky ME. Plasmid-mediated antibiotic resistance and virulence in gram-negatives: the Klebsiella pneumoniae paradigm. Microbiol Spectr. 2014;2:1. https://doi.org/10.1128/microbiolspec.PLAS-0016-2013.
18. Sharma D, Misba L, Khan AU. Antibiotics versus biofilm: an emerging battleground in microbial communities. Antimicrob Resist Infect Control. 2019;8:76. https://doi.org/10.1186/s13756-019-0533-3.

19. Kadirvelu L, Sivaramalingam SS, Jothivel D, Chithiraiselvan DD, Karaiyagowder Govindarajan D, Kandaswamy K. A review on antimicrobial strategies in mitigating biofilm-associated infections on medical implants. Curr Res Microb Sci. 2024;6:100231. https://doi.org/10.1016/j.crmicr.2024.100231.
20. Khatoon Z, McTiernan CD, Suuronen EJ, Mah T-F, Alarcon EI. Bacterial biofilm formation on implantable devices and approaches to its treatment and prevention. Heliyon. 2018;4:e01067. https://doi.org/10.1016/j.heliyon.2018.e01067.
21. Ramasamy SK. Structure and functions of blood vessels and vascular niches in bone. Stem Cells Int. 2017;2017:5046953. https://doi.org/10.1155/2017/5046953.
22. Mandell JC, Khurana B, Smith JT, Czuczman GJ, Ghazikhanian V, Smith SE. Osteomyelitis of the lower extremity: pathophysiology, imaging, and classification, with an emphasis on diabetic foot infection. Emerg Radiol. 2018;25:175–88. https://doi.org/10.1007/s10140-017-1564-9.
23. Cierny G, Mader JT, Penninck JJ. A clinical staging system for adult osteomyelitis. Clin Orthop. 2003;7–24 https://doi.org/10.1097/01.blo.0000088564.81746.62.
24. Pineda C, Espinosa R, Pena A. Radiographic imaging in osteomyelitis: the role of plain radiography, computed tomography, ultrasonography, magnetic resonance imaging, and scintigraphy. Semin Plast Surg. 2009;23:80–9. https://doi.org/10.1055/s-0029-1214160.
25. Hatzenbuehler J, Pulling TJ. Diagnosis and management of osteomyelitis. Am Fam Physician. 2011;84:1027–33.
26. Fritz JM, McDonald JR. Osteomyelitis: approach to diagnosis and treatment. Phys Sportsmed. 2008;36:nihpa116823. https://doi.org/10.3810/psm.2008.12.11.
27. Kapoor A, Page S, LaValley M, Gale DR, Felson DT. Magnetic resonance imaging for diagnosing foot osteomyelitis: a meta-analysis. Arch Intern Med. 2007;167:125–32. https://doi.org/10.1001/archinte.167.2.125.
28. Shemesh S, Kosashvili Y, Groshar D, Bernstine H, Sidon E, Cohen N, Luria T, Velkes S. The value of 18-FDG PET/CT in the diagnosis and management of implant-related infections of the tibia: a case series. Injury. 2015;46:1377–82. https://doi.org/10.1016/j.injury.2015.03.002.
29. Brinkmann J, Zeißler E-C, Scharrenberg JS, Schenk J, Majjouti M, Oberste M, Yagdiran A, Scheyerer MJ, Jung N, Siewe J, Mahabir E. The diagnostic value of cytokines for the discrimination of vertebral osteomyelitis and degenerative diseases of the spine. Cytokine. 2022;150:155782. https://doi.org/10.1016/j.cyto.2021.155782.
30. Saravolatz LD, Labalo V, Fishbain J, Szpunar S, Johnson LB. Lack of effect of antibiotics on biopsy culture results in vertebral osteomyelitis. Diagn Microbiol Infect Dis. 2018;91:273–4. https://doi.org/10.1016/j.diagmicrobio.2018.02.017.
31. Crisologo PA, La Fontaine J, Wukich DK, Kim PJ, Oz OK, Lavery LA. The effect of withholding antibiotics prior to bone biopsy in patients with suspected osteomyelitis: a meta-analysis of the literature. Wounds Compend Clin Res Pract. 2019;31:205–12.
32. Sybenga AB, Jupiter DC, Speights VO, Rao A. Diagnosing osteomyelitis: a histology guide for pathologists. J Foot Ankle Surg. 2020;59:75–85. https://doi.org/10.1053/j.jfas.2019.06.007.
33. Kurpad AV. The requirements of protein & amino acid during acute & chronic infections. Indian J Med Res. 2006;124:129–48.
34. Blackburn GL. Nutritional assessment and support during infection. Am J Clin Nutr. 1977;30:1493–7. https://doi.org/10.1093/ajcn/30.9.1493.
35. Navigating the spectrum and intricacies of osteomyelitis: organisms, hosts, antibiotics, and surgery. https://www.aaos.org/aaosnow/2024/jun/clinical/clinical10/. Accessed 15 Aug 2024.
36. Wagner RK, Guarch-Pérez C, van Dam AP, Zaat SA, Kloen P. Antimicrobial mechanisms and preparation of antibiotic-impregnated cement-coated locking plates in the treatment of infected non-unions. Strateg Trauma Limb Reconstr. 2023;18:73–81. https://doi.org/10.5005/jp-journals-10080-1586.
37. Roeder B, Van Gils CC, Maling S. Antibiotic beads in the treatment of diabetic pedal osteomyelitis. J Foot Ankle Surg. 2000;39:124–30. https://doi.org/10.1016/s1067-2516(00)80037-x.
38. Bor N, Dujovny E, Rinat B, Rozen N, Rubin G. Treatment of chronic osteomyelitis with antibiotic-impregnated polymethyl methacrylate (PMMA)—the Cierny approach: is the

second stage necessary? BMC Musculoskelet Disord. 2022;23:38. https://doi.org/10.1186/s12891-021-04979-y.
39. Tanwar YS, Ferreira N. The role of bioactive glass in the management of chronic osteomyelitis: a systematic review of literature and current evidence. Infect Dis Lond Engl. 2020;52:219–26. https://doi.org/10.1080/23744235.2019.1695059.
40. Papineau LJ. Excision-graft with deliberately delayed closing in chronic osteomyelitis. Nouv Press Med. 1973;2:2753–5.
41. Masquelet AC. Muscle reconstruction in reconstructive surgery: soft tissue repair and long bone reconstruction. Langenbeck's Arch Surg. 2003;388:344–6. https://doi.org/10.1007/s00423-003-0379-1.
42. Walter N, Rupp M, Baertl S, Hinterberger T, Alt V. Prevalence of psychological comorbidities in bone infection. J Psychosom Res. 2022;157:110806. https://doi.org/10.1016/j.jpsychores.2022.110806.
43. Conterno LO, Turchi MD. Antibiotics for treating chronic osteomyelitis in adults. Cochrane Database Syst Rev. 2013:CD004439. https://doi.org/10.1002/14651858.CD004439.pub3.
44. Pandey M, Kumar P, Khanna AK. Marjolin's ulcer associated with chronic osteomyelitis. J Wound Care. 2009;18:504–6. https://doi.org/10.12968/jowc.2009.18.12.45607.
45. Heimes D, Kämmerer PW. Bisphosphonate-treatment of secondary chronic osteomyelitis of the jaw—a case report. J Surg Case Rep. 2023;2023:rjad270. https://doi.org/10.1093/jscr/rjad270.
46. Kumar JK. Lysostaphin: an antistaphylococcal agent. Appl Microbiol Biotechnol. 2008;80:555–61. https://doi.org/10.1007/s00253-008-1579-y.
47. Geredew Kifelew L, Mitchell JG, Speck P. Mini-review: efficacy of lytic bacteriophages on multispecies biofilms. Biofouling. 2019;35:472–81. https://doi.org/10.1080/08927014.2019.1613525.

Septic Arthritis of the Native Joint

11

Avinash Kumar and Swayam Prakash Das

Abstract

Septic arthritis of native joint may be monoarticular, oligoarticular, or polyarticular. Pathogenesis of the same encompasses various mechanisms apart from decreased immunological response. A thorough differential diagnosis be made and looked for in case of septic arthritis of native joint. For a good yield of causative microorganism, correct and efficient investigative method for synovial fluid analysis should be used to enhance the yield of positive results. This will help in accepting best antibiotic protocol for the positive result obtained on investigation else an empirical antibiotic policy may be required. Surgical treatment ranges from arthroscopic to open surgeries and the trend to treat septic arthritis is shifting toward the minimal invasive technique.

Keywords

Septic arthritis · Native joint · Pathogenesis · Synovial fluid analysis · Antibiotic Arthroscopic

A. Kumar (✉)
Orthopedics, All India Institute of Medical Sciences, Patna, India
e-mail: dravinashk@aiimspatna.org

S. P. Das
Orthopedics, All India Institute of Medical Sciences, New Delhi, India

P. Kumar et al. (eds.), *Textbook of Orthopedic Infections*,
https://doi.org/10.1007/978-981-95-5029-6_11

Learning Objectives

- Irrespective of presence of fever, acute monoarthritis should raise the suspicion of septic arthritis. Oligo- or polyarticular involvement is not rare for septic arthritis.
- Synovial fluid analysis in blood culture bottles give better yield. At least two pairs of blood cultures should be performed before initiating antibiotic therapy, even in the absence of a fever.
- Ultrasound on the joint is useful to confirm the presence of intra-articular effusion and pus pocket in case of clinical uncertainty and can be useful to assist in diagnostic and therapeutic aspiration.
- The total duration of antibiotic therapy (IV then oral) should be 4–6 weeks for pyogenic bacterial septic arthritis. A total duration of 7 days is sufficient in cases of Neisseria gonorrhoeae arthritis.
- Percutaneous needle aspiration and arthroscopic lavage (for larger joints) are preferred over arthrotomy surgical drainage.

11.1 Introduction

Septic arthritis (SA) is defined as infection and inflammation of a joint. The incidence ranges from 4 to 12/100,000 person-years (PY). SA of native (nonperiprosthetic) joint is a rare condition. The incidence varies with age and ethnicity. It is positively associated with poor socio-economic conditions [1].

According to Newman's definition [2] in 1976, if a patient meets any one of the four criteria for having an inflammatory joint, they have SA.

1. Positive synovial fluid cultures
2. Positive blood cultures with negative synovial fluid cultures
3. Negative cultures due to prior use of antibiotics, but with purulent drainage from the joint
4. Definite radiological or postmortem confirming the diagnosis of septic arthritis

Forty years later, these criteria hold true. A significant drawback is that SA can exist even in cases that do not meet Newman's criteria.

11.2 Sites Affected

- The knee is the primary site for septic arthritis, accounting for 45% of cases in adults. This prevalence is likely due to the evolution of humans to bipedal walking, which forces the knee joint to a significant mechanical stress, making it very susceptible to injury.
- Other large joints frequently affected include the hip (15%), ankle (9%), elbow (8%), wrist (6%), and shoulder (5%).

- Polyarticular involvement is seen in about 10–20% of patients. Polyarticular septic arthritis is more common with gonococcal, pneumococcal, group B streptococcal, and gram-negative bacteria. It typically affects around four joints asymmetrically, with at least one knee is involved in almost 72% of the patients. Major risk factors for polyarticular SA include steroid therapy, rheumatoid arthritis, systemic lupus erythematosus, and diabetes mellitus [3].

11.3 Etiology

- Gram-positive organisms are most common causes for septic arthritis. Enteric gram-negative rods accounts for 43% of community-acquired infections in comparison to only 10% of septic arthritis. The discrepancy is probably due to the greater capacity of gram-positive bacteria to adhere to the extracellular matrix proteins and the connective tissue. Staphylococcus aureus, the leading cause of septic arthritis, produces different adhesins that adhere to extracellular matrix proteins [4].
- Intravenous drug use or compromised integrity of the gastrointestinal or urinary tracts may cause SA due to gram-negative bacteria.
- Septic arthritis may be due to direct penetrating trauma, such as bites (human/animal) or injection drug use, most commonly seen for the small joints of the hands and feet.

11.4 Pathogenesis

- Minor breaches in the mucous membranes or skin can facilitate the entry of staphylococci and streptococci into the bloodstream and to the vascular synovium. The synovium lacks a protective basement membrane, moreover it is highly vascular structure thereby susceptible to bacterial inoculation during bacteremia. Bacteria colonize the synovial fluid and multiply quickly, causing an immediate inflammatory reaction.
- Interleukin 1b (IL-1b) and IL-6 produced help in opsonization and complement system activation.
- When the host possesses immunocompetence, macrophages, synoviocytes, and polymorphonuclear cells eradicate infections by inducing a protective inflammatory response.
- Bacterial enzymes and toxins damage the cartilage along with the lysosomal proteases secreted by host neutrophils which autodigest the cartilage. Purulent exudates inside the joint increases the cavity pressure tamponading the synovial blood flow which leads to decreased oxygen supply and nutrition to the cartilage [5].

11.5 Risk Factors

- Around 47% of individuals with bacterial arthritis have a previous history of joint issues. Septic arthritis should be thought of in patients with other rheumatological conditions, including rheumatoid arthritis (RA), systemic lupus erythematosus, osteoarthritis, gout, pseudogout, recent trauma, and previous joint surgery. Among these, RA is the most prevalent and is associated with worse prognosis. The risk of SA in RA patients is doubled by the use of tumor necrosis factor blockers and are prone to intracellular bacteria like Salmonella and Listeria.
- In gout, the patients who develop SA, presence of synovial micro tophi hinders the diagnosis of SA. Therefore, all patients with suspected gouty joints should undergo Gram stain and culture to rule out presence of concurrent septic arthritis.
- Dermatological diseases such as psoriasis, eczema, and skin ulcers may predispose to SA too.
- Intravenous drug use, and immunocompromised conditions like diabetes mellitus, chronic renal failure, liver cirrhosis, and the use of immunosuppressive drugs are also important risk factors for SA.
- Despite all risk factors, about 22% of the patients don't have any risk factors or underlying joint diseases to cause SA.
- During long hospitalization, patients develop SA more commonly with antibiotic-resistant organisms, due to presence of preexisting comorbidities. The in-patients' mortality rate is around 2.6% due to nosocomial and other hospitalization-related SA [4].

11.6 Clinical Features

In setting of acute (<2 weeks) monoarthritis, characterized by painful swelling and stiff joints, SA needs to be meticulously evaluated. In situations of acute arthritis, several differential diagnoses are conceivable as in Table 11.1. Only 58% of the patients experience high-grade fever while almost 90% of them complain of low-grade fever. Therefore, it is prudent to not rule out SA, if the patient is not having high-grade fever. Polyarticular affection (in 10–17% of the patients) indicates poor prognosis. Such patients frequently succumb to sepsis or septic shock [6].

Third international guidelines updated the definition of sepsis and septic shock in 2016 [7]. The Sequential Organ Failure Assessment (SOFA) is a scoring system for sepsis in adult patients which evaluates the multi-organ involvement/function. Higher the score, poorer the prognosis of sepsis. Assessing the instant severity score of the SOFA is necessary if at least two of the three Quick SOFA indicators are present. The three indicators are (1) respiratory rate >22/min; (2) confusion or reduced alertness; (3) systolic blood pressure <100 mmHg (Table 11.2).

Table 11.1 Differential diagnosis for situations of acute septic arthritis

1. Soft tissue inflammation and infections	Bursitis (septic or microcrystalline) Acute resorption of apatite calcification Infectious dermohypodermitis (erysipelas)
2. Microcrystalline and metabolic arthropathies	Acute arthritis with monosodium urate deposits (gout) Calcium pyrophosphate dihydrate (CPPD) crystal deposition disease(chondrocalcinosis) Acute resorption of apatite calcification
3. Inflammatory rheumatic disorders	Peripheral spondylarthritis including psoriatic arthritis and Rheumatoid arthritis Auto-inflammatory diseases (AOSD, FMF, CAPS, etc.) Vasculitis (Henoch Schoenlein Purpura, Behcet's disease)
4. Infectious or post-infectious arthropathies	Post-venereal or post-dysenteric reactive arthritis Post-streptococcal arthritis or rheumatic fever Fungal or parasitic arthritis Viral arthritis (hepatitis A, B, C, rubella, parvovirus B19, HIV, arbovirus)
5. Other arthropathies	Episodic attacks of synovitis (intermittent hydrarthrosis) Hemarthrosis

Table 11.2 SOFA (Sequential Organ Failure Assessment) immediate severity score

Scores	0	1	2	3	4
PaO_2/FiO_2, mmHg (kPa)[a]	≥400/ −53.3 SaO2 ≥ 95%	<400/53.3 SaO_2 90–94%	<300/40 SaO2 < 90%	<200/ 26.7 with ventilators assistance	<100/13.3 with ventilators assistance
Platelets (G/L)	≥150	<150	<100	<50	<20
Bilirubin (mol/L)	<20	21–32	33–101	102–204	>204
Cardiovascular	MAP ≥ 70 mm Hg	MAP ≥ 70 mm Hg	Dopamine <5 or Dobutamine (any dose)	Dopamine 5.1–15 or adrenaline ≤0.1 or Noradrenaline ≤0.1	Domaine >15 or Adrenaline >0.1 or Noradrenaline >0.1
Glasgow score	15	13–14	10–12	6–9	<6
Creatinine (mol/L)	<110	110–170	171–299	300–440	>440
Urine output (mL/24 h)	≥500	≥500	≥500	<500	<200

Should be calculated if quick-SOFA ≥ 2 (confusion or respiratory rate >22/min, or SBP < 100 mmHg)

11.7 Investigations

11.7.1 Synovial Fluid Analysis

- Prior antibiotic therapy decreases the sensitivity of identifying the microorganism from the synovial fluid (SF) [8]. Purulent SF may be seen even in metabolic or reactive arthritis, therefore, it is not specific for SA [9].
- Suspected SA may have negative cultures of synovial fluid on solid media in almost 20% of the patients. It is suggested that inoculating SF in a blood culture vial will enhance the microbiological detection by 20%, specially when prior antibiotic treatment is involved [10].
- Blood culture bottles are recommended because they can dilute the antibiotics and other bacterial inhibitors (like complement). Secondly, lytic agents in such culture media, like saponin, may release intracellular bacteria rendering them available for detection. Thirdly, blood culture media support the growth of fastidious bacteria like Kingella and streptococci. Lastly, a larger amount of synovial fluid can be inoculated into blood cultures.
- Currently, no biochemical markers in synovial fluid (such as lactate or glucose) are considered reliable and effective for systematic diagnosis of septic arthritis.
- Broad range 16S rDNA PCR testing of synovial fluid has shown poor yield in diagnosing SA. It had low sensitivity than the synovial fluid or blood cultures or direct examination as per Coiffier et al. [11]. Hence, a negative 16S rDNA PCR testing of synovial fluid does not rule out the diagnosis of SA.

11.7.2 Blood Culture and Sensitivity

- Positive blood cultures seen in 9–36% of the patients with septic arthritis, may many a times be the only way to recognize the bacteria [12]. Using at least two different pairs of aerobic and anaerobic containers is important. Samples should preferably, whenever feasible, should be taken prior to start of any antibiotics.
- There's no established justification for prioritizing blood cultures during fever spikes [13]. To minimize false negatives, blood culture bottles should contain an adequate volume (≥8 mL/bottle).

11.7.3 Radiological Investigations

- Radiographs are not good tool in diagnosing septic arthritis as the signs do not appear on X-rays till 10 days or so after the onset of illness [6].
- Magnetic Resonance Imaging (MRI) can discreetly show soft tissue collections/abscesses and bony erosions in SA [14]. Howsoever, due to poor availability and

accessibility, MRI is not used for diagnosis of SA in emergency situations. For the less voluminous joints and/or which are not so easily accessible to normal imaging, like sacroiliac joints, sternoclavicular joints, pubic symphysis; and many a times, hip and shoulder joints, MRI is the gold standard imaging tool for SA diagnosis.

- There is no much reported literature regarding use of 18FDG PET/CT for diagnosing SA in native joints. Again, it is not so affordable and accessible, that's why it is hardly used for SA diagnosis [15].
- Ultrasound examination shows joint effusion and/or synovitis [16]. However, it alone cannot differentiate SA from other arthritis. It can indirectly diagnose metabolic form of arthritis by identifying features such as crystals (tophi), double contour sign/snowstorm appearance [17]. It also helps in diagnostic or therapeutic joint aspiration or in localizing pocket of pus for aspiration.

11.8 Treatment

An algorithm outlining clinical situations requiring antibiotic therapy is provided (see Fig. 11.1).

Synovial fluid analyses have low specificity to diagnose septic arthritis, therefore the threshold to initiate antibiotics should be low. Broad spectrum antibiotics is preferred till the microorganism is identified from the cultures to prevent the catastrophe of SA. Such antibiotics must include one against MRSA like Vancomycin, as MRSA is one of the commonest cases of SA. Cefazolin may be used in regions with low prevalence of MRSA. Cefepime or antipseudomonal beta-lactam (against gram-negative bacilli) must be included for critically ill patients, elderly patients or the immunocompromised, or intravenous drug users. Dual antibiotic is not recommended initially except for Pseudomonas infections. Aminoglycosides may be added in cases of septic shock (for Enterococcus sp. or Pseudomonas aeruginosa), else they are not warranted [18].

Table 11.3 tabulates the first-line intravenous antibiotics and the oral antibiotics according to the main bacteria identified.

11.8.1 Antimicrobial Therapy

In cases of septic arthritis with quick SOFA ≥ 2, it's prudent not to wait for microorganisms to start antibiotic therapy and, therefore, first-generation injectable cephalosporin (cefazolin) should be started for patients below 70 years of age, and third-generation injectable cephalosporin (ceftriaxone or cefotaxime) should be started for patients above 70 years of age. Suspecting the probability of Gram-negative rods in geriatric patients with SA [19]. If multiple, repeated tests also don't yield the microorganisms, it is better to continue with IV β-lactams throughout the treatment and should not switch to the oral drugs.

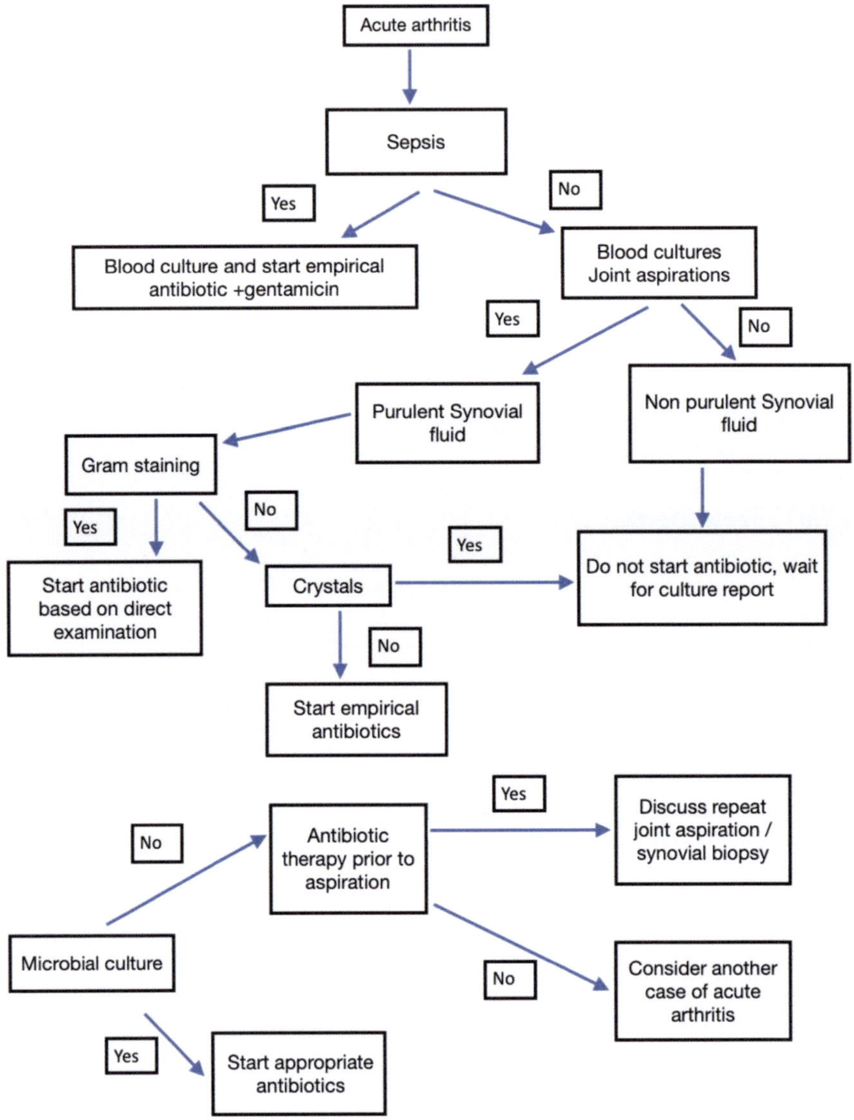

Fig. 11.1 Algorithm to manage septic arthritis (medical management)

Table 11.3 Antibiotic of choice for different microorganisms

Bacterial species	First line IV antibiotic	Switch to oral antibiotic
Methicillin sensitive Staph. Aureus	Cefazolin or Cloxacillin	Rifampicin[a] + Fluoroquinolone (FQ)[b] or FQ + Clindamycin[c]
Methicillin resistant Staph. Aureus	Vancomycin or Teicoplanin	Rifampicin + Fluoroquinolone (FQ) or FQ + Clindamycin
Streptococci	Amoxicillin	Amoxicillin
Enterococci	Amoxicillin + Gentamicin[d] or Amoxicillin + Ceftriaxone	Amoxicillin
Group 1 & 2 Enterobacteriaceae	Cefotaxime or Ceftriaxone	FQ (if sensitive to nalidixic acid)
Group 3 Enterobacteriaceae[e]	Cefepime	According to sensitivity
Pseudomonas aeruginosa	Ceftazidime + ciprofloxacin[f]	According to sensitivity
Anaerobes	Amoxicillin if sensitive or Metronidazole	Clindamycin OR Amoxicillin
Neisseria gonorrhea	Cefotaxime or Ceftriaxone	FQ

[a]Rifampicin should not be used as a monotherapy

[b]FQ: the following fluoroquinolones can be used in the treatment of septic arthritis: ofloxacin, levofloxacin, ciprofloxacin, and moxifloxacin. All of these FQs are effective against staphylococci, Enterobacteriaceae, and gonococci. Levofloxacin and moxifloxacin are effective against streptococci. Ciprofloxacin and levofloxacin are effective against Pseudomonas aeruginosa. Moxifloxacin should be used with caution due to its cardiac toxicity (heart rhythm disorders) and potential liver toxicity

[c]Clindamycin monotherapy can be proposed as an alternative (second-line treatment), according to US recommendations, in staph infections sensitive to erythromycin and clindamycin, in particular, if resistant to FQ and/or rifampicin

[d]Gentamicin is offered for a period of 3–5 days in the absence of concomitant endocarditis

[e]Group 3 Enterobacteriaceae (Enterobacter sp., Citrobacter freundii, Serratia sp., Morganella sp., Providencia sp.) should not be treated using a 3GC antibody (cephalosporinase is induced, making the antibiotic inactive), but with a fourth-generation cephalosporin such as cefepime

[f]A dual therapy comprised of Ceftazidime + amikacin can be used for the first 48 h (decrease in bacterial inoculum) pending the final bacterial sensitivity test (sensitivity to ciprofloxacin)

11.8.2 Duration of Antibiotic Course

The generally accepted duration for antibiotic therapy in treating a native joint infection ranges from 4 to 6 weeks.

- A 4-week treatment regimen is recommended for streptococcal septic arthritis (SA), while a 6-week therapy is recommended for Staphylococcus infections [11]. Bernard et al. have shown that 6 weeks of antibiotics is not inferior to 12 weeks of therapy for treating pyogenic spondylodiscitis [20]. Still, there is lack of literature regarding adequate duration of antibiotic course.
- Relapse or recurrence rate is higher with 2 weeks of antibiotic therapy in comparison to 3–6 weeks of antibiotics for septic arthritis involving large joints [1].

- A seven-day antibiotic therapy is enough for Neisseria gonorrhoeae or other Neisseria species infections [21]. A recent randomized controlled study has shown that even early switch to oral antibiotics as early as after 7 days may be effective in few conditions like infective endocarditis, S. Aureus, P. aeruginosa, MRSA or in case without sepsis but SOFA ≥ 2 [22].

11.8.3 Surgical Management

There are two phases seen in septic arthritis:

1. Initial congestive phase: where the collector can be aspirated from the joint minimally hyper vascularized synovitis.
2. Synovial phase: where synovial tissue is grossly hypertrophied and hypervascularized without any aspiratable fluid [23].

11.8.4 Surgical Drainage

- During the congestive phase, aspiration reduces the bacterial load enhancing the efficacy of the antibiotics and thereby minimizing the cartilage damage. Incomplete or partial drainage is an independent risk factor for the failure of the treatment [24]. Mortality rates don't increase if joint drainage is done at least 48 h after starting treatment compared to early drainage [25].
- Early surgical lavage or synovectomy has not shown functional benefits [26], and no longitudinal studies have proven early surgery to be superior to needle aspiration drainage for treating SA in a native joint [27].
- Percutaneous joint drainage has shown better functional recovery and less mortality in comparison to surgical drainage (open surgery or arthroscopy) [24]. Repeated percutaneous synovial fluid (SF) drainage till the joint is dry is now preferred guideline rather than arthroscopic drainage if percutaneous drainage is not complete.
- Arthroscopic lavage is recommended in failed repeat percutaneous aspiration, specially if cultures remain positive despite 5–7 days of antibiotic course or still purulent fluid is aspirable after antibiotic course.

11.8.5 Synovectomy

- Synovectomy is never a first-line treatment for SA in a native joint, more so during the congestive phase, because apart from joint stiffness, it may decrease the chances of functional recovery and prognosis [28].
- Synovectomy should be thought of in cases of persistent hypertrophy of synovial tissues despite appropriate and adequate antibiotic course, where infection is not controlled, after ruling out other differential diagnoses.

- Arthroscopic synovectomy has superior mid-term functional recovery and prognosis than open synovectomy [29].

Odio et al. have shown dexamethasone therapy to be effective in preventing morbidity and disability in children with septic arthritis. But same does not hold true for adults with SA in the literature [30].

11.8.6 Physiotherapy

- The primary goal of physical therapy is to prevent joint contractures and recover or maintain joint range of motion, thereby preventing muscle disuse atrophy too.
- The literature does not recommend complete immobilization. Animal studies have shown more chondrolysis and joint stiffness in animal models with SA in comparison to passive continuous movement. Early non-weight bearing may be allowed in acutes phase of infection till there is pain. Rehabilitation and continuous passive range of motion will prevent contracture and disuse muscular atrophy [31].
- From initial non-weight-bearing mobilization to weight-bearing mobilization be encouraged over 4–6 weeks [32].

11.8.7 Follow-up

- The parameters to follow up should include fever, pain, range of movement across joints, swelling around joint, muscle atrophy, and functional outcomes. This follow up should continue at least for 6 months.
- Structural joint erosion or damage may be seen in almost 50% of such patients even after complete infection control, therefore only poor functional result does not mean there is recurrence or relapse of septic arthritis or infection or the treatment has failed.

References

1. McBride S, Mowbray J, Caughey W, Wong E, Luey C, Siddiqui A, et al. Epidemiology, management, and outcomes of large and small native joint septic arthritis in adults. Clin Infect Dis. 2020;70(2):271–9.
2. Newman JH. Review of septic arthritis throughout the antibiotic era. Ann Rheum Dis. 1976;35(3):198–205.
3. Dubost JJ, Fis I, Denis P, et al. Polyarticular septic arthritis. Medicine (Baltimore). 1993;72:296–310.
4. Ross JJ. Septic arthritis of native joints. Infect Dis Clin N Am. 2017;31(2):203–18.
5. Roerdink RL, Huijbregts HJTAM, van Lieshout AWT, Dietvorst M, van der Zwaard BC. The difference between native septic arthritis and prosthetic joint infections: a review of literature. J Orthop Surg (Hong Kong). 2019;27(2):2309499019860468.

6. Couderc M, Pereira B, Mathieu S, Schmidt J, Lesens O, Bonnet R, et al. Predictive value of the usual clinical signs and laboratory tests in the diagnosis of septic arthritis. CJEM. 2015;17(4):403–10.
7. Singer M, Deutschman CS, Seymour CW, Shankar-Hari M, Annane D, Bauer M, Bellomo R, Bernard GR, Chiche JD, Coopersmith CM, Hotchkiss RS, Levy MM, Marshall JC, Martin GS, Opal SM, Rubenfeld GD, van der Poll T, Vincent JL, Angus DC. The third international consensus definitions for sepsis and septic shock (Sepsis-3). JAMA. 2016;315(8):801–10.
8. Hindle P, Davidson E, Biant L. Septic arthritis of the knee: the use and effect of antibiotics prior to diagnostic aspiration. Ann R Coll Surg Engl. 2012;94(5):351–5.
9. Ferrand J, El Samad Y, Brunschweiler B, Grados F, Dehamchia-Rehailia N, Séjourne A, et al. Morbimortality in adult patients with septic arthritis: a three-year hospital-based study. BMC Infect Dis. 2016;16:239.
10. Hughes JG, Vetter EA, Patel R, Schleck CD, Harmsen S, Turgeant LT, et al. Culture with BACTEC Peds Plus/F bottle compared with conventional methods for detection of bacteria in synovial fluid. J Clin Microbiol. 2001;39(12):4468–71.
11. Coiffier G, David C, Gauthier P, Le Bars H, Guggenbuhl P, Jolivet-Gougeon A, et al. Broad-range 16 s rDNA PCR in synovial fluid does not improve the diagnostic performance of septic arthritis in native joints in adults: cross-sectional single-center study in 95 patients. Clin Rheumatol. 2019;38(7):1985–92.
12. Clerc O, Prod'hom G, Greub G, Zanetti G, Senn L. Adult native septic arthritis: a review of 10 years of experience and lessons for empirical antibiotic therapy. J Antimicrob Chemother. 2011;66(5):1168–73.
13. Habib G, Lancellotti P, Antunes MJ, Bongiorni MG, Casalta JP, Del Zotti F, et al. 2015 ESC guidelines for the management of infective endocarditis: the Task Force for the Management of Infective Endocarditis of the European Society of Cardiology (ESC)Endorsed by: European Association for Cardio-Thoracic Surgery (EACTS), the European Association of Nuclear Medicine (EANM). Eur Heart J. 2015;36(44):3075–128.
14. MRI findings of septic arthritis and associated osteomyelitis in adults [Internet]. [cited 2024 Jun 3]. Available from: https://www.ajronline.org/doi/epdf/10.2214/ajr.182.1.1820119.
15. Akaike G, Akaike T, Fadl SA, Lachance K, Nghiem P, Behnia F. Imaging of Merkel cell carcinoma: what imaging experts should know. Radiographics. 2019;39(7):2069–84.
16. Gaigneux E, Cormier G, Varin S, Mérot O, Maugars Y, Le Goff B. Ultrasound abnormalities in septic arthritis are associated with functional outcomes. Joint Bone Spine. 2017;84(5):599–604.
17. Clin Exp Rheumatol [Internet]. [cited 2024 Jun 3]. Ultrasound in crystal-related arthritis. Available from: https://www.clinexprheumatol.org/abstract.asp?a=7642.
18. Coiffier G, Albert JD. Do aminoglycosides still have a role in acute osteoarticular infections in adults in 2012? Joint Bone Spine. 2012;79(3):212–5.
19. Coiffier G, Albert JD. Is ceftriaxone 2g once daily a valid treatment option for osteoarticular infections due to Staphylococcus spp., Streptococcus spp., and Gram-negative rods? Joint Bone Spine. 2014;81(3):200–2.
20. Bernard L, Dinh A, Ghout I, Simo D, Zeller V, Issartel B, et al. Antibiotic treatment for 6 weeks versus 12 weeks in patients with pyogenic vertebral osteomyelitis: an open-label, non-inferiority, randomised, controlled trial. Lancet. 2015;385(9971):875–82.
21. Bardin T. Gonococcal arthritis. Best Pract Res Clin Rheumatol. 2003;17(2):201–8.
22. Lieber SB, Fowler ML, Zhu C, Moore A, Shmerling RH, Paz Z. Clinical characteristics and outcomes in polyarticular septic arthritis. Joint Bone Spine. 2018;85(4):469–73.
23. Riegels-nielsen P, Frimodt-Möller N, Jensen JS. Rabbit model of septic arthritis. Acta Orthop Scand. 1987;58(1):14–9.
24. Maneiro JR, Souto A, Cervantes EC, Mera A, Carmona L, Gomez-Reino JJ. Predictors of treatment failure and mortality in native septic arthritis. Clin Rheumatol. 2015;34(11):1961–7.
25. Kodumuri P, Geutjens G, Kerr HL. Time delay between diagnosis and arthroscopic lavage in septic arthritis. Does it matter? Int Orthop. 2012;36(8):1727–31.
26. Lauper N, Davat M, Gjika E, Müller C, Belaieff W, Pittet D, et al. Native septic arthritis is not an immediate surgical emergency. J Infect. 2018;77(1):47–53.

27. Ravindran V, Logan I, Bourke BE. Medical vs surgical treatment for the native joint in septic arthritis: a 6-year, single UK academic centre experience. Rheumatology. 2009;48(10):1320–2.
28. Coakley G, Mathews C, Field M, Jones A, Kingsley G, Walker D, et al. BSR & BHPR, BOA, RCGP and BSAC guidelines for management of the hot swollen joint in adults. Rheumatology. 2006;45(8):1039–41.
29. Böhler C, Pock A, Waldstein W, Staats K, Puchner SE, Holinka J, et al. Surgical treatment of shoulder infections: a comparison between arthroscopy and arthrotomy. J Shoulder Elb Surg. 2017;26(11):1915–21.
30. Odio CM, Ramirez T, Arias G, et al. Double blind, randomized, placebo-controlled study of dexamethasone therapy for hematogenous septic arthritis in children. Pediatr Infect Dis J. 2003;22:883–9.
31. Salter RB. The biologic concept of continuous passive motion of synovial joints. The first 18 years of basic research and its clinical application. Clin Orthop Relat Res. 1989;242:12–25. PMID: 2650945.
32. Peres LR, Marchitto RO, Pereira GS, Yoshino FS, De Castro FM, Matsumoto MH. Arthrotomy versus arthroscopy in the treatment of septic arthritis of the knee in adults: a randomized clinical trial. Knee Surg Sports Traumatol Arthrosc. 2016;24(10):3155–62.

Periprosthetic Joint Infection: Lower Limb

12

Rajesh Kumar Rajnish, Sandeep Kumar Yadav, and Nitesh Gahlot

Abstract

Periprosthetic joint infection (PJI) is a major complication of arthroplasty and poses challenges to surgeons. This is associated with several grave complications, functional loss, and even mortality. Choosing an efficient management protocol for modern diagnostic techniques and treatment for eradicating pathogens is viable for many individuals. In this chapter, we will discuss the current knowledge of the diagnosis, prevention, and treatment of the PJI of the lower limb.

Keywords

Periprosthetic joint infection · PJI · Lower limb · Total knee arthroplasty · Total hip arthroplasty

12.1 Introduction

Infection involving the prosthetic implant following joint arthroplasty is known as PJI [1]. The estimated incidence of PJI following primary arthroplasty is about 1%. The rate is approximately five times higher following secondary aseptic arthroplasty and around ten times higher after revision arthroplasty performed for PJI [1, 2]. PJI is the leading cause of failure of arthroplasty and causes significant morbidity and mortality in patients who undergo arthroplasty [2]. Recent understanding regarding the PJI has helped surgeons standardize the approaches to handle this complex disease process. The effective and practical preventive methods available for PJI are on the rise, and the introduction of several identifying criteria for PJI has drastically improved early diagnosis with improved accuracy [3, 4]. Additionally, the prior risk

R. K. Rajnish (✉) · S. K. Yadav · N. Gahlot
Department of Orthopedics, All India Institute of Medical Sciences, Jodhpur, India

P. Kumar et al. (eds.), *Textbook of Orthopedic Infections*,
https://doi.org/10.1007/978-981-95-5029-6_12

calculation and implementation of evidence-based medicine treatment protocol have led to individualized treatment and selection of more appropriate and effective treatment options for patients with PJI [5]. This chapter will bring forth the current evidence on the clinical profile, diagnosis, and management of PJI.

12.2 Prevention

Prevention of PFI starts with identifying the risk factors that cause an increased incidence of PJI or predispose some patients to a higher risk of developing infection. These factors can be considered under the following three headings: preoperative, intraoperative, and postoperative factors.

Preoperative Factors There are several host-related modifiable and non-modifiable risk factors like obesity, malignancy, diabetes, smoking, and so on, which are all associated with an increased risk of infection in patients undergoing arthroplasty [6], as shown in Table 12.1. Diabetes mellitus is one of the common risk factors associated with these patients. HbA1c is considered the gold standard test for evaluating glycemic control over the last 90 days; however, a recent multicentric study suggested that fructosamine, a glucose intermediate, outperformed HbA1c at predicting 90-day outcomes [3, 7]. Other than diabetes, obesity is also a well-established risk factor for peri- and postoperative medical-surgical complications. However, recent literature suggested that obesity is a risk for PJI, but implementing the body mass index threshold was not effective in decreasing the PJI [8].

Intraoperative Factors Perioperative prophylactic first- or second-generation cephalosporin antibiotic administration before skin incision as part of routine care [9]. In certain high-risk patients who need additional antibiotics coverage, dual antibiotics comprising cephalosporin and vancomycin have been commonly practiced in patients who are at increased risk of developing methicillin-resistant Staphylococcus aureus infection, but the nephrotoxicity should be considered [10]. Another method is the use of an antiseptic agent for cleaning, for which evidence is

Table 12.1 Modifiable and non-modifiable risk factors for the PJI

Modifiable risk factors	Non-modifiable risk factors
Obesity	Age
Diabetes	Genetic predisposition
Smoking	Previous local infection
Alcoholism	Revision arthroplasty
Corticosteroid use	Urinary colonization
Poor hygiene	Nasal carrier
Oral dent infections	Immunosuppression
Anemia	Hemodialysis
Intravenous drugs	Malignancy
Anticoagulants	
Rheumatoid arthritis	

in favor of a povidone-iodine irrigation solution, which is used at most institutions [11]

Postoperative Factors Meticulous wound closure with subarticular sutures and silver-impregnated occlusive dressing has effectively reduced the rate of superficial infection drainage from the wound in the postoperative period [3, 12]. Additionally, the use of a more potent anticoagulant for DVT prophylaxis may lead to prolonged wound drainage, which in turn increases the risk of infection; recent data suggests that the use of less potent anticoagulation, such as aspirin, can effectively decrease the risk of DVT without interfering with wound drainage [3, 13].

12.3 Diagnosis

12.3.1 Stepwise Diagnostic Approach

Serological Markers

Although blood serological markers like quantitative C-reactive protein (CRP) and erythrocyte sedimentation rate (ESR) are universally accepted screening tests to evaluate the PJI in patients with painful prostheses [14]. However, literature has suggested that the specificity of ESR and CRP is poor for diagnosing PJI, which can miss the diagnosis in cases of low-virulence organisms [15]. Recently, the use of serum D-dimer levels in screening suspected PJI has shown promising results [16].

Synovial Fluid Markers

The aspiration of synovial fluid and its analysis of biomarkers from the suspected PJI is the next step [3, 14]. Literature suggests that the synovial fluid white blood cell (WBC) count and polymorphonuclear (PMN) cell percentage are important in diagnosing PJI [14]. Another synovial fluid alpha defensin marker has gained particular interest in recent years. However, its diagnostic utility is comparable to conventional synovial fluid markers like WBC count and PMN cell percentage [14, 17].

Identification of Pathogen

Although the culture and sensitivity analysis of the obtained sample is considered the gold standard for identifying pathogens in PJI patients, the rise in culture-negative PJI is of great concern [3, 18]. It has been recommended that at least three or more samples be taken intraoperatively to maximize the chances of having a positive culture and isolating a pathogen [18]. Molecular techniques like polymerase chain reaction and next-generation sequencing have recently attracted researchers' interest. In such cases, next-generation sequencing can find at least one or more organisms in up to 82% of culture-negative PJI [18].

Diagnostic Criteria

The International Consensus Meeting (ICM) on musculoskeletal infection in 2018 recommended the first evidence-based and validated definition for the PJI [19]. The

Table 12.2 MSIS criteria for diagnosis of prosthetic joint infection [21]

Major criteria	Minor criteria
Communicating	Raised level of erythrocyte sedimentation rate / C-reactive protein
Isolated organism in two different tissue/fluid culture	Raised synovial leukocyte counts
	Raised synovial polymorphonuclear neutrophil percentage.
	Purulent material
	Isolated organism in one tissue or fluid culture
	> 5 neutrophils/high power field histological tissue analysis 400 magnification

A Single Major, or 4 out of 6 minor criteria, are needed to establish the diagnosis
CRP C-reactive protein, *ESR* erythrocyte sedimentation rate, *PMN%* polymorphonuclear neutrophil

2018 ICM criteria have shown a diagnostic sensitivity of 97.7% and a specificity of 99.5% for PJI. The diagnostic utility of the different serological markers has been evaluated using the random forest plot analysis, and each variable was given a score and weight based on its performance. Following this, patients were categorized into three groups based on the scores of ICM: (i) infected (6), (ii) inconclusive (4–5), or (iii) aseptic (0–3).

The ESR and CRP levels in the blood are basic screening tests for any infection after joint arthroplasty. The cut-off values of the ESR and CRP have been defined by Ghanem et al. ESR more than 30 mm/h. and CRP > 10 mg/l were reported to have sensitivity >94% and 91%, respectively, which, in combination with both, gives a sensitivity of more than 97% [20]. However, the Musculoskeletal Infection Society (MSIS) gave a new definition of PJI with a cut-off point for ESR being 48.5 mm/h. and 36.5 mm/h. for hip and knee replacements, respectively. The cut-off values for CRP were 13.5 mg/L and 23.5 mg/L for hip and knee replacements, respectively [21], as shown in Table 12.2.

12.4 Management

12.4.1 Acute PJI

The commonly used treatment strategy for acute PJI is debridement, antibiotics, and implant retention (DAIR) [22]. However, the result of DAIR is influenced by several factors. Raised CRP-positive blood culture, elderly patients, and PJI due to MRSA have higher rates of failure, and the literature has suggested no role for subsequent irrigation and debridement in patients that fail an initial DAIR procedure [23].

12.4.2 Chronic PJI

Two-stage exchange arthroplasty is considered the gold standard procedure for chronic PJI [24]. The downside of these procedures is that, to date, we have yet to identify a single marker that can predict the infection control optimal timing of reimplantation of the implants. Hence, the decision-making for the reimplantation is difficult to determine, and it relies on several other factors [25]. In recent years, single-stage exchange arthroplasty has shown promising results [26]. Similarly, the success rate of the single-stage procedure is dependent on several host and pathogen-related factors, like concomitant associated comorbidities of the patient and PJI, because the resistant organisms are a big no for the single-stage exchange arthroplasty [3, 26, 27].

12.5 Emerging Technologies

1. *Prevention of PJI:* Recent literature has suggested that drug-eluting implants can have a role in preventing PJI. Recent animal studies have shown that antibiotics eluting from polyethylene materials have shown absolute eradication of infection due to Staphylococcus aureus [28]. Special attention has been given to silver-coated hip implants as a preventive measure and has shown promising results; in contrast to antimicrobial therapy, silver-impregnated have several mechanisms of action against the microorganisms, hence, less risk of antibiotic resistance than the conventional method [29].
2. *Diagnosis of PJI:* Advances in technology have led to the identification of several novel diagnostic biomarkers for PJI. Synovial calprotectin is one of those biomarkers that gain attention and have demonstrated perfect accuracy in diagnosing PJI [30]. Further, the widespread use of genomic sequence testing has led to more use of technologies, one of them being shotgun metagenomics; however, concern regarding the specificity of these technologies for diagnosing PJI is still under scrutiny [31].

   Leukocyte esterase: This test is performed using a colorimetric strip of joint fluid and is based on detecting an enzyme secreted by activated neutrophils at the infection site. The result comes out as negative, trace, +, or ++. The ++ test outcome has been shown to give 80.6% sensitivity and 100 specificity for joint infection. The advantage of this test is the ease of doing it, but a drawback is the requirement for clear fluid without blood stains [32].
3. *Treatment of PJI*: Current literature suggests no accurate matrix to determine and eradicate the infection in patients with PJI. Additionally, PJI has been shown to suppress the host's immune status through an unknown mechanism [32]. Warren et al. suggested that overexpression of the programmed cell death receptor, a protein that downregulates the immune system, is commonly seen in

infected tissues [33]. The data from the literature suggest that monoclonal antibodies, cationic peptides, bacteriophage therapy, and lysins effectively eradicate the infection and can be used to manage PJI in the near future [3, 34].

12.6 Conclusion

PJI of the lower limb tremendously impacts the patient and the healthcare industry worldwide. Although fewer arthroplasty joints get infected, they need appropriate early recognition and management to preserve the implant, restore adequate joint function, and prevent morbidity.

12.7 Illustrative case example (Cases 12.1, 12.2, 12.3, 12.4, 12.5, 12.6, and 12.7)

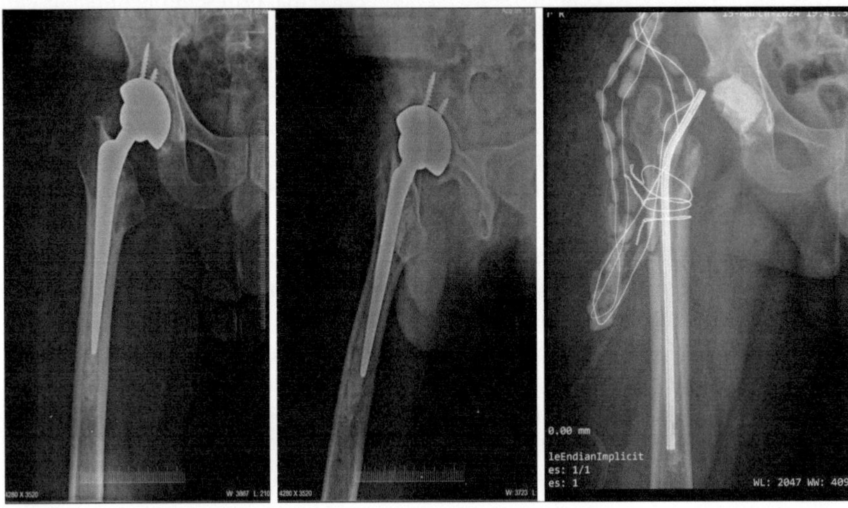

Case 12.1 Radiographs of infected total hip arthroplasty

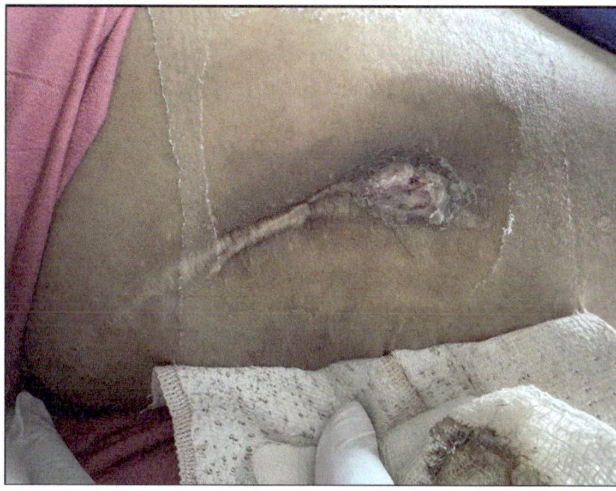

Case 12.2 Infected total hip arthroplasty with discharging sinus

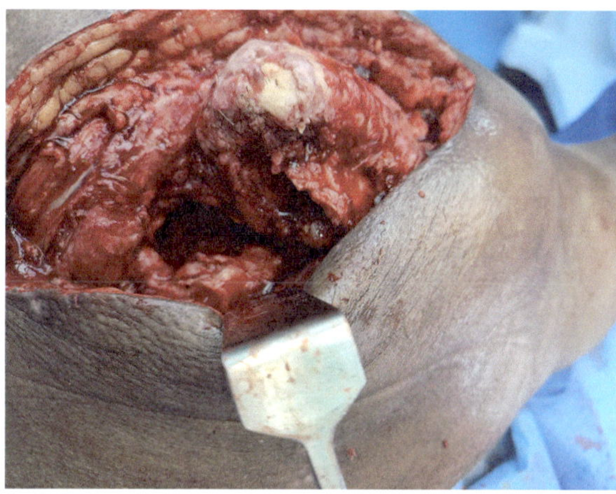

Case 12.3 Infected total hip arthroplasty with complete loss of abductor musculature

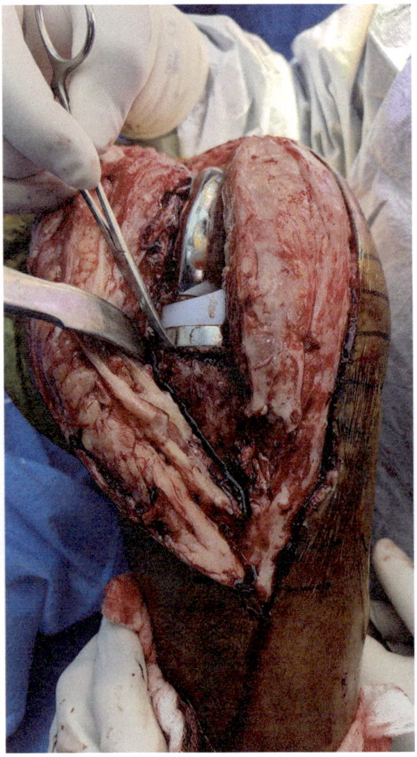

Case 12.4 Infected total knee replacement with patellar tendon damage and bone loss

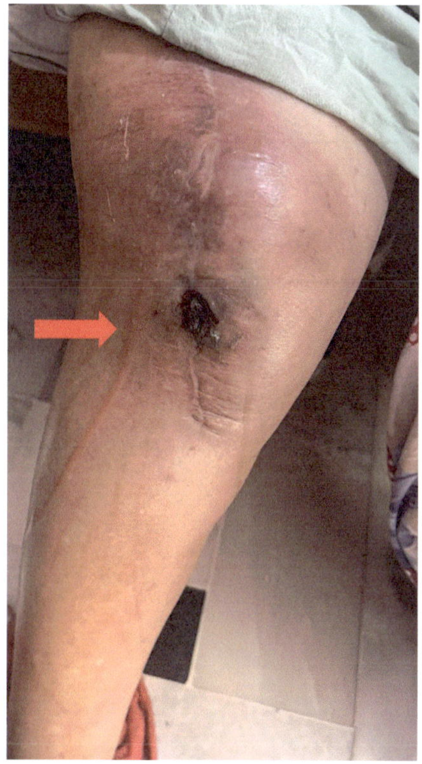

Case 12.5 Infected total knee replacement with pus discharge

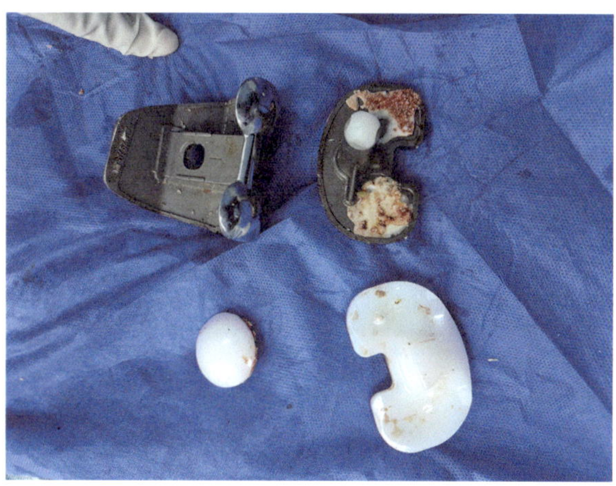

Case 12.6 Removed infected implant of total knee replacement

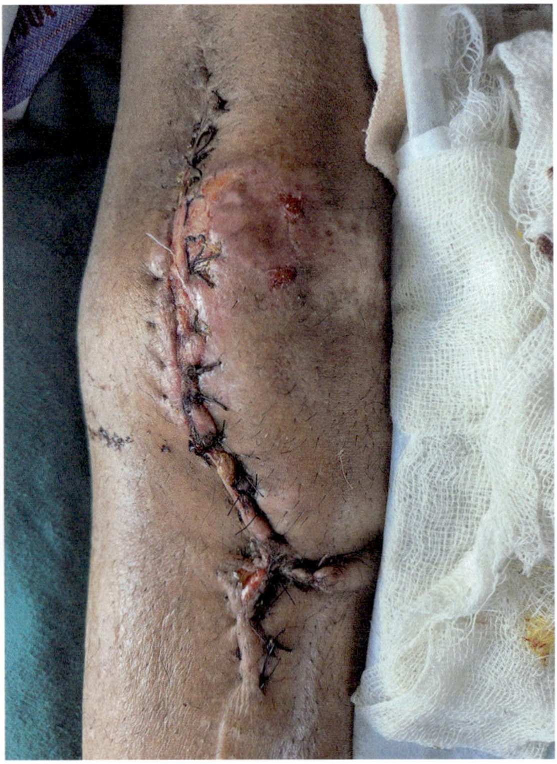

Case 12.7 Flap coverage is done for skin loss

Declarations by All the Authors

Ethical Approval Not Applicable.

Consent to Participate Not applicable.

Consent to Publish Not applicable.

Authors' Contributions All the authors mentioned above have contributed substantially to drafting the article or revising it critically for important intellectual content, as well as to the final approval of the version to be submitted.

Funding None.

Competing Interests The authors declare no competing interests.

Availability of Data and Materials No repositories were used for data.

References

1. Perni S, Prokopovich P. Risk equations for prosthetic joint infections (PJIs) in UK: a retrospective study using the Clinical Practice Research Datalink (CPRD) AURUM and GOLD databases. BMJ Open. 2024;14(5):e082501. https://doi.org/10.1136/bmjopen-2023-082501.
2. Perni S, Bojan B, Prokopovich P. A retrospective study of risk factors, causative microorganisms and healthcare resources consumption associated with prosthetic joint infections (PJI) using the Clinical Practice Research Datalink (CPRD) Aurum database. PLoS One. 2023;18(3):e0282709. https://doi.org/10.1371/journal.pone.0282709.
3. Tarabichi S, Chen AF, Higuera CA, Parvizi J, Polkowski GG. 2022 American Association of Hip and Knee Surgeons Symposium: Periprosthetic joint infection. J Arthroplast. 2023;38(7 Suppl 2):S45–9. https://doi.org/10.1016/j.arth.2023.01.045.
4. Parvizi J, Tan TL, Goswami K, Higuera C, Della Valle C, Chen AF, Shohat N. The 2018 definition of Periprosthetic hip and knee infection: an evidence-based and validated criteria. J Arthroplast. 2018;33(5):1309–1314.e2. https://doi.org/10.1016/j.arth.2018.02.078.
5. Shohat N, Goswami K, Tan TL, Yayac M, Soriano A, Sousa R, Wouthuyzen-Bakker M, Parvizi J, ESCMID Study Group of Implant Associated Infections (ESGIAI) and the Northern Infection Network of Joint Arthroplasty (NINJA). 2020 Frank Stinchfield Award: Identifying who will fail following irrigation and debridement for prosthetic joint infection. Bone Joint J. 2020;102-B(7_Supple_B):11–9.
6. Marmor S, Kerroumi Y. Patient-specific risk factors for infection in arthroplasty procedure. Orthop Traumatol Surg Res. 2016;102(1 Suppl):S113–9. https://doi.org/10.1016/j.otsr.2015.05.012.
7. Shohat N, Tarabichi M, Tan TL, et al. 2019 John Insall award: Fructosamine is a better glycaemic marker compared with glycated haemoglobin (HbA1C) in predicting adverse outcomes following total knee arthroplasty: a prospective multicentre study. Bone Joint J. 2019;101-B(7_Supple_C):3–9.
8. Shohat N, Fleischman A, Tarabichi M, Tan TL, Parvizi J. Weighing in on body mass index and infection after Total joint arthroplasty: is there evidence for a body mass index threshold? Clin Orthop Relat Res. 2018;476(10):1964–9. https://doi.org/10.1007/s11999.0000000000000141.
9. Aboltins CA, Berdal JE, Casas F, et al. Hip and knee section, prevention, antimicrobials (systemic): proceedings of international consensus on orthopedic infections. J Arthroplast. 2019;34(2S):S279–88. https://doi.org/10.1016/j.arth.2018.09.012.
10. Courtney MP, Melnic CM, Zimmer Z, Anari J, Lee G-C. Addition of vancomycin to cefazolin prophylaxis is associated with acute kidney injury after primary joint arthroplasty. Clin Orthop Relat Res. 2015;473(7):2197–203. https://doi.org/10.1007/s11999-014-4062-3.
11. Siddiqi A, Abdo ZE, Rossman SR, Kelly MA, Piuzzi NS, Higuera CA, Schwarzkopf R, Springer BD, Chen AF, Parvizi J. What is the optimal irrigation solution in the management of periprosthetic hip and Knee Joint Infections? J Arthroplast. 2021;36(10):3570–83. https://doi.org/10.1016/j.arth.2021.05.032.
12. Grosso MJ, Berg A, LaRussa S, Murtaugh T, Trofa DP, Geller JA. Silver-impregnated occlusive dressing reduces rates of acute Periprosthetic joint infection after Total joint arthroplasty. J Arthroplast. 2017;32(3):929–32. https://doi.org/10.1016/j.arth.2016.08.039.
13. Parvizi J, Huang R, Restrepo C, Chen AF, Austin MS, Hozack WJ, Lonner JH. Low-dose aspirin is effective chemoprophylaxis against clinically important venous thromboembolism following Total joint arthroplasty: a preliminary analysis. J Bone Joint Surg Am. 2017;99(2):91–8. https://doi.org/10.2106/JBJS.16.00147.
14. Yilmaz MK, Abbaszadeh A, Tarabichi S, Azboy I, Parvizi J. Diagnosis of periprosthetic joint infection: the utility of biomarkers in 2023. Antibiotics (Basel). 2023;12(6):1054. https://doi.org/10.3390/antibiotics12061054.
15. Kheir MM, Tan TL, Shohat N, Foltz C, Parvizi J. Routine diagnostic tests for periprosthetic joint infection demonstrate a high false-negative rate and are influenced by the infecting organism. J Bone Joint Surg Am. 2018;100:2057e65. https://doi.org/10.2106/JBJS.17.01429.

16. Shahi A, Kheir MM, Tarabichi M, Hosseinzadeh HRS, Tan TL, Parvizi J. Serum D dimer test is promising for the diagnosis of periprosthetic joint infection and timing of reimplantation. J Bone Joint Surg Am. 2017;99:1419e27. https://doi.org/10.2106/JBJS.16.01395.
17. Kleeman-Forsthuber LT, Johnson RM, Brady AC, Pollet AK, Dennis DA, Jennings JM. Alpha-defensin offers limited utility in routine workup of periprosthetic joint infection. J Arthroplast. 2021;36(5):1746–52. https://doi.org/10.1016/j.arth.2020.12.018.
18. Goh GS, Parvizi J. Diagnosis and treatment of culture-negative Periprosthetic joint infection. J Arthroplast. 2022;37(8):1488–93. https://doi.org/10.1016/j.arth.2022.01.061.
19. Schwarz EM, Parvizi J, Gehrke T, et al. 2018 international consensus meeting on musculoskeletal infection: research priorities from the general assembly questions. J Orthop Res. 2019;37(5):997–1006. https://doi.org/10.1002/jor.24293.
20. Della Valle C, Parvizi J, Bauer TW, Dicesare PE, Evans RP, Segreti J, American Academy of Orthopaedic Surgeons, et al. Diagnosis of periprosthetic joint infections of the hip and knee. J Am Acad Orthop Surg. 2010;18:760–70.
21. Aggarwal VK, Rasouli MR, Parvizi J. Periprosthetic joint infection: current concept. Indian J Orthop. 2013;47(1):10–7. https://doi.org/10.4103/0019-5413.106884.
22. Longo UG, De Salvatore S, Bandini B, Lalli A, Barillà B, Budhiparama NC, Lustig S. Debridement, antibiotics, and implant retention (DAIR) for the early prosthetic joint infection of total knee and hip arthroplasties: a systematic review. J ISAKOS. 2024;9(1):62–70. https://doi.org/10.1016/j.jisako.2023.09.003.
23. Veerman K, Raessens J, Telgt D, Smulders K, Goosen JHM. Debridement, antibiotics, and implant retention after revision arthroplasty: antibiotic mismatch, timing, and repeated DAIR associated with poor outcome. Bone Joint J. 2022;104-B(4):464–71. https://doi.org/10.1302/0301-620X.104B4.BJJ-2021-1264.R1.
24. Lazic I, Scheele C, Pohlig F, von Eisenhart-Rothe R, Suren C. Treatment options in PJI – is two-stage still gold standard? J Orthop. 2021;23:180–4. https://doi.org/10.1016/j.jor.2020.12.021.
25. Aalirezaie A, Bauer TW, Fayaz H, Griffin W, et al. Hip and knee section, diagnosis, Reimplantation: proceedings of international consensus on orthopedic infections. J Arthroplast. 2019;34(2S):S369–79. https://doi.org/10.1016/j.arth.2018.09.021.
26. Abdelaziz H, Grüber H, Gehrke T, Salber J, Citak M. What are the factors associated with re-revision after one-stage revision for periprosthetic joint infection of the hip? A case-control study. Clin Orthop Relat Res. 2019;477:2258–63.
27. Dombrowski ME, Wilson AE, Wawrose RA, O'Malley MJ, Urish KL, Klatt BA. A low percentage of patients satisfy typical indications for single-stage exchange arthroplasty for chronic Periprosthetic joint infection. Clin Orthop Relat Res. 2020;478(8):1780–6. https://doi.org/10.1097/CORR.0000000000001243.
28. Suhardi VJ, Bichara DA, Kwok S, Freiberg AA, Rubash H, Malchau H, Yun SH, Muratoglu OK, Oral E. A fully functional drug-eluting joint implant. Nat Biomed Eng. 2017;1:0080. https://doi.org/10.1038/s41551-017-0080.
29. Wyatt MC, Foxall-Smith M, Roberton A, Beswick A, Kieser DC, Whitehouse MR. The use of silver coating in hip megaprostheses: a systematic review. Hip Int. 2019;29(1):7–20. https://doi.org/10.1177/1120700018811070.
30. Warren J, Anis HK, Bowers K, et al. Diagnostic utility of a novel point-of-care test of calprotectin for Periprosthetic joint infection after Total knee arthroplasty: a prospective cohort study. J Bone Joint Surg Am. 2021;103(11):1009–15. https://doi.org/10.2106/JBJS.20.01089.
31. Tarabichi M, Alvand A, Shohat N, Goswami K, Parvizi J. Diagnosis of *streptococcus canis*periprosthetic joint infection: the utility of next-generation sequencing. Arthroplast Today. 2017;4(1):20–3. https://doi.org/10.1016/j.artd.2017.08.005.
32. (Parvizi J, Jacovides C, Antoci V, Ghanem E. Diagnosis of periprosthetic joint infection: the utility of a simple yet unappreciated enzyme. J Bone Joint Surg Am 2011;93:2242–2248).
33. Warren SI, Charville GW, Manasherob R, Amanatullah DF. Immune checkpoint upregulation in periprosthetic joint infection. J Orthop Res. 2022;40(11):2663–9. https://doi.org/10.1002/jor.25276.
34. Akanda ZZ, Taha M, Abdelbary H. Current review-the rise of bacteriophage as a unique therapeutic platform in treating peri-prosthetic joint infections. J Orthop Res. 2018;36(4):1051–60. https://doi.org/10.1002/jor.23755.

Prosthetic Joint Infection: Upper Limb

13

Inese Breide, Dace Vīgante, and Dmitrijs Grigorjevs

Abstract

Periprosthetic joint infection (PJI) of the upper extremity, although uncommon, represents a serious complication following joint arthroplasty. The increasing utilisation of shoulder and elbow replacements has correspondingly elevated the incidence of infection. Distinct anatomical and microbiological characteristics of upper limb joints necessitate a management approach differing from lower limb PJI. Reported infection rates range from approximately 0.8–1.4% for shoulder arthroplasty and around 1.5% for elbow arthroplasty. PJI may arise from intraoperative contamination, contiguous spread from adjacent tissues, or haematogenous dissemination. Treatment options include one- or two-stage reimplantation, debridement with prosthesis retention, or resection arthroplasty, though evidence remains limited. Further research is warranted to determine optimal diagnostic and therapeutic strategies for upper limb PJI.

Keywords

Periprosthetic Joint Infection · Upper limb arthroplasty · Shoulder arthroplasty · Elbow arthroplasty · Arthroplasty complications · Infection diagnosis · Debridement · Prosthesis retention · PJI treatment · Resection arthroplasty

I. Breide (✉)
Hospital of Traumatology and Orthopedics, Head of upper extremity division, Chief of the Outpatient and Short-Term Surgery Department, Riga, Latvia

D. Vīgante
Hospital of Traumatology and Orthopedics, Infectious diseases specialist, Riga, Latvia

D. Grigorjevs
Deputy Chief of Infectious department, Riga, Latvia

P. Kumar et al. (eds.), *Textbook of Orthopedic Infections*,
https://doi.org/10.1007/978-981-95-5029-6_13

Learning Objectives
1. Evaluate pathogenesis and risk factors associated with upper limb PJI.
2. Develop diagnostic and management strategies for upper limb PJI.
3. Formulate comprehensive treatment protocols for affected patients.

13.1 Introduction

Upper limb periprosthetic joint infection, though infrequent, can lead to severe functional impairment and morbidity. The increasing indications for arthroplasty have expanded the population at risk, and anatomical and microbiological differences compared with lower limb joints suggest that management of upper limb PJI may require tailored strategies. Shoulder arthroplasty remains the most frequently performed upper limb joint replacement. Epidemiological data suggest an infection incidence of 0.8–1.4% following shoulder arthroplasty and approximately 1.5% after elbow arthroplasty [1, 2].

PJI may develop through intraoperative contamination, direct spread from contiguous tissues, or haematogenous seeding from distant infection sites. Management strategies encompass one- or two-stage revision, debridement with retention of the prosthesis, or resection arthroplasty; however, clinical experience is comparatively limited, and the evidence base remains modest.

13.2 Diagnosis and Clinical Manifestations

Diagnosing upper limb PJI is challenging due to the absence of a single definitive test. A thorough approach incorporating patient history, clinical examination, imaging, histopathology, culture, and inflammatory markers is essential. Preoperative diagnostic testing is critical before any revision procedure, as identification of infection significantly influences therapeutic decisions [1, 3, 4].

Clinical presentation may include pain, warmth, erythema, joint effusion, and fever, though these signs are not universally observed (Fig. 13.1). Pain and restricted range of motion are almost always present. Consequently, any painful shoulder arthroplasty should be investigated comprehensively for potential infection [1, 3, 4].

Radiographic assessment may demonstrate progressive radiolucent lines along the bone–prosthesis interface, osteolysis, or osteopenia; however, these findings are nonspecific. Joint aspiration is recommended for all suspected infections, regardless of implant stability. Synovial fluid analysis should include leukocyte count with differential, Gram stain, and culture for aerobic, anaerobic, fungal, and mycobacterial organisms.

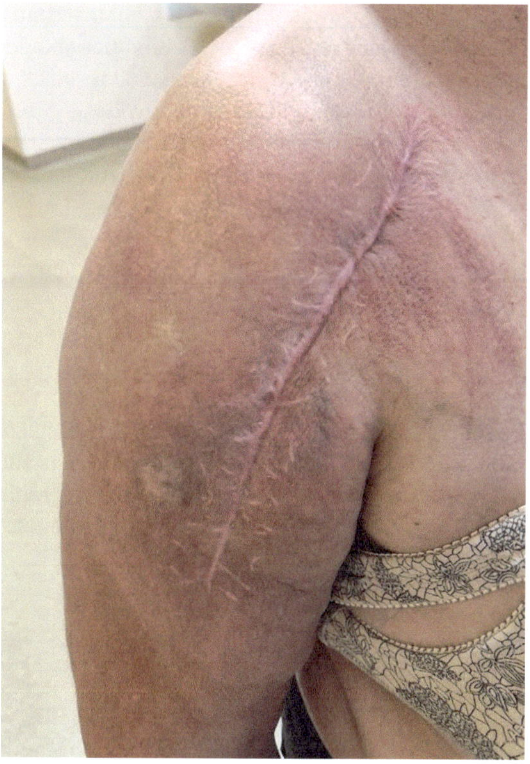

Fig. 13.1 Clinical presentation of infected shoulder PJI in a patient with multiple prior surgeries

13.2.1 Synovial Leukocyte Count

Synovial biomarkers, including white blood cell (WBC) count and percentage of polymorphonuclear (PMN) cells, assist in identifying periprosthetic infections. The 2018 International Consensus Meeting (ICM) minor criteria suggest that a synovial WBC count exceeding 3000 cells/μL and neutrophil proportion above 80% is indicative of infection [3, 5]. However, WBC and PMN percentages may remain elevated for up to 3 months postoperatively, limiting diagnostic utility in the first 6 weeks after arthroplasty, particularly for the shoulder [5].

13.2.2 Microbiological Culture

Accurate microbiological assessment is crucial. Synovial fluid and tissue samples should be incubated for a minimum of 14 days, as Cutibacterium species, common in shoulder PJI, grow slowly. Laboratories must ensure samples are not prematurely discarded. Pottinger et al. reported Cutibacterium acnes as the pathogen in 70% of infected shoulder revisions [6]. Antibiotics should be withheld for at least 14 days before aspiration to avoid false-negative results.

Intraoperative sampling should involve 4–5 separate tissue specimens collected using sterile instruments and individual containers. Synovial fluid may be inoculated into aerobic and anaerobic blood culture bottles [1, 3, 7]. Gram staining provides rapid diagnosis if positive but has low sensitivity (< 26%) despite high specificity (> 97%). Cultures for fungi and mycobacteria should be considered based on epidemiological and clinical risk factors.

13.2.3 Molecular Investigations

Polymerase chain reaction (PCR) techniques can detect microbial DNA in synovial fluid within hours and identify antibiotic resistance. PCR is particularly useful in culture-negative cases or when prior antimicrobial therapy may have suppressed bacterial growth. Limitations include potential false positives due to the detection of non-viable bacteria [4].

13.2.4 Blood Tests

Preoperative serological markers, including WBC count, C-reactive protein (CRP), and erythrocyte sedimentation rate (ESR), are frequently used. These markers typically rise rapidly after arthroplasty, peaking within days, and return to baseline around 6 weeks in the absence of infection [3–5]. Low-virulence infections, such as those caused by Cutibacterium acnes, may not elevate systemic markers; Dodson et al. found CRP > 10 mg/L in only 72% of patients with periprosthetic shoulder infections [6, 8].

13.2.5 Sonication of Removed Implants

Biofilms on prosthetic surfaces allow microorganisms to persist despite standard treatment. Sonication dislodges these biofilms, improving microbial detection. Trampuz et al. demonstrated higher sensitivity for sonicated fluids compared with periprosthetic tissue biopsies (75% versus 45%) in patients recently treated with antibiotics [26]. Culture of sonication fluid is particularly beneficial in patients receiving antibiotics prior to surgery.

13.3 Treatment

Successful management of upper limb PJI requires meticulous surgical debridement and excision of all devitalised tissue. Incomplete debridement substantially increases the likelihood of treatment failure, irrespective of antibiotic regimen. In certain cases, treatment goals may shift from eradication to long-term infection suppression.

Treatment choice is influenced by several factors:

1. Interval since initial arthroplasty
2. Infecting microorganism(s)
3. Patient-specific considerations (age, comorbidities, functional demands, compliance)
4. Local anatomical factors, including bone and soft tissue integrity [9]

The *two-stage revision* remains the most commonly adopted strategy, comprising complete implant removal, placement of an antibiotic-loaded spacer, systemic antibiotic therapy, and delayed reimplantation following infection control. Spacers may be prefabricated or custom-made intraoperatively, with antibiotics selected according to preoperative culture results to achieve local infection control [10]. Routine aspiration of the joint prior to second-stage reimplantation is debated due to high rates of "dry taps" and false-negative cultures.

One-stage revision can yield superior functional outcomes and cost-effectiveness but carries a higher risk of reinfection and should be performed only in specialised centres [9, 11]. Its limitations are largely related to insufficient preoperative identification of the infecting organism.

Some centres have described *three-stage revision protocols*, incorporating implant removal and spacer insertion, 6 weeks of antibiotics, a 4-week antibiotic-free interval with repeat biopsies to confirm eradication, and, if negative, final prosthesis implantation [12, 13].

Debridement with implant retention is generally reserved for early infections, ideally within 2 weeks of symptom onset. Modular components should be exchanged to enhance visualisation and allow thorough removal of biofilms [14]. Late infections (> 12 weeks) are poorly controlled by debridement alone. Early intervention in haematogenous infections may also permit retention, with acceptable recurrence rates [14, 21].

For *chronic infection in low-demand patients* or those unsuitable for revision surgery, options include:

- Debridement, implant removal, and antibiotic spacer placement (Fig. 13.2)
- Resection arthroplasty (Fig. 13.3) [9, 11]

Resection arthroplasty provides effective pain relief but yields limited functional recovery [11]. In select high-risk patients, long-term suppressive antibiotic therapy may be considered following initial intravenous treatment; duration remains variable, often guided by clinical response [14].

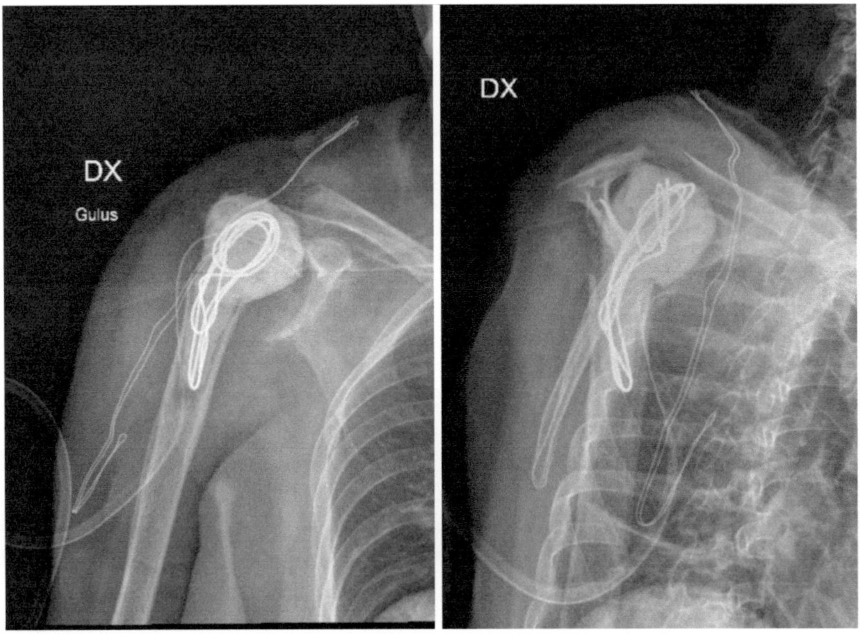

Fig. 13.2 Debridement, implant removal, and cement spacer implantation

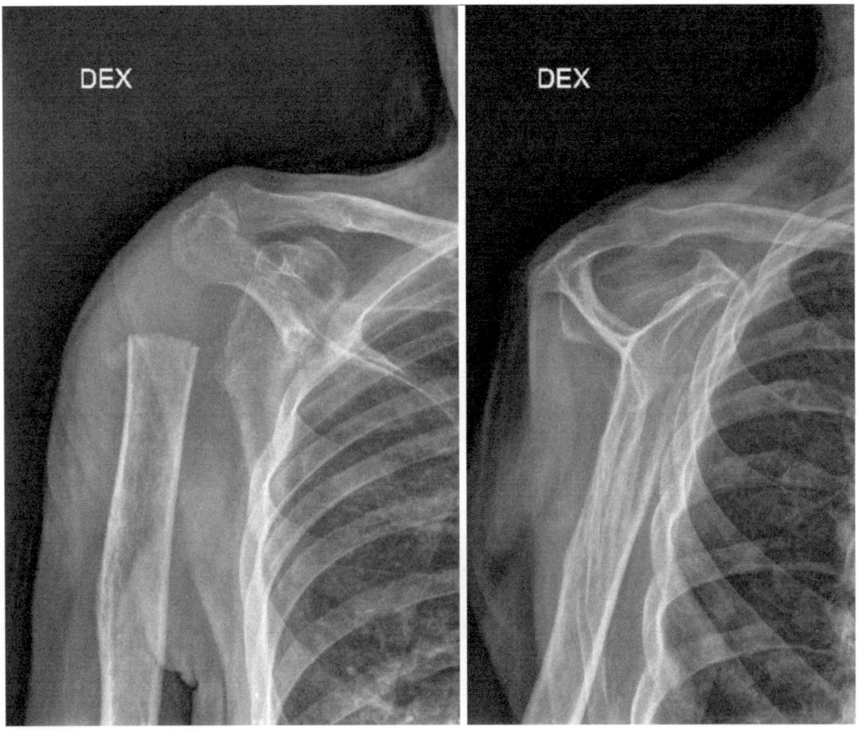

Fig. 13.3 Resection arthroplasty

Table 13.1 Pathogen-specific first-choice antibiotic therapies [25]

Microorganism	Recommended antibiotic
Staphylococcus spp. (methicillin-susceptible)	Cefazolin or oxacillin ± fosfomycin for 2 weeks, then oral rifampin + levofloxacin/cotrimoxazole/doxycycline/fusidic acid
Staphylococcus spp. (methicillin-resistant)	Vancomycin or daptomycin ± fosfomycin for 2 weeks, then oral rifampin combination as above
Streptococcus spp.	Penicillin G or ceftriaxone 2–4 weeks, then amoxicillin or doxycycline
Enterococcus spp. (ampicillin-susceptible)	Ampicillin + gentamicin 2–3 weeks, then amoxicillin or doxycycline
Enterococcus spp. (ampicillin-resistant)	Vancomycin or daptomycin ± fosfomycin 2–4 weeks, then linezolid (max 4 weeks)
Gram-negative Enterobacterales	Ciprofloxacin
Gram-negative non-fermenters	Piperacillin/tazobactam, meropenem, or ceftazidime ± aminoglycosides, then ciprofloxacin
Anaerobes (gram-positive)	Penicillin G or ceftriaxone 2 weeks, then rifampin + levofloxacin/amoxicillin/doxycycline
Anaerobes (gram-negative)	Ampicillin/sulbactam 2 weeks, then metronidazole
Candida spp. (fluconazole-susceptible)	Caspofungin/anidulafungin 1–2 weeks, then fluconazole ≥1 year
Candida spp. (fluconazole-resistant)	Suppression or implant removal with alternative antifungal
Culture-negative	Ampicillin/sulbactam ± vancomycin 2 weeks, then rifampin + levofloxacin

13.4 Antimicrobial Treatment

Antimicrobial strategies for upper limb PJI align with principles used in lower limb arthroplasty. Antibiotics without surgery are generally discouraged except in patients refusing surgery or when operative risk is prohibitive. Critically ill patients receive broad-spectrum empirical therapy prior to surgery, while stable patients may await definitive microbiological identification for targeted therapy.

Empirical regimens commonly include β-lactams with gram-negative coverage (e.g., piperacillin–tazobactam or ceftriaxone) and agents effective against gram-positive cocci, including MRSA (e.g., vancomycin) [22]. Antibiotic therapy is initiated intraoperatively after obtaining culture specimens, initially intravenously. Once pathogens are identified, therapy should be de-escalated to targeted agents (Table 13.1).

13.5 Unexpected Positive Cultures

Unexpected positive cultures (UPC) are frequently detected during shoulder arthroplasty even in the absence of clinical or radiographic signs of infection, with a prevalence of ~15%. Cutibacterium acnes is the most commonly implicated organism. In most cases, UPCs do not significantly alter patient outcomes or reoperation rates. Antibiotic strategies vary, but reinfection rates are generally unaffected. Approximately 10% of UPC cases may represent persistent infection [23, 24].

13.6 Prevention

Preoperative skin decontamination with chlorhexidine gluconate showers and topical benzoyl peroxide reduces positive skin cultures; however, evidence for routine topical prophylaxis in reducing PJI is limited. Optimal skin preparation includes 2% chlorhexidine gluconate with 70% isopropyl alcohol [14]. Blue light therapy shows in-vitro efficacy against C. acnes, though clinical evidence remains preliminary [10].

All patients undergoing primary or revision shoulder arthroplasty should receive perioperative intravenous antibiotics covering both gram-positive and gram-negative organisms. Standard regimens include weight-based cefazolin, with MRSA-colonised patients receiving glycopeptides. Patients allergic to cefazolin may receive vancomycin or clindamycin. Postoperative antibiotics for primary arthroplasty are not recommended beyond surgery; for revision procedures, antibiotics should not exceed 24 h unless infection is suspected preoperatively [7, 15–17].

Intrawound agents, such as vancomycin powder or diluted antiseptic irrigation, may be considered in high-risk patients, though supporting data are limited [14]. Use of closed-suction drains has not been shown to increase infection risk [18].

Certain demographic and comorbidity factors increase infection risk: male sex, younger age, HIV positivity, hepatitis C infection, rheumatoid arthritis, poorly controlled diabetes (HbA1c >8.0 mg/dL), chronic corticosteroid use, obesity (BMI > 35 kg/m^2), malnutrition, smoking, drug abuse, and prior corticosteroid injections within 3 months before arthroplasty [10, 12, 19, 20]. Previous shoulder surgery also elevates infection risk.

13.7 Conclusion

Periprosthetic joint infection of the upper limb is rare but potentially devastating, with unique anatomical and microbial considerations that distinguish it from lower limb infections. Diagnosis requires a comprehensive approach integrating clinical assessment, imaging, synovial analysis, cultures, and molecular techniques. Treatment should be individualised, balancing surgical options with patient comorbidities and functional demands. Two-stage revision remains the standard, while one-stage revision may offer improved functional outcomes in specialised settings. Early intervention, meticulous debridement, and targeted antimicrobial therapy are critical to optimise outcomes. Preventive strategies, including perioperative skin preparation, appropriate antibiotic prophylaxis, and careful patient selection, are essential in minimising the risk of PJI. Further studies are needed to refine diagnostic thresholds, treatment protocols, and preventive measures for upper limb PJI.

Take-Home Messages

- Upper limb PJI is uncommon but can have severe consequences.
- Microbial flora and soft tissue considerations in the upper limb differ from lower limb PJI.

- Slow-growing pathogens, particularly Cutibacterium spp., require prolonged culture incubation.
- One-stage revision may offer superior function but carries higher reinfection risk relative to two-stage revision.

References

1. Rangan A, Falworth M, Watts AC, Scarborough M, Thomas M, Kulkarni R, Rees J. Investigation and Management of Periprosthetic Joint Infection in the Shoulder and Elbow: Evidence and consensus based guidelines of the British Elbow and Shoulder Society. Shoulder Elbow. 2018;10(1 Suppl):S5–S19. https://doi.org/10.1177/1758573218772976. Epub 2018 May 16. Erratum in: Shoulder Elbow. 2018 Oct;10(4):NP1. doi: 10.1177/1758573218790123. PMID: 29796102; PMCID: PMC5958475
2. Samuel Schick, Joseph Elphingstone, Sudarsan Murali, Karen Carter, William Davis, Gerald McGwin, Thomas Evely, Brent Ponce, Amit Momaya, Eugene Brabston. The incidence of shoulder arthroplasty infection presents a substantial economic burden in the United States: a predictive model. JSES Int. 2023;7(4):636–41., ISSN 2666-6383. https://doi.org/10.1016/j.jseint.2023.03.013.
3. Ochsner PE, Borens O, Bodler P-M, Schweizerische Gesellschaft für Orthopädie und Traumatologie. Infections of the musculoskeletal system : basic principles, prevention, diagnosis and treatment. 1st ed. Swiss Orthopaedics in-house-publisher; 2016.
4. Fink B, Sevelda F. Periprosthetic joint infection of shoulder arthroplasties: diagnostic and treatment options. Biomed Res Int. 2017;2017:4582756. https://doi.org/10.1155/2017/4582756. Epub 2017 Dec 20. PMID: 29423407; PMCID: PMC5750516. 2017 Apr 27;2(4):104–109
5. Bonnevialle N, Dauzeres F, Toulemonde J, Elia F, Laffose JM, Mansat P. Periprosthetic shoulder infection: an overview. EFORT Open Rev. 2017;2(4):104–9. https://doi.org/10.1302/2058-5241.2.160023.
6. Pottinger P, Butler-Wu S, Neradilek MB, Merritt A, Bertelsen A, Jette JL, et al. Prognostic factors for bacterial cultures positive for Propionibacterium acnes and other organisms in a large series of revision shoulder arthroplasties performed for stifness, pain, or loosening. J Bone Joint Surg Am. 2012;94:2075–83.
7. Berrios-Torres SI, Umscheid CA, Bratzler DW, Leas B, Stone EC, Kelz RR, et al. Centers for Disease Control and Prevention guideline for the prevention of surgical site infection, 2017. JAMA Surg. 2017;152:784–91. https://doi.org/10.1001/jamasurg.2017.0904.
8. Dodson CC, Craig EV, Cordasco FA, et al. Propionibacterium acnes infection after shoulder arthroplasty: a diagnostic challenge. J Shoulder Elb Surg. 2010;19(2):303–7.
9. Marcheggiani Muccioli GM, Guerra E, Roberti di Sarsina T, Alesi D, Fratini S, Cammisa E, Rinaldi VG, Lullini G, Rotini R, Zaffagnini S. Diagnosis and treatment of infected shoulder arthroplasty. Curr Concepts Rev Joints. 2018;6(3):173–6. https://doi.org/10.1055/s-0038-1675800. PMID: 30582106; PMCID: PMC6301844
10. Markes AR, Bigham J, Ma CB, Iyengar JJ, Feeley BT. Preventing and treating infection in reverse total shoulder arthroplasty. Curr Rev Musculoskelet Med. 2023;16(8):371–80. https://doi.org/10.1007/s12178-023-09843-1. Epub 2023 May 25. PMID: 37227587; PMCID: PMC10382412
11. Weber P, Utzschneider S, Sadoghi P, Andress HJ, Jansson V, Müller PE. Management of the infected shoulder prosthesis: a retrospective analysis and review of the literature. Int Orthop. 2011;35(3):365–73. https://doi.org/10.1007/s00264-010-1019-3. Epub 2010 Apr 20. PMID: 20405287; PMCID: PMC3047637
12. Tseng W-J, Lansdown DA, Grace T, Zhang AL, Feeley BT, Hung L-W, et al. Outcomes of revision arthroplasty for shoulder periprosthetic joint infection: a three-stage revision protocol. J Shoulder Elb Surg. 2019;28:268–75.

13. Zhang AL, Feeley BT, Schwartz BS, Chung TT, Ma CB. Management of deep postoperative shoulder infections: is there a role for open biopsy during staged treatment? J Shoulder Elb Surg. 2015;24:e15–20. https://doi.org/10.1016/j.jse.2014.04.007.
14. Garrigues GE, Zmistowski B, Cooper AM, Green A, Abboud J, Beasley J, et al. Proceedings from the 2018 international consensus meeting on orthopedic infections: management of periprosthetic shoulder infection. J Shoulder Elb Surg. 2019;28:S67–99.
15. Allegranzi B, Zayed B, Bischoff P, Kubilay NZ, de Jonge S, de Vries F, et al. New WHO recommendations on intraoperative and postoperative measures for surgical site infection prevention: an evidence-based global perspective. Lancet Infect Dis. 2016;16:e288–303. https://doi.org/10.1016/S1473-3099(16)30402-9.
16. Perez-Prieto D, Portillo ME, Puig-Verdie L, Alier A, Gamba C, Guirro P, et al. Preoperative antibiotic prophylaxis in prosthetic joint infections: not a concern for intraoperative cultures. Diagn Microbiol Infect Dis. 2016;86:442–5. https://doi.org/10.1016/j.diagmicrobio.2016.09.014.
17. Padegimas EM, Lawrence C, Narzikul AC, Zmistowski BM, Abboud JA, Williams GR, et al. Future surgery after revision shoulder arthroplasty: the impact of unexpected positive cultures. J Shoulder Elbow Surg. 2017;26:975–81. https://doi.org/10.1016/j.jse.2016.10.023.
18. Erickson BJ, Campbell K, Jain A, Cvetanovich GL, Higgins JD, Frank RM, et al. Are postoperative drains beneficial in total and reverse total shoulder arthroplasty?. Openventio Publishers, https://openventio.org/are-postoperative-drains-beneficial-in-total-and- reverse-total-shoulder-arthroplasty/. Accessed 16 Jan 16 2019.
19. Werner BC, Cancienne JM, Burrus MT, Griffin JW, Gwathmey FW, Brockmeier SF. The timing of elective shoulder surgery after shoulder injection affects postoperative infection risk in Medicare patients. J Shoulder Elb Surg. 2016;25:390–7. https://doi.org/10.1016/j.jse.2015.08.039.
20. Gates S, Nguyen I, Del Core M, Nakonezny PA, Bradley H, Khazzam M. Incidence and predictors of positive intraoperative cultures in primary shoulder arthroplasty following prior ipsilateral shoulder surgery. JSES Int. 2020;4:366–71.
21. Dennison T, Alentorn-Geli E, Assenmacher AT, Sperling JW, Sanchez-Sotelo J, Cofield RH. Management of acute or late hematogenous infection after shoulder arthroplasty with irrigation, debridement, and component retention. J Shoulder Elbow Surg. 2017;26:73–8. https://doi.org/10.1016/j.jse.2016.05.018.
22. Le Vavasseur B, Zeller V. Antibiotic therapy for prosthetic joint infections: an overview. Antibiotics. 2022;11:486. https://doi.org/10.3390/antibiotics11040486.
23. Hodakowski AJ, Cohn MR, Mehta N, Menendez ME, McCormick JR, Garrigues GE. An evidence-based approach to managing unexpected positive cultures in shoulder arthroplasty. J Shoulder Elb Surg. 2022;31(10):2176–86. https://doi.org/10.1016/j.jse.2022.03.019. Epub 2022 May 2
24. Foruria AM, Fox TJ, Sperling JW, Cofield RH. Clinical meaning of unexpected positive cultures (UPC) in revision shoulder arthroplasty. J Shoulder Elb Surg. 2013;22(5):620–7. https://doi.org/10.1016/j.jse.2012.07.017. Epub 2012 Sep 13
25. Pocket Guide to Diagnosis & Treatment for the Periprosthetic Joint Infection (PJI), Version 11:November 2023, PRO-IMPLANT Foundation (www.pro-implantfoundation.org).
26. Trampuz A, Piper KE, Jacobson MJ, Hanssen AD, Unni KK, Osmon DR, Mandrekar JN, Cockerill FR, Steckelberg JM, Greenleaf JF, Patel R. Sonication of removed hip and knee prostheses for diagnosis of infection. N Engl J Med. 2007;357(7):654–63. https://doi.org/10.1056/NEJMoa061588.

Fracture-Related Infections 14

Ansh Gupta, Prasoon Kumar, Benjamin Petry, Markus Süß, and Rohit Arora

Abstract

- Fracture-related infection (FRI) is a known and dreaded complication of fracture fixation with a very high socio-economic burden.
- Identification of the risk factors, clinical and biological markers associated with FRI can help in its early diagnosis and prevention.
- Biofilm formation over the implant can protect the microbe from host defences and antibiotics making eradication without surgical debridement difficult.
- Treatment varies due to various host, injury, surgical and microbial factors and requires multidisciplinary approach.

Keywords

Fracture · Osteomyelitis · Biofilm · Early diagnosis

14.1 Epidemiology

Infection rates of fractures vary greatly with rates as high as 40% [1]. With advances such as prophylactic antibiotics before surgery, the trend is decreasing. The infection rate between 1955 and 1960 was 12% and between 1961 and 1968 was 5%. It further decreased to 2.5% for the duration between 1969 and 1973 [1–3]. The rate

A. Gupta · P. Kumar
Department of Orthopedics, PGIMER, Chandigarh, India

B. Petry (✉) · M. Süß · R. Arora
Department of Orthopedic and Trauma Surgery, Medical University of Innsbruck, Innsbruck, Austria
e-mail: benjamin.petry@tirol-kliniken.at

P. Kumar et al. (eds.), *Textbook of Orthopedic Infections*,
https://doi.org/10.1007/978-981-95-5029-6_14

of infection of closed fractures and open fractures of Gr I is 0–1%, Gr II is 5.7%, Gr IIIA is 8.3%, Gr IIIB is 17.9%, and Gr IIIC is 38.5% [4].

The incidence of FRI differs amongst different fracture sites. The various risk factors for FRI have been tabulated in Table 14.1 [5, 6]. Anatomical sites which have relatively poor blood supply such as the distal leg tend to have a higher incidence of FRI. Open fractures due to soft tissue compromise are at a higher risk of development of FRI. Soft tissue coverage acts as an antimicrobial barrier preventing further contamination in the compromised region.

14.2 Pathogenesis

Microbial contamination for FRI can occur via the following mechanisms: exogenously due to trauma, during fixation surgery, wound dehiscence post-operatively, delayed wound closure in case of open fractures and rarely hematogenous [7]. The most commonly implicated organism is Staphylococcus aureus [8–10] (Table 14.2). However, microbial contamination doesn't always lead to FRI. The bacteria need to adhere to the implant, evade the host immune response and initiate the formation of the biofilm, a concept described as "Race to the surface" by Gristina et al., which eventually decides the fate of the implant [11].

Biofilms are organized communities, often polymicrobial, embedded in an extracellular matrix composed of proteins and polysaccharides. Maturation of the

Table 14.1 Risk factors of FRI

Risk factors for FRI
Old age
Male sex
Smoking
Diabetes
Obesity
Alcohol consumption
Lower socio-economic status
Malnutrition (serum albumin <3 g/dL indicative of malnutrition)
Open fracture (risk increases with increasing grade)
Lower limb injury (tibia > ankle > femur)
High energy injury
American Society of Anesthesiology (ASA) grade > 2
Delayed soft tissue coverage
Need for muscle/skin flaps
Previous application of external fixator
Multiple incisions and plates required

Table 14.2 Common microorganisms causing FRI

Microbe	Frequency
Staphylococcus aureus	30–40%
CONS	20–40%
Enterobacteriaceae	15–25%
Anaerobes	15%
Streptococci	10%

biofilm takes 1–2 weeks and involves four steps: adherence, accumulation, maturation, and detachment [12]. The adherence stage is by non-specific forces and thus reversible. Accumulation of bacteria is brought about by polysaccharide intercellular adhesin (PIA) and helps them avoid phagocytosis by leucocytes. Maturation phase is associated with secretion of the glycocalyx, which provides the biofilm structural integrity and protection. The glycocalyx helps the bacteria develop an acidic milieu in its vicinity, entraps minerals from surrounding environment and promotes bacterial growth. It enables trans-colony communication through extracellular DNA transfer and other signalling molecules. This is termed as quorum sensing and is responsible for rapid transfer and development of antibiotic resistance. This diverts the host responses from a bone-healing course to an inflammatory and antibacterial course that can hinder the bone from healing. Mature biofilms are mostly metabolically inactive, due to the nutrient gradient created by the superficial zone. The microbes in the superficial zones are active, use aerobic metabolism and have the potential to detach from the biofilm to become streamers or planktonic forms which then transport to adjacent areas and create new foci of biofilms.

The biofilm offers the bacteria multiple advantages. Active components of humoral immunity like complement protein and antibodies cannot penetrate the biofilm. Macrophages too cannot phagocytose bacteria embedded in the deep zones, called the persisters or sedentary forms, leading to the phenomenon of "frustrated phagocytosis". Higher concentration of bacterial leukotoxins inside the biofilm has been associated with poor polarity of macrophages and weaker inflammatory response. Systemically administered antibiotics have poor penetrance into the biofilm. Quorum sensing helps in rapid gene transfer and antibiotic resistance. Any residual biofilm after debridement serves as a seed for recurrence of infection.

14.3 Investigations and Diagnosis

Until recently, there was no consensus on the definition of FRI. However, in 2018, Metsemekers et al. [13] formulated guidelines to define and diagnose FRI. This included certain confirmatory and suggestive criteria which have been included in Table 14.3 and Fig. 14.1. Since patients with FRI often present with unspecific symptoms, two levels of certainty regarding the diagnostic criteria were created.

Therefore, diagnosis of FRI is based on history, clinical examination, radiological and serological tests, microbiological and histopathological tests. The patients

Table 14.3 Diagnostic criteria of FRI by Metsemekers et al.

Confirmatory criteria
Fistula, sinus or wound breakdown (with communication to the bone or the implant) (Fig. 14.3).
Purulent drainage from the wound or presence of pus during surgery.
Phenotypically indistinguishable pathogens identified by culture from at least two separate deep tissue/implant (including sonication-fluid) specimens taken during an operative intervention. In case of tissue, multiple specimens (≥ 3) should be taken, each with clean instruments (not superficial or sinus tract swabs). In cases of joint effusion, arising in a joint adjacent to a fractured bone, fluid samples obtained by sterile puncture may be included as a single sample.
Presence of microorganisms in deep tissue taken during an operative intervention, as confirmed by histopathological examination using specific staining techniques for bacteria or fungi.
Suggestive criteria
Clinical signs—Any one of: a. Pain (without weight bearing, increasing overtime, new-onset) b. Local redness c. Local swelling d. Increased local temperature e. Fever (single oral temperature measurement of ≥38.3 °C [101 °F])
Radiological signs—Any one of: a. Bone lysis (at the fracture site, around the implant) (Fig. 14.2) b. Implant loosening c. Sequestration (occurring over time) d. Failure of progression of bone healing (i.e. non-union) e. Presence of periosteal bone formation (e.g. at localizations other than the fracture site or in case of a consolidated fracture)
A pathogenic organism identified by culture from a single deep tissue/implant (including sonication-fluid) specimen taken during an operative intervention. In case of tissue, multiple specimens (≥ 3) should be taken, each with clean instruments (not superficial or sinus tract swabs). In cases of joint effusion arising in a joint adjacent to a fractured bone, a fluid sample obtained by sterile puncture is permitted.
Elevated serum inflammatory markers: In musculoskeletal trauma, these should be interpreted with caution. They are included as suggestive signs in case of a secondary rise (after an initial decrease) or a consistent elevation over a period in time, and after exclusion of other infectious foci or inflammatory processes: a. Erythrocyte sedimentation rate (ESR) b. White blood cell count (WBC) c. C-reactive protein (CRP)
Persistent, increasing or new-onset wound drainage, beyond the first few days postoperatively, without solid alternative explanation.
New-onset of joint effusion in fracture patients. Surgeons should be aware that FRI can present as an adjacent septic arthritis in the following cases: a. Implant material which penetrates the joint capsule (e.g. femoral nailing) b. Intra-articular fractures

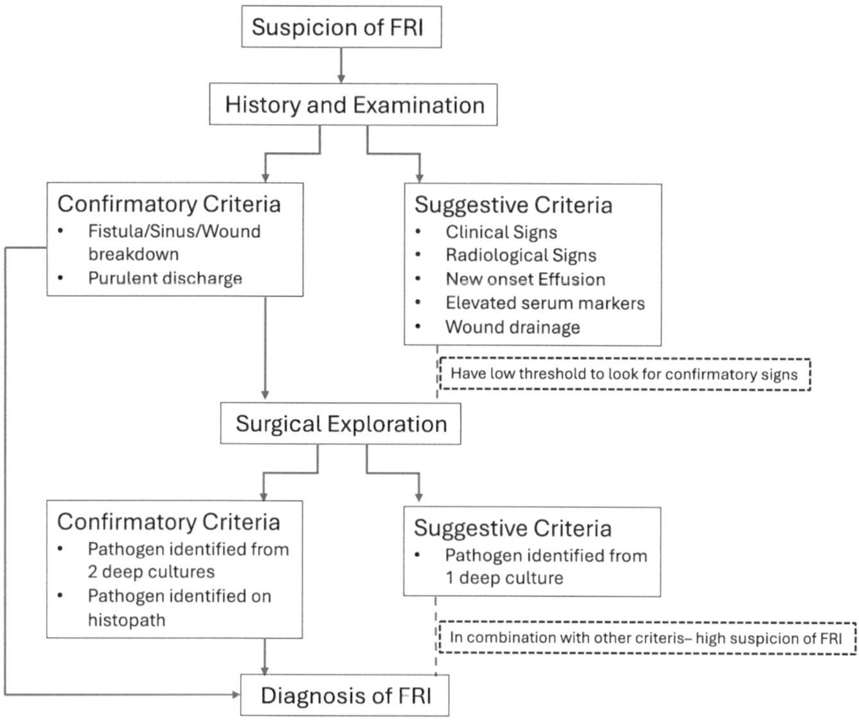

Fig. 14.1 The diagnostic criteria of FRI.

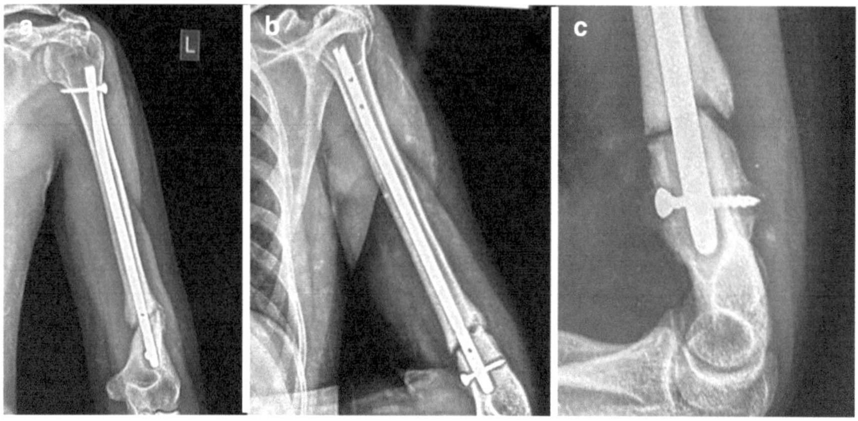

Fig. 14.2 X-rays suggestive of FRI in a humerus fracture fixed with interlocking nail. (**a**) AP view and (**b**) Lateral view. (**c**) Focused view of the distal humerus. Note the osteolysis at the distal lock and radiolucency around the nail

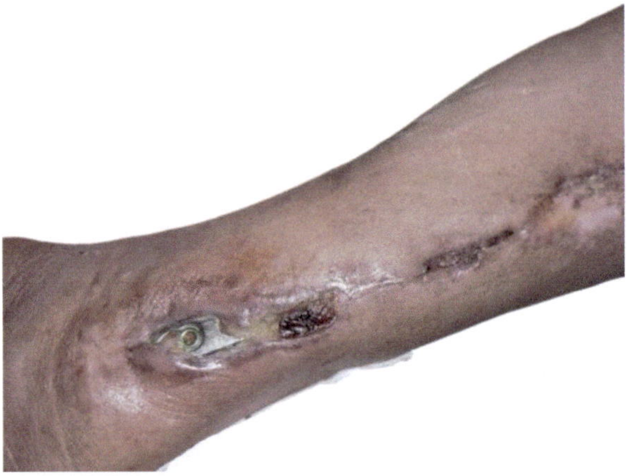

Fig. 14.3 FRI in tibia after attempted osteosynthesis with plating with pus discharge from multiple sinuses and wound dehiscence distally with exposed implant

can present with a wide variety of symptoms including pain, fever, swelling, discharge, wound dehiscence or generalized symptoms like weakness, night sweats, weight loss. Early signs, like pain, redness, and swelling, can overlap with normal healing. Examination should focus on localization of pain. Pain originating at the fracture site could also be because of implant prominence, bursitis over the metalware, poor reduction of an intraarticular fracture or sarcopenia. Serological tests include a complete cell count with a differential leucocyte count to check for lymphocytosis in chronic infections. Inflammatory biomarkers such as ESR and CRP are also commonly used. However, they have poor specificity (70%). ESR takes approximately 3 weeks to return to normal due to long half-life of fibronectin. CRP especially hs-CRP has high sensitivity (76%) and a quicker return to baseline levels in 5–7 days. Newer biomarkers like interleukin-6, alpha defensin have a role for early diagnosis of FRI. Kumar et al. [14] found that alpha-defensin is raised by >2.5 times in early FRI at post-op day 2 before other clinical signs set in. However, these tests are expensive and need further research to establish cut-off values. D-dimer and Procalcitonin are other markers raised in acute orthopedic infections.

Radiological tests include X-rays, CT scan, MRI and radionucleotide imaging. X-rays may show nonunion, osteopenia, osteolysis, sequestered bone, implant loosening and enhanced soft tissue shadows. CT scans can be used to check for cortical thickness and continuity, which is necessary while planning for implant exchange. MRI is a useful tool to check for soft tissue extension of the infection, intramedullary involvement, any localized collections and joint involvement, however, is limited by metal artifacts from the implant. Radionucleotide scans like positron emission tomography (PET), triple-phase bone scintigraphy (BS) and leucocyte scan (WBC labelled scan) are useful in identifying indolent infections and extent of disease. These tests are a feasible strategy in cases of recent trauma and surgery where conventional markers are usually elevated.

Microbial cultures are indispensable for diagnosis of the offending microbe and antibiotic stewardship. Superficial cultures taken in the outpatient setting are usually false positive due to contaminants and shouldn't be used. Deep cultures taken during debridement, usually multiple, are more representative. It must be remembered that atypical organisms like Cutibacterium acnes and Mycobacterium tuberculosis are fastidious, require special media for growth and take over 2–3 weeks. Hence extended cultures should be performed for suspected cases. It is recommended to avoid antibiotics for as long as 2 weeks before surgical debridement to prevent bacterial growth inhibition in-vitro. Cultures from implant surface obtained via sonication and from sequestered bone are more sensitive and specific and should be used if available. Histopathology to identify neutrophils or polymorphs per high power field (NP/HPF) has a high positive and negative predictive value. >5 NP/HPF is indicative of infection while 0 NP/HPF rules out infection and points towards aseptic nonunion.

New molecular methods using polymerase chain reaction are coming up for diagnosing FRI. However, since they are based on nucleic acid amplification, they can be positive even if the pathogen is dead creating false positives and this should be interpreted with caution.

According to the duration from fracture or fracture intervention to the onset of infection, FRI is classified as early (shorter than 2 weeks), delayed (2–10 weeks), and late (over 10 weeks) infections [13]. The Cierny–Mader (C-M) classification for OM is often selected, especially for those in the chronic stage.

14.4 Treatment

Treatment of FRI requires an interdisciplinary approach involving the orthopedic surgeon, plastic surgeon, microbiologist and infectious disease specialist (Figs. 14.4 and 14.5). Treatment is dictated by host condition, pathogen virulence and infection site and extent and patient's expectations. FRI, unlike PJI, is a heterogenous entity, with cases differing in anatomical location, articular communication, type of implant used, fixation achieved, status of soft tissue coverage and is the consequence of an emergency surgery.

Once the diagnosis of FRI is established, time of onset of infection plays a key role to determine the correct treatment. Implants in FRI are only necessary until fracture healing has occurred. As opposed to PJI, once the fracture has healed, implants can be removed.

14.4.1 Early FRI (< 2 Weeks)

In early FRI, the bone hasn't healed yet so fracture stability is not expected, necessitating fixation. Also, the pathogen is commonly a virulent organism. Biofilm formation and features of osteomyelitis usually are not fully established. The primary treatment comprises of DAIR (Debridement, antibiotics and implant retention) which has a good success rate. However, certain factors like intramedullary implants, implant loosening, secondary fracture displacement, compromised soft tissue may warrant an implant removal. If the implant is removed, the fracture needs stabilization either via implant exchange or a less invasive implant like an external fixator.

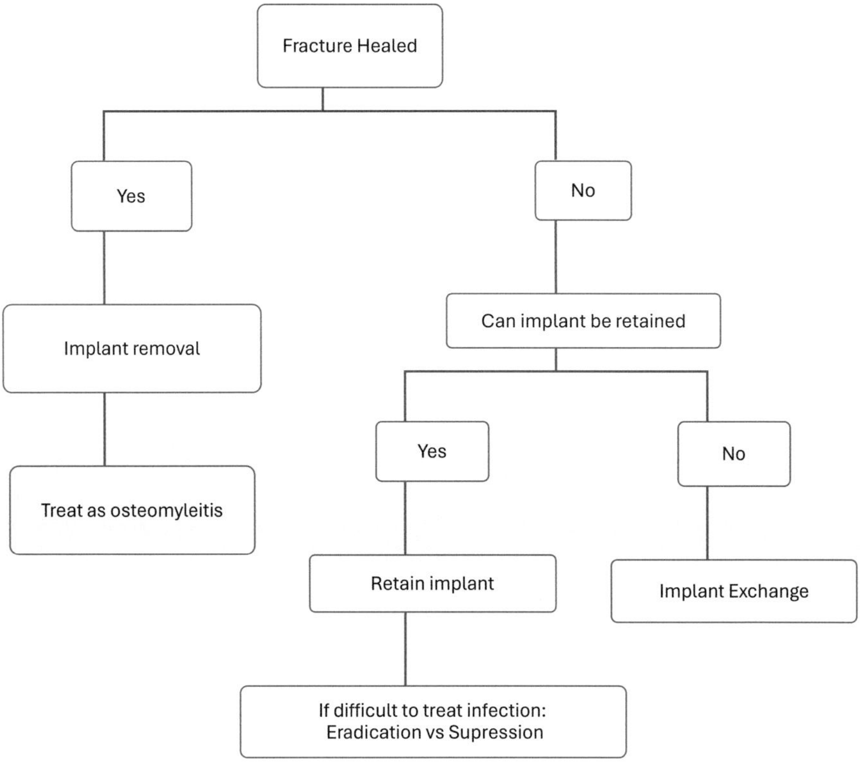

Fig. 14.4 Management algorithm for FRI

Antibiotic treatment should be commenced as soon as culture reports are available. Empirical antibiotics should be avoided unless the patient is in sepsis. Antibiotics can be administered intravenously or orally. Previously, intravenous antibiotics were recommended for the initial 2–3 weeks followed by oral antibiotics for the same duration. Recent evidence suggest that both have similar efficacies, while oral route is cheaper and not associated with risk of infection and thrombophlebitis [15]. Antibiotics were continued for 12 weeks in cases of implant retention. However, recent evidence suggests the total duration of antibiotics be restricted at 4–6 weeks since longer durations have no additional benefit but are associated with side effects and patient non-compliance. Infections associated with biofilm formation are intrinsically resistant to systemic antibiotics. However, Rifampicin and Fluroquinolones have shown to have ability to penetrate such biofilms and are useful in gram positive and gram negative bacterial infections, respectively [16]. Local administration of antibiotics after debridement helps achieve concentrations several times higher than systemic route and have lesser side effects. This can be done with cement (polymethylmethacrylate), poly-lactide, collagen sponges and hydrogels.

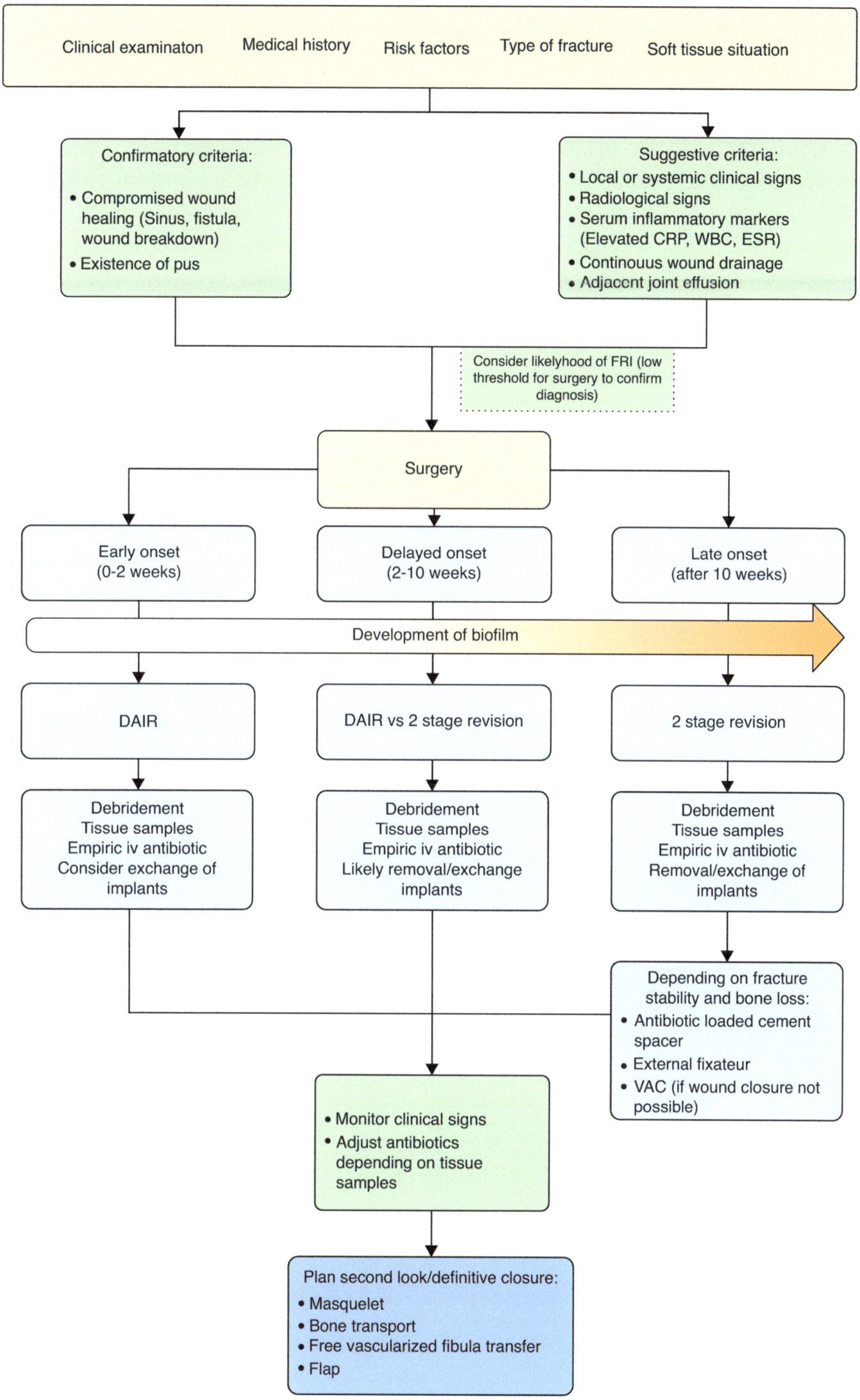

Fig. 14.5 Detailed algorithm for management of FRI

14.4.2 Late FRI (> 10 Weeks)

Late FRI can present with less distinctive symptoms. The fracture may or may not have healed. Infection creates a catabolic milieu regressing healing.

If the fracture has healed, implant removal, radical debridement along with wound coverage is usually sufficient to eradicate the infection. Removal of implant should always be favoured, so as soon as the fracture seems radiologically stable and bony healing is intraoperatively or radiologically confirmed, removal of implant is recommended. Effort should be made to remove the entire implant including any broken or cold-welded screws to reduce the risk of recurrence. All devitalized tissue including bone should be removed until good vascular tissue is reached. At least five samples of deep-tissue or fluid suspicious for infection, ideally taken from proximity to fracture and/or implant, are recommended. A standardized sampling protocol with separate, unused instruments placing specimen directly into sterile sample container should be used. Superficial samples, and sinus tracts should not be considered. Swabs are obsolete due to inferior sensitivity [17]. Intramedullary long bone infections can be reamed, and curettage can be used for metaphyseal infections and small bones. Antibiotic wash has no role in treatment but intra-operative addition of antibiotic-eluting substances like via calcium phosphate granules, ceramics, collagen sponges and post-op antibiotic irrigation systems are useful (Fig. 14.6) [18]. Primary closure of the wound may not always be possible, especially over bony prominences such as the elbow and knee with the patient requiring soft tissue flaps. The removed implant must undergo sonication and the fluid be sent for culture. Systemic antibiotics need to be administered based on culture sensitivity.

In cases where the bone hasn't healed, it is important to check for the construct stability [9]. If the fixation is stable, the implant can be retained. Implant removal is recommended in the following conditions: open fractures, intramedullary nail

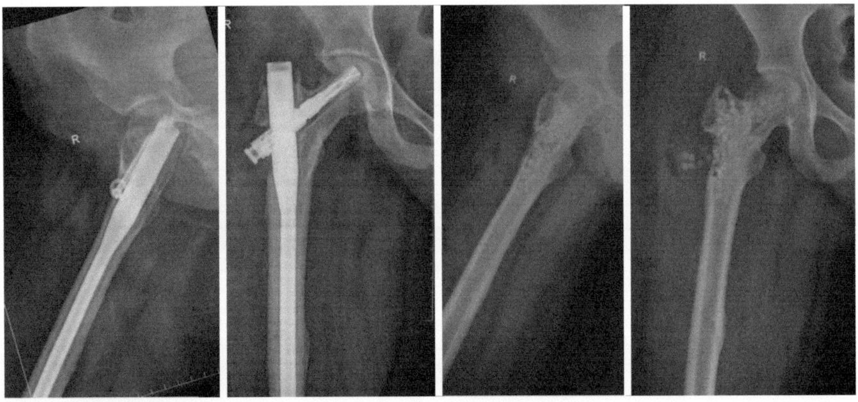

Fig. 14.6 A case of intertrochanteric fracture femur fixed with proximal femoral nail with osteolysis suggestive of infection. However bony union was achieved. Hence it was treated with implant removal and dead space was managed with antibiotic-impregnated calcium phosphate beads

fixation, poor fracture reduction or unstable fixation, poor soft tissue condition, highly virulent organisms, poor host immunity which is unlikely to recover in a short time, and if the patient is a smoker or drug addict [18, 19]. The new modality of fixation depends on the site of infection. Intramedullary infections can be treated with antibiotic-coated nails. External fixators and Ilizarov ring fixators can be used to decrease the implant load at the site of infection while providing stability. Bone defects and dead space after radical debridement may be treated with Masquelet technique (Figs. 14.7 and 14.8). A PMMA spacer is moulded into the resulting defect. This creates a foreign-body reaction, and a membrane is "induced" around the spacer. During secondary surgery, longitudinal membrane opening and spacer removal is performed. The cavity is then filled with morselized autologous bone graft and closed. The secondary surgery is possible from 4 to 8 weeks. Bone grafting is not recommended in the primary surgery since the graft undergoes osteolysis. Hybrid fixators and Illizarov fixators may serve as definitive management in certain cases.

Infection eradication is desired in cases where implant is retained, however, it may not always be possible. Unique to the treatment of FRI is infection suppression. Antibiotics may suppress bacterial proliferation and biofilm growth, preventing the local milieu from becoming acidic and catabolic. This promotes bone growth and fracture healing. Since implants used for fixation can be removed after union, unlike prosthesis, infection suppression can serve as a viable option in FRI, unlike prosthetic joint infection (PJI).

14.4.3 Delayed FRI (2–10 Weeks)

Delayed FRI can show aspects of either early or late stage infections. Pathogens are expected to be less virulent (i.e. Staphylocuccus epidermidis). Biofilm is more resistant to systemic antibiotic therapy. Progressive tissue invasion starts to be present, and bones can show signs of osteomyelitis. Management is as explained above.

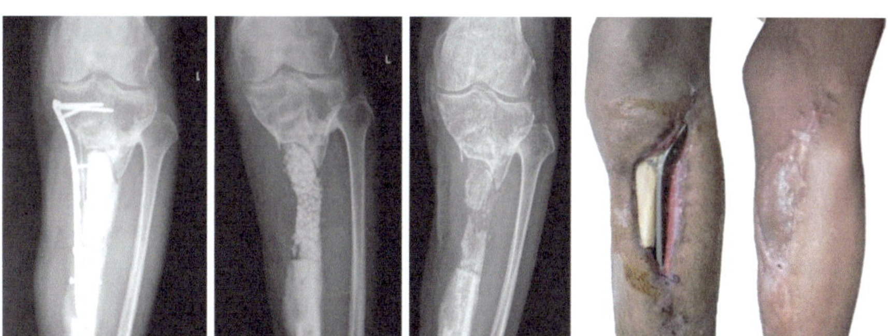

Fig. 14.7 A proximal tibia fracture which was treated via open reduction and fixation was infected with wound dehiscence. The implants were exchanged with antibiotic beads and soft tissue cover was obtained using a flap

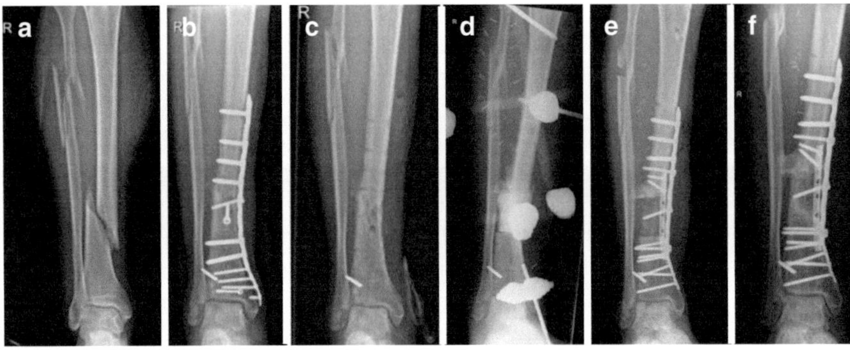

Fig. 14.8 Pre Op X-ray (**a**); Initial fixation (**b**); Implant removal due to infection (**c**); Temporizing external fixator with cement spacer for bone gap after sequestrectomy (**d**); Final fixation with bone graft (**e**); 2-year follow up (**f**)

14.5 Prevention of FRI

Strategies consist of management of surgical site contamination in open fractures and reducing the risk of iatrogenic microbial contamination. These include:

- Prompt management of open fractures with early irrigation, debridement and fracture stabilization along with early empirical antibiotics.
- Maintaining an aseptic environment in the operation theatre and following sterile protocols.
- Optimizing patient risk factors such as perioperative glycemic control, quitting smoking, and treating malnutrition. These may not always be possible in the emergency setting, but should always be tried.

14.6 Implications of FRI

FRI is associated with a large health cost, including social, mental, and economic. They have poorer pain scores and worse physical function even after completion of treatment. Patients with FRI require a large volume of healthcare resources, have longer operative and admission durations. The cost of treatment is three to six times that of an average fracture fixation. The average length of stay for FRI is five to eight times and the rate of readmission is also five times higher. Patients with FRI have shown to have a higher risk of substance use. They are also more susceptible to mental health disorders like depression [8]. Apart from the above, the economic burden in terms of loss of productivity for the patient due to prolonged morbidity is much larger and cannot be estimated. Despite this, resources which are often applied for elective arthroplasty are virtually nonexistent for preventing, monitoring, and accounting for FRI.

Many steps can be taken to prevent FRI. Early administration of antibiotics has proven to be the most effective method to reduce the incidence of infections in open fractures. Through wash with copious amounts of saline in the emergency as well as in the operating room, surgery under antibiotic cover with the drug being administered before tourniquet inflation, staged surgery with external fixator primarily followed by definitive fixation 5–7 days later (conversion osteosynthesis), early soft tissue coverage, vacuum-assisted closure are other important ways to decrease the risk of FRI.

Bibliography

1. Gustilo RB, Anderson JT. Prevention of infection in the treatment of one thousand and twenty-five open fractures of long bones: retrospective and prospective analyses. JBJS. 1976;58(4):453.
2. Jorge-Mora A, Amhaz-Escanlar S, González IC, Teso CLD, Gómez R, Jorge-Mora T, et al. Management of open fracture [internet]. In: Trauma surgery. IntechOpen; 2018. [cited 2023 Mar 12]. Available from: https://www.intechopen.com/chapters/59356.
3. Garner MR, Sethuraman SA, Schade MA, Boateng H. Antibiotic prophylaxis in open fractures: evidence, evolving issues, and recommendations. J Am Acad Orthop Surg. 2020;28(8):309–15.
4. Ye Z, Zhao S, Zeng C, Luo Z, Yuan S, Li R. Study on the relationship between the timing of conversion from external fixation to internal fixation and infection in the treatment of open fractures of extremities. J Orthop Surg Res. 2021;16(1):662.
5. Castillo RC, Bosse MJ, MacKenzie EJ, Patterson BM, LEAP Study Group. Impact of smoking on fracture healing and risk of complications in limb-threatening open tibia fractures. J Orthop Trauma. 2005;19(3):151–7.
6. Morris BJ, Unger RZ, Archer KR, Mathis SL, Perdue AM, Obremskey WT. Risk factors of infection after ORIF of bicondylar tibial plateau fractures. J Orthop Trauma. 2013;27(9):e196–200.
7. Depypere M, Morgenstern M, Kuehl R, Senneville E, Moriarty TF, Obremskey WT, et al. Pathogenesis and management of fracture-related infection. Clin Microbiol Infect. 2020;26(5):572–8.
8. Foster AL, Warren J, Vallmuur K, Jaiprakash A, Crawford R, Tetsworth K, et al. A population-based epidemiological and health economic analysis of fracture-related infection. Bone Joint J. 2024;106-B(1):77–85.
9. Kuehl R, Tschudin-Sutter S, Morgenstern M, Dangel M, Egli A, Nowakowski A, et al. Time-dependent differences in management and microbiology of orthopaedic internal fixation-associated infections: an observational prospective study with 229 patients. Clin Microbiol Infect. 2019;25(1):76–81.
10. Zimmerli W. Bone and joint infections: from microbiology to diagnostics and treatment. Wiley; 2021. p. 466.
11. Gristina AG, Naylor P, Myrvik Q. Infections from biomaterials and implants: a race for the surface. Med Prog Technol. 1988;14(3–4):205–24.
12. Rozis M, Evangelopoulos DS, Pneumaticos SG. Orthopedic implant-related biofilm pathophysiology: a review of the literature. Cureus. 13(6):e15634.
13. Metsemakers WJ, Morgenstern M, McNally MA, Moriarty TF, McFadyen I, Scarborough M, et al. Fracture-related infection: a consensus on definition from an international expert group. Injury. 2018;49(3):505–10.
14. Kumar P, Mittal A, Bansal P, Aggarwal S, Rajnish RK, Dadra A, et al. Wound alpha defensin levels are significantly higher in patients with fracture related infection: a pilot, prospective cohort study. Injury. 2023;54(2):416–21.
15. Li HK, Rombach I, Zambellas R, Walker AS, McNally MA, Atkins BL, et al. Oral versus intravenous antibiotics for bone and joint infection. N Engl J Med. 2019;380(5):425–36.

16. Depypere M, Kuehl R, Metsemakers WJ, Senneville E, McNally MA, Obremskey WT, et al. Recommendations for systemic antimicrobial therapy in fracture-related infection: a consensus from an international expert group. J Orthop Trauma. 2020;34(1):30–41.
17. Hellebrekers P, Rentenaar RJ, McNally MA, Hietbrink F, Houwert RM, Leenen LPH, et al. Getting it right first time: The importance of a structured tissue sampling protocol for diagnosing fracture-related infections. Injury 2019;50:1649–55. https://doi.org/10.1016/j.injury.2019.05.014.
18. He SY, Yu B, Jiang N. Current concepts of fracture-related infection. Int J Clin Pract [Internet]. 2023; [cited 2024 Jul 27]. Available from: https://www.ncbi.nlm.nih.gov/pmc/articles/PMC10154639/
19. Nan Jiang, Bo-Wei Wang. Chinese expert consensus on diagnosis and treatment of infection after fracture fixation. Injury. 2019;50(11):1952–8.

Spinal Infections: Understanding, Diagnosis, and Treatment

15

Aditya Gupta and Vishal Kumar

Abstract

Spinal infections occur as a result of either bacterial or fungal invasion of the spine. It is most commonly caused by staphylococcus aureus, as a result of direct contamination from surgery or trauma, spread from another infected site in the body, or through the bloodstream, or as a result of spinal procedures such as spinal injections or surgery. Early recognition and diagnosis is crucial for successful treatment. A thorough evaluation including blood tests, imaging studies such as X-rays, CT scans, or MRI scans, and obtaining a sample of the infected spinal fluid must be conducted to confirm the diagnosis.

Keywords

Spine · Infections · Tuberculosis · Diagnosis · Investigations, · Management

15.1 Introduction

Spinal infections represent a challenging medical condition that presents with significant pain, immobility, and other severe consequences if not promptly diagnosed and appropriately managed. These infections can affect any part of the spine, including the vertebrae, intervertebral discs, and surrounding soft tissues [1]. It can lead to significant morbidity and neurological deficits. Extrapolating the causes, clinical implications, approach to diagnosis, and different modalities of treatment is crucial for healthcare providers to effectively manage spinal infections. It is a serious and potentially life-threatening condition that can affect individuals of all ages. It can be

A. Gupta · V. Kumar (✉)
PGIMER, Chandigarh, India

P. Kumar et al. (eds.), *Textbook of Orthopedic Infections*,
https://doi.org/10.1007/978-981-95-5029-6_15

caused by bacteria, viruses, or fungi and may lead to severe complications if not promptly diagnosed and treated.

15.2 Pathogenesis

The pathogenesis typically involves the introduction of microorganisms into the spinal tissues, followed by their proliferation and the host's inflammatory response [2]. Several factors can predispose individuals to spinal infections, which include immunocompromised status caused by immunosuppressive drugs, IV drug abuse, Diabetes Mellitus, or smoking, malnutrition, history of systemic infection (UTI, pneumonia), malignancy, and obesity.

15.2.1 Inoculation Can Occur Via

(a) Hematogenous seeding: The microbes can travel through the arterial or venous systems to reach the endplates and intervertebral discs. These low-flow regions at vascular anastomosis at the endplates aid in inoculation. Microbes first involve a single endplate followed by intervertebral disc and then the adjacent endplate.
(b) Direct inoculation: It usually occurs due to surgical procedure or open fracture.
(c) Associated with local infection: Most commonly caused by retropharyngeal and retroperitoneal abscesses.

15.3 Clinical Manifestations

The clinical presentation of spinal infections can differ based on the affected structures, the causative microorganism, and the patient's overall health status [3]. Common symptoms may include:

- Localised Pain: Persistent and localised back pain, which may worsen with movement or palpation, is a hallmark feature of spinal infections.
- Fever: It is a systemic response to the infection.
- Neurological Deficits: In 10–20%, patients may develop neurodeficits like weakness, numbness, or involvement of bowel and bladder, secondary to spinal cord compression or nerve root involvement. Compression from instability of the spine can also lead to progressive neurodeficit.
- Limited Mobility: Patients may experience reduced range of motion in the spine and stiffness.
- Soft Tissue Swelling: Epidural abscess can present as swelling, erythema, and warmth over the affected spinal region. Nearly 50% of patients with an epidural abscess will have neurologic symptoms. Psoas abscess may also be present.

15.4 Types and Causes of Spinal Infections

Spinal infections can be broadly categorised into three main types: Vertebral osteomyelitis, Discitis, Spinal Tuberculosis, Spinal Epidural Abscess and Spine Surgical Site Infection [4]. Vertebral osteomyelitis refers to the infection of the vertebral bodies, while discitis involves the infection of the intervertebral discs. Spinal epidural abscesses are collections of pus located within the epidural space, which can cause pressure on the spinal cord, leading to neurological deficits.

Adult Pyogenic Vertebral Osteomyelitis or spondylodiskitis includes discitis, vertebral osteomyelitis, and epidural abscess. It is usually seen in adults in the sixth and seventh decade of life. Most cases involve lumbar spine followed by thoracic spine (Fig. 15.1).

The most common causative agents of spinal infections are bacteria, with Staphylococcus aureus being the predominant pathogen in 60–65% patients followed by Staph epidermidis [5]. Other bacteria, such as Streptococcus species, Escherichia coli, and Pseudomonas aeruginosa, can also cause spinal infections, especially in patients with predisposing factors such as IV drug use, immunocompromised states, diabetes mellitus, or recent spinal procedures [6]. Fungal and atypical bacterial pathogens, including Mycobacterium tuberculosis, can also cause spinal infections, particularly in certain geographic regions or patient populations. Approximately 18% of patients with spondylodiscitis are present with spinal epidural abscess.

Spinal Epidural Abscess is caused by a collection of pus or inflammatory granulation tissue between the dura mater and surrounding adipose tissue. It is usually seen in adults >60 years of age. Early diagnosis is critical and is made with MRI

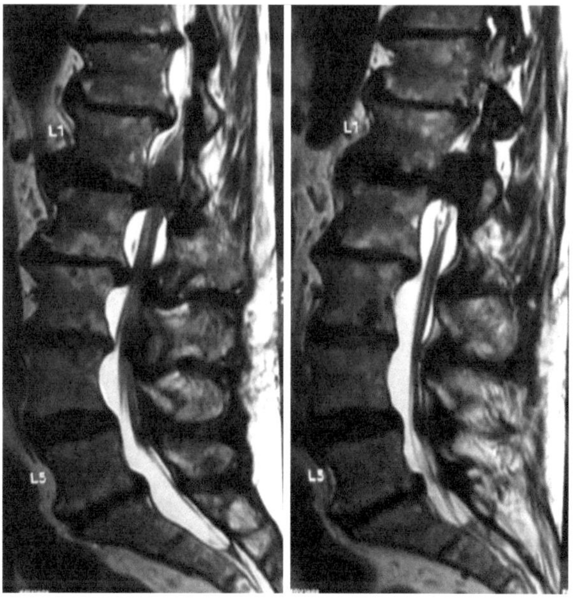

Fig. 15.1 Discitis with endplate erosion

studies with contrast and involves dorsal part of thoracolumbar spine. Treatment is usually aggressive surgical decompression and long-term administration of IV antibiotics (Fig. 15.2).

Spinal Tuberculosis (Pott's Disease) incidence is also increasing due to increased immunocompromised population. Pott's spine usually manifests as kyphotic deformity due to destruction and osteomyelitis of vertebral body leading to progressive instability. The diagnosis is confirmed with biopsy (preferably CT guided) and the tissue sample sent for acid-fast bacilli. Anti-tubercular drugs are given (HRZE for 2 months) followed by HR for 9–18 months. Surgical intervention is done if there is worsening or severe neurological deficits, increasing kyphotic deformity $>80^\circ$ or presence of mechanical instability (Fig. 15.3).

Infection starts in the metaphysis of the vertebral body and spreads under the anterior longitudinal ligament leading to involvement at multilevels, formation of skip lesion or paraspinal abscess. Compared to pyogenic osteomyelitis, disc space involvement occurs later.

Chronic infection manifests as severe kyphosis. The diagnosis is often delayed due to sub-acute clinical presentation and delayed presentation owing generally to the poor socio-economic status of the patients or misdiagnosis as simple backache. There is often much more severe kyphosis in granulomatous spinal infections compared to pyogenic infections. The kyphosis stays static after healing in adults but progress in 40% of children due to growth spurt.

Rajasekaran classification of progression: [7]

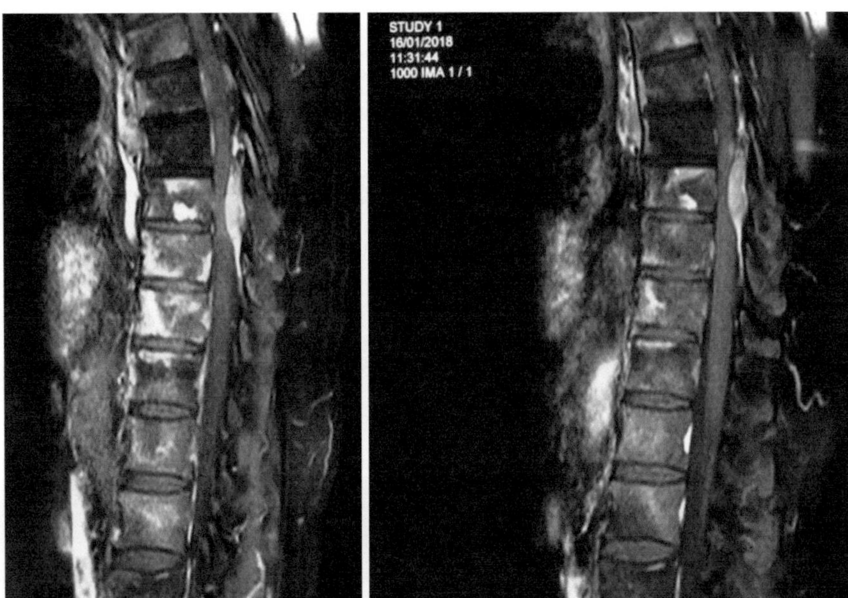

Fig. 15.2 Epidural abscess

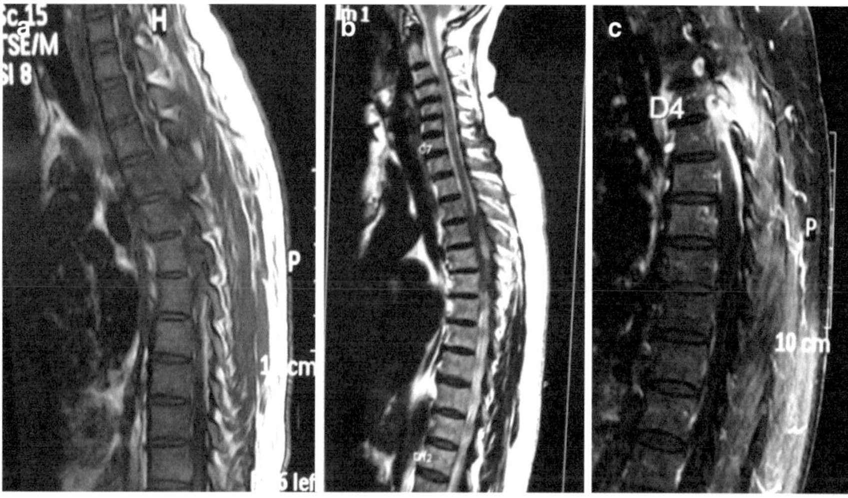

Fig. 15.3 (**a**) T1WI shows vertebral body destruction and epidural abscess in Pott's spine. (**b**)-T2WI shows canal involvement and abscess in Pott's spine. (**c**) CE MRI shows paraspinal muscle involvement and active infection

Type-I: Increase in deformity until cessation of growth, treated with surgery.
Type-II: Decreasing progression with growth.
Type-III: Minimal change during either active/healed phases.

Constitutional symptoms include chronic illness, malaise, night sweats, weight loss, and back pain. Back pain occurs later in the course after significant bony destruction and deformity. Radiographs show involvement of anterior vertebral body with sparing of the disc space in early stages. Disk space destruction, lucency, and compression of adjacent vertebral bodies, and development of severe kyphosis are seen in later stages.

"Spine at risk signs": They include retropulsion, subluxation, lateral translation, and toppling. These indicate risk factors for buckling collapse.

Treatment of Pott's spine consists of the "middle path regime" proposed by S. M. Tuli. The key principles of this regime are:

- Combination of Medical and Surgical Treatment:
  - Initiate with ATT to control the infection.
  - Reserve surgery for cases with specific indications such as significant spinal deformity, neurological deficits, or lack of response to medical therapy.
- Indications for Surgery:
  - Progressive neurological deficit.
  - Severe spinal instability or deformity.
  - Abscess formation that does not resolve with medical treatment.

- Failure of medical management (persistent or worsening infection despite adequate ATT).

- Surgical Goals:
  - Decompression of neural elements to prevent or address neurological damage.
  - Debridement of necrotic and infected tissue.
  - Stabilisation of the spine to prevent or correct deformity.
- Advantages of the Middle Path Regime:
  - Reduces the morbidity associated with extensive surgical procedures.
  - Minimises the risk of drug resistance and recurrence through adequate ATT.
  - Balances the need for surgical intervention with the benefits of conservative treatment.
- Postoperative Care:
  - Continued ATT for a sufficient duration to ensure complete eradication of the infection.
  - Regular monitoring and follow-up to assess the patient's response to treatment and adjust the plan as needed.

Operative treatment is indicated with worsening neurological deficit, acute severe paraplegia, presence of instability or worsening kyphotic deformity and includes anterior decompression with or with our corpectomy, and posterior-instrumented stabilisation along with strut grafting. Minimally Invasive Techniques like Video-Assisted Thoracoscopic Surgery (VATS) or endoscopic techniques for debridement and decompression in select cases. Percutaneous or open drainage of large paravertebral or psoas abscesses is indicated for large abscesses not responding to ATT Drugs.

15.5 Diagnosis

The diagnosis of spinal infections requires a systematic approach, incorporating clinical evaluation, imaging studies, and laboratory tests [8]. Key steps in the diagnostic process include:

1. Clinical Assessment: Medical history combined with physical examination can help in diagnosing the presence of spinal infection, including risk factors, symptom duration, and neurological findings.
2. Laboratory Tests: Blood tests showing lymphocytosis with neutrophilia, elevated Erythrocyte Sedimentation Rate (ESR), C-Reactive Protein (CRP) can help support the diagnosis of spinal infection and blood cultures can identify the causative microorganism. ESR is elevated in most cases but is less reliable than CRP. CRP can be monitored serially to track success of treatment. Blood culture is indicated prior to antibiotic administration in all patients infected with

unknown infectious agent as identification of organism is mandatory for treatment. It is the least invasive method to determine a diagnosis. In Potts' spine, there is relative lymphocytosis, low haemoglobin, and elevated ESR.

3. Imaging Studies: Radiological imaging (X-rays), Magnetic Resonance Imaging (MRI), and Computed Tomography (CT) scans, are essential for visualising spinal anatomy and identifying signs of infection, such as bone destruction, disc space narrowing, or abscess formation.

X-ray findings including narrowing and destruction of disc space is seen earliest by 7–10 days. CT scan is useful to show bony abnormalities, abscess formation, and extent of bony involvement.

MRI is the gold standard for diagnosis with high sensitivity (96%) and specificity (93%). MRI findings of spondylodiscitis include epidural inflammation, paraspinal inflammation, which enhances with gadolinium. T2-weighted MRI images show hyper-intensity of the disc and endplate rim enhancement. Technetium (Tc99m) and bone scans are indicated in patients who cannot obtain an MRI. Pott's spine shows reduced signal on T1-weighted images and high-intensity signal on T2-weighted images. A smooth-walled abscess with a subligamentous extension and breaching of the epidural space can be seen. Other features include endplate disruption, paravertebral soft tissue shadow. Spinal cord may show edema, myelomalacia, atrophy, and syringomyelia (Fig. 15.4).

4. Biopsy: Biopsy is used to confirm the diagnosis and is done in all patients with positive findings on MRI. CT-guided biopsy is primary modality of diagnosis in patients who have negative blood cultures. It can provide diagnosis in 68–86% of patients. It can be guided by fluoroscopy or by CT scan. The cultures are sent for aerobic, anaerobic, fungal, and acid-fast cultures. A tissue biopsy may be performed to obtain samples for microbial culture and sensitivity testing to isolate the micro-organism. Diagnosis of Pott's spine is confirmed with cultures and staining. The TB microbes should be tested for Acid-Fast bacilli (AFB). PCR allows for faster identification with 94% sensitivity and 92% accuracy.

15.6 Treatment

The management of spinal infections is a multifaceted process that aims to eradicate the infection, relieve pain, preserve spinal stability, prevent neurological dysfunction, and promote bone fusion in the affected segments. Conservative treatment goals include eradicating the microbial agent, preserving neurological function, restoring spinal stability and morphology, debriding and decompressing the spinal canal in the presence of epidural abscess, and promoting bone fusion. Surgical intervention in spinal infections involves obtaining an organism culture, debriding the infection, and maintaining neurological and mechanical stability. Early detection and aggressive treatment are crucial in managing post-procedural spinal infections to limit long-term sequelae.

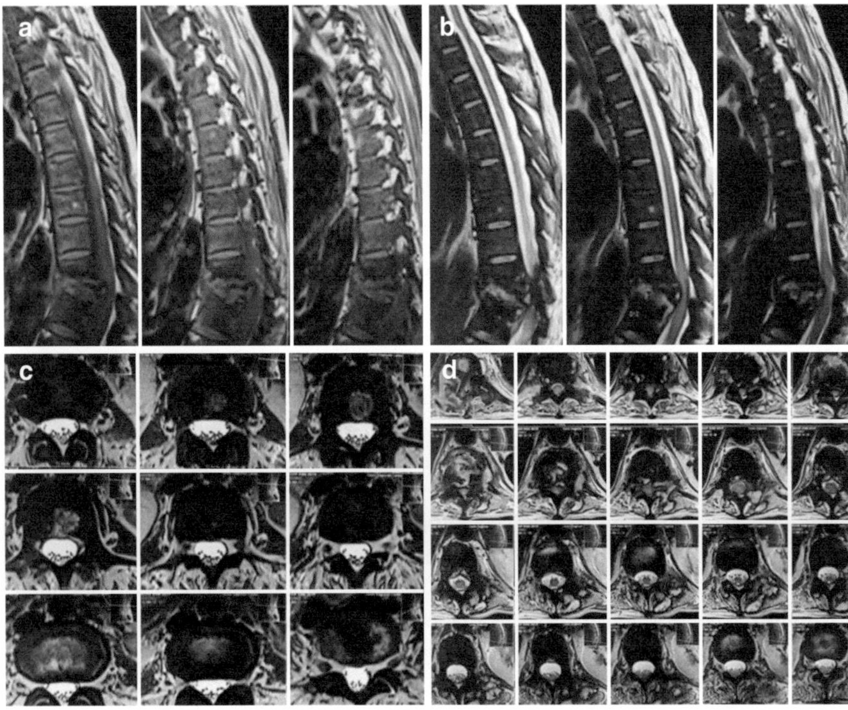

Fig. 15.4 Pott's spine. Slow signal on T1-weighted images (**a**) and bright signal on T2-weighted images (**b**). Presence of subligamentous extension and endplate disruption, paravertebral soft tissue shadow can be seen. Spinal cord shows edema and myelomalacia (**c**, **d**)

For specific types of spinal infections, such as spinal implant infections, early onset of cases can be successfully treated with debridement, implant retention, and antimicrobial therapy. In cases of infections caused by pathogens, like Staphylococcus aureus or Coxiella burnetii, a combination of antibiotic therapy and surgical intervention is essential for successful treatment. Disseminated spinal infections, such as those caused by Coccidioidomycosis, may require antifungal drugs and surgical treatment.

The management of spinal infections continues to evolve with the advancement of diagnostic tools and surgical techniques. Hyperbaric oxygen therapy, antibiotic therapy, debridement, decompression of the spinal canal, and fixation of affected segments are key principles for successful treatment. Surgical management may involve minimal debridement of infected tissue, which has shown to be a safe and effective method. The duration of antibiotic therapy post-debridement in spinal implant infections is still a topic of debate, with some advocating for long-term antimicrobial therapy.

In conclusion, the treatment of spinal infections requires a multidisciplinary approach that combines conservative and surgical interventions tailored to the specific type of infection. Early detection, aggressive treatment, and adherence to established guidelines are crucial in achieving successful outcomes and preventing long-term complications.

15.6.1 Nonoperative

In septic, critically ill patients with spinal abscess or discitis, broad spectrum antibiotics are administered to the patient immediately, otherwise gram stains and cultures are first obtained before starting the antibiotic. CT-guided aspiration before administration of culture-specific IV antibiotics is the ideal recommended protocol.

Vancomycin remains the drug of choice for penicillin-resistant and gram-positive bacteria. Third-generation cephalosporin is used for coverage of gram-negative organism. Organism-specific antibiotic for 6–12 weeks with or without bracing can eradicate the infection in majority of the cases. However, some advocate surgical debridement to improve pain and prevent deformity. Rigid cervicothoracic orthosis or halo traction is used for stabilisation of spine and reduce muscle spasm in cervical osteomyelitis. Culture-specific antibiotics are administered intravenously until signs of improvement are seen and then converted to oral antibiotics. There is an increase in anti-microbial resistance to antibiotics. The most common example is Staph aureus-MRSA (methicillin-resistant Staph aureus), VRSA (vancomycin-resistant Staph aureus), and VRE (vancomycin-resistant enterococcus). Linezolid and daptomycin are newer generation of antibiotics for antibiotic resistant organisms. [9]

15.6.2 Operative

Operative treatment is indicated if there is worsening neurodeficit, refractory cases, formation of large spinal abscess or increase in deformity. Anterior debridement and strut grafting with or without posterior instrumentation is the treatment of choice with anterior debridement having better results.

Bone grafts have been used to increase the stability of the spinal column. They are usually effective and safe to use even in the presence of acute infection. Autograft obtained from tricortical iliac crest, ribs or fibula strut grafts have better incorporation and lesser chances of failure and rejection compared to allograft. The bone grafts can be supplemented with mesh cages filled with autograft. These cages are made of PEEK (Polyether Ether Ketone), titanium, or stainless steel. Pedicle screw fixation and posterior fixation can also augment the stability of the construct and are safe to use. It is recommended to carry out debridement, bone grafting, and fixation in a single procedure in the presence of an active infection [10]. Titanium is preferred over stainless steel. Posterior instrumentation is indicated when severe kyphotic deformity or a multilevel anterior construct is noticed. Spinal epidural abscess requires immediate surgical decompression and administration of long-term IV antibiotics (Fig. 15.5).

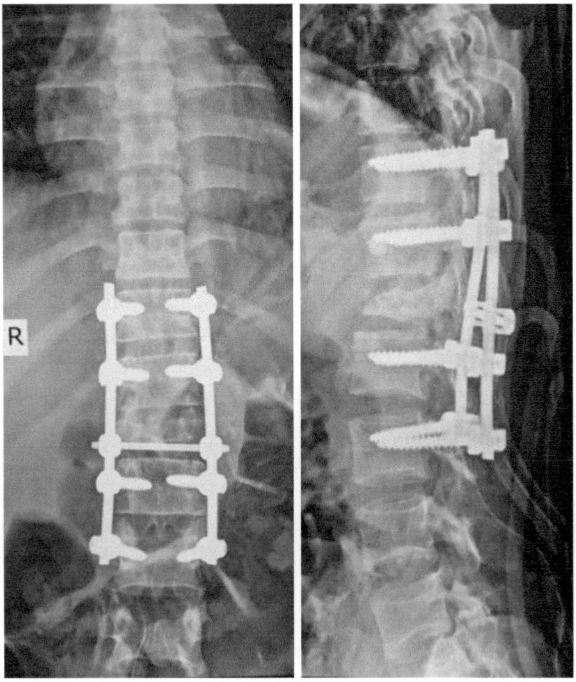

Fig. 15.5 Anterior decompression + posterior instrumented stabilization

15.7 Prevention

Preventing spinal infections involves strategies aimed at reducing the risk of microbial contamination and optimising patient outcomes following spinal procedures [11].

- Aseptic Technique: Healthcare providers should adhere to strict sterile protocols during spinal surgeries, including hand hygiene, use of sterile drapes and instruments, and appropriate peri-operative antimicrobial prophylaxis.
- Patient Optimisation: Preoperative optimisation of modifiable risk factors, such as diabetes control, smoking cessation, and nutritional supplementation, can improve surgical outcomes and reduce the risk of postoperative infections.
- Surveillance and Education: Healthcare facilities should implement surveillance programmes to monitor for surgical site infections and provide education to healthcare providers and patients regarding infection prevention strategies.

Take-Home Message

Spinal infections represent a significant clinical challenge, requiring early recognition and active management to prevent complications. By knowing the causes, clinical symptoms, diagnostic approaches, and treatment modalities associated with spinal infections, healthcare providers can optimise patient outcomes and reduce the burden of this debilitating condition. Continued research efforts aimed at elucidating the pathogenesis, improving diagnostic techniques, and developing novel therapeutic strategies are essential for advancing the field of spinal infection management.

References

1. Tsantes AG, Papadopoulos DV, Vrioni G, et al. Spinal infections: an update. Microorganisms. 2020;8(4):476. Published 2020 Mar 27. https://doi.org/10.3390/microorganisms8040476.
2. Alpantaki K, Katonis P, Hadjipavlou AG. Microbiological findings in spinal infections. Spine J. 2007;7(3):325–30.
3. Weng LM, Zheng Y, Qu B. Clinical characteristics and surgical treatment of thoracolumbar spinal tuberc. 2017.
4. Tschöke SK, Oberle J, Sellenschloh K, Kobbe P, Pishnamaz M, Pfeifer R. Spinal infections: diagnosis and treatment. Dtsch Arztebl Int. 2020;117(8):123–30.
5. Rutges JP, Kempen DH, van Dijk M, Oner FC, Leenen LP. Outcome of conservative and surgical treatment of pyogenic spondylodiscitis: a systematic literature review. Eur Spine J. 2014;23(1):120–31.
6. Gouliouris T, Aliyu SH, Brown NM. Spondylodiscitis: update on diagnosis and management. J Antimicrob Chemother. 2010;65(suppl_3):iii11–24. ulosis: a retrospective analysis of 30 cases. Pakistan Journal of Medical Sciences, 33(4), 848
7. Rajasekaran S. The natural history of post-tubercular kyphosis in children. Radiological signs which predict late increase in deformity. J Bone Joint Surg Br. 2001;83(7):954–62. https://doi.org/10.1302/0301-620x.83b7.12170.
8. Saeed K, Eschweiler J. Diagnosis and management of pyogenic spinal infections. Biomed Res Int. 2018;2018
9. Hogan JI, Hurt JB. Practical management of spinal infections. Phys Sportsmed. 2016;44(4):399–406.
10. Kasliwal MK, Tan LA, Traynelis VC. Infection with spinal instrumentation: review of pathogenesis, diagnosis, prevention, and management. Surg Neurol Int. 2013;4(Suppl 5):S392–403. Published 2013 Oct 29. https://doi.org/10.4103/2152-7806.120783.
11. Sanjari MA, Azimian J, Ebrahimi A, Mousavi SM. Prevention and treatment of postoperative spondylodiscitis. J Orthop Surg Res. 2019;14(1):45.

Diabetic Foot Infection

16

Uttam Chand Saini, Singh Akashdeep, and Ashu Rastogi

Abstract

Septic arthritis is an uncommon but potentially destructive joint infection, most often caused by *Staphylococcus aureus*. It typically presents as acute monoarthritis, most frequently involving the knee, but can also affect other large joints or occur in a polyarticular form. Pathogenesis involves bacterial seeding of the synovium, leading to rapid inflammation, cartilage destruction, and potential systemic complications. Risk factors include rheumatoid arthritis, diabetes, immunosuppression, skin disease, prior joint pathology, and injection drug use, though cases may arise without predisposing conditions. Diagnosis relies on a high index of suspicion, supported by synovial fluid analysis, cultures, and clinical assessment. Early recognition and prompt treatment are essential to preserve joint function and reduce morbidity and mortality.

Keywords

Septic arthritis · Joint Infection · *Staphylococcus aureus* · Monoarthritis · Synovial fluid

U. C. Saini (✉) · S. Akashdeep
Department of Orthopedic Surgery, PGIMER, Chandigarh, India

A. Rastogi
Department of Endocrinology and Metabolism, Post-Graduate Institute of Medical Education and Research (PGIMER), Chandigarh, India

P. Kumar et al. (eds.), *Textbook of Orthopedic Infections*,
https://doi.org/10.1007/978-981-95-5029-6_16

Table 16.1 Categories of diabetic foot infections

Infection type	Affected tissue or structure
Paronychia	Soft tissue surrounding the toe nail
Cellulitis	Skin (dermis) and underlying fat
Myositis	Muscle tissue
Abscess	Accumulation of inflammatory fluid
Necrotizing soft tissue infection	Fat, muscle, and/or fascia
Septic arthritis	Joint cavity
Tendonitis	Tendon
Osteomyelitis	Bone

16.1 Introduction

Diabetes has become a widespread issue, bringing with it an increased risk of related complications. According to the International Diabetes Federation, nearly 700 million people are projected to be living with diabetes by 2045 [1]. The term "Diabetic Foot" encompasses a range of conditions such as diabetic neuropathy, peripheral vascular disease, Charcot's neuroarthropathy, foot ulcers, osteomyelitis, and in some cases, limb amputation, which could often be prevented [2]. Approximately 15% of people with diabetes will develop foot ulcers, and of those, 14–24% may face the need for amputation due to bone infection or complications from the ulcer [3]. Given the significant morbidity associated with osteomyelitis and amputations in diabetic foot infection (DFI) patients, addressing the root causes is critical. Some common types of DFIs are given in Table 16.1. This review aims to offer a new perspective on the epidemiology of DFIs, summarize key aspects of their development, highlight challenges like antimicrobial resistance, explore diagnostic and management strategies, and identify important treatment-related complications relevant to healthcare providers.

16.2 Pathophysiology of Diabetic Foot Infection

The pathogenesis of diabetic foot infection is explained by a triad: neuropathy, vascular insufficiency, and secondary infection from foot trauma [4].

Neuropathy Diabetes-induced sensory neuropathy results from hyperglycaemia, which up-regulates aldose reductase and sorbitol dehydrogenase, producing sorbitol and fructose. These compounds cause osmotic stress, reducing nerve cell myoinositol synthesis and impairing nerve conduction [5]. Additionally, advanced glycation end-products (AGEs) form due to elevated glucose, exacerbating diabetic complications [6]. Autonomic neuropathy leads to reduced sweat production, resulting in dry, cracked skin that is prone to fissures [7]. Motor neuropathy contributes to muscle atrophy and foot deformities, increasing plantar pressure points and ulcer risk [8, 9].

Impaired Wound Healing Chronic DFIs fail to progress through the normal phases of healing—hemostasis, inflammation, proliferation, and remodeling [10, 11]. Hyperglycemia disrupts these processes by inducing excessive neutrophil extracellular trap (NET) formation (NETosis), triggering an overproduction of pro-inflammatory cytokines and superoxide [12–14]. AGEs interact with the receptor for advanced glycation end-products (RAGE), activating nuclear factor kappa-B (NF-κB), and prolonging inflammation [15–17]. This self-sustaining inflammatory cascade delays healing and promotes apoptosis.

Extracellular Matrix (ECM) Dysregulation The ECM, crucial for wound repair, becomes highly disorganized in DFUs due to hyperactive matrix metalloproteinases (MMPs), which degrade collagen and create a proteolytic environment [18–20]. AGEs further impair ECM repair by reducing fibroblast growth factor (FGF) and transforming growth factor-beta (TGF-β), promoting fibroblast apoptosis, and decreasing collagen synthesis [21–23].

Impaired Angiogenesis Angiogenesis, essential for granulation tissue formation and nutrient delivery, is significantly impaired in DFUs [24]. Key growth factors like vascular endothelial growth factor (VEGF) and fibroblast growth factor-2 (FGF-2), which mediate endothelial proliferation and migration, are reduced [25–27]. Endothelial progenitor cells (EPCs), vital for expressing pro-angiogenic factors, are deficient in type 2 diabetes due to AGE accumulation [28–31]. This impairs new blood vessel formation and contributes to chronic non-healing ulcers.

16.3 Classification of Diabetic Foot Infections

Wagner's classification is a widely used system for grading DFI based on six wound grades (0–5) that assess ulcer depth [32]. However, it does not independently account for ischemia or infection as risk factors in all grades [33]. For instance, ischemia is only recognized in the most severe stages (grades 4 and 5), while infection and osteomyelitis (OM) are limited to grade 3, addressing only deep wounds (Figs. 16.1 and 16.2).

The University of Texas Health Science Center San Antonio (UT) classification system offers a more detailed matrix with four grades of wound depth, supplemented by subgroups to denote infection, ischemia, or both (33). Infection is defined by purulence or at least two local signs of inflammation, such as erythema, pain, or edema. Ischemia is diagnosed through clinical signs like claudication, absent pulses, or pallor, supported by non-invasive tests such as a $TCPO_2 < 40$ mmHg, ABI < 0.8, or toe systolic pressure < 45 mmHg.

The Infectious Diseases Society of America (IDSA) classification, developed in 2004, categorizes infections into four levels of severity [34]. While this system distinguishes infection severity—mild (< 2 cm erythema), moderate (> 2 cm erythema), and severe (systemic toxicity)—it does not address local wound conditions. Combining the IDSA and UT systems may provide a comprehensive evaluation (e.g., UT 3B with IDSA moderate infection).

16.4 Evaluation of Diabetic Foot Infections

Patients present with complaints ranging from local to systemic signs of infection. Local symptoms include pain, erythema, edema, purulent drainage, and malodor. Systemic symptoms include anorexia, nausea, vomiting, fever, chills, night sweats, mental status changes, and worsening glycemic control. A thorough diabetic history should cover disease duration, insulin dependence, previous complications, and recent glycemic control. Comorbidities like renal, liver, cardiovascular disease, neuropathy, and retinopathy should also be assessed. Social history, including tobacco/alcohol use, weight-bearing ability, ambulation level, diet, exercise, and home support, is vital. A comprehensive review of systems helps gauge infection severity (Fig. 16.3).

16.4.1 Physical Examination

Initial evaluation includes vital signs, BMI, and overall well-being. Signs like hypothermia (< 36 °C), fever (> 38 °C), hypotension, tachycardia, and tachypnea may indicate severe infection or sepsis 34. Diabetic patients may lack typical inflammatory responses. Nearly 82% of patients admitted for osteomyelitis (OM) are afebrile [35]. Secondary infection signs such as exudate, delayed healing, or wound breakdown should be noted. Document wound dimensions, drainage characteristics, and wound-based condition (granular, fibrous, or necrotic). Erythema from infection typically does not resolve with leg elevation. Visible or palpable bone in an ulcer suggests OM.

16.4.2 Vascular and Neurological Assessment

Edema, lower extremity pulses, and capillary refill should be evaluated. Use a hand-held Doppler for faint pulses and consider ankle-brachial index (ABI) for peripheral artery disease (PAD). Elevated ABI values may necessitate further vascular studies. High PAD suspicion warrants vascular consultation or angiography for ischemic infections. Neurological exams should check sensory, motor, and autonomic neuropathy, Achilles reflex, foot deformities, range of motion, and gait abnormalities.

16.4.3 Imaging Studies

Plain radiography is critical for identifying soft tissue and osseous infection, deformities, or foreign bodies. Soft tissue emphysema requires immediate treatment. OM appears as radiolucencies or destructive changes after 30–50% bone mineral loss [36]. Plain films are 67% specific and 60% sensitive for OM [37]. MRI is more sensitive and specific, especially for abscesses or sinus tracts [38].

Bone scans like Indium-111 or Technetium-99 m HMPAO can differentiate acute from chronic infections, particularly OM from Charcot neuroarthropathy [39].

16.4.4 Laboratory Investigations

Baseline lab tests help monitor treatment response. Studies observed fewer than 50% of diabetic foot infection (DFI) patients had elevated WBC counts, with a mean of $11.9 \pm 5.4 \times 10^3$ cells/mm^3 35. Metabolic panels assess renal function, electrolytes, and glycemic control. Acute-phase reactants like ESR and CRP are inflammation markers. Studies found ESR > 70 mm/hr. increased OM likelihood and determined CRP > 3.2 mg/dL helped differentiate OM from cellulitis [40, 41]. Elevated post-treatment CRP and ESR levels are linked with increased amputation risk [42]. Serum albumin and prealbumin levels, indicators of nutritional status, are often low in inflammation. Lower serum albumin patients require amputation [42]. Diabetic patients with serum albumin ≥3.5 g/dL heals better post-amputation and similarly lower albumin levels correlated with treatment failure [43, 44].

16.4.5 Microbiological Analysis

Diabetic foot ulcers are colonized by bacteria, potentially leading to infections characterized by tissue invasion and inflammation. Deep tissue cultures are preferred over superficial swabs, which risk false results due to colonizing organisms [45]. Studies have shown that patients with severe DFI have 83% of cultures polymicrobial, averaging 2.8 species per specimen, with an aerobic-to-anaerobic ratio of 3:1 [46]. Common organisms include Staphylococcus aureus, Staphylococcus epidermidis, and Streptococcus species. Anaerobes like Peptostreptococcus magnus and Bacteroides fragilis were noted.

16.5 Management Strategies

The management of DFI includes preventive care and treatment modalities, both non-invasive and invasive.

16.5.1 Preventive Care

DFIs are often asymptomatic until advanced stages due to underlying peripheral vascular disease. Neuropathy can mask ischemia, and vice versa, necessitating regular diabetic foot screening. Early detection avoids complications like gangrene and amputation. Screening includes daily self-checks and routine healthcare visits.

16.5.2 Non-invasive Care

(a) Local Care

Local care involves wound dressings, human skin equivalents (HSEs), pressure offloading, total-contact casting (TCC), hyperbaric oxygen therapy (HBOT), maggot therapy, topical growth factors, shockwave therapy, and stem cell therapy.

- Wound Dressings: Basic but limited in effectiveness compared to adjunctive methods.
- Human Skin Equivalents (HSEs): A randomized controlled trial (RCT) highlighted an 18% increase in complete healing with Graft skin compared to saline-moistened gauze [33]. Accessibility remains a limitation [47].
- Offloading & TCC: Pressure offloading treats neuropathic ulcers, while ischemic ulcers require revascularization. TCC has a 91% healing rate versus 32% for dressing changes in 65 days, with a 0% infection rate compared to 26% in controls [35]. TCC use is limited due to its complexity [48].
- Hyperbaric Oxygen Therapy (HBOT): Systemic HBOT reduces amputation risk, with studies reporting success in advanced DFI cases. Sessions last 45–120 min at pressures of 1.5–3.0 ATA [36, 49].
- Maggot Therapy: Effective for debridement, faster granulation tissue formation, and wound surface reduction, though it does not improve disinfection or complete healing [37, 50].
- Topical Growth Factors: Platelet-derived growth factors enhance ulcer healing. Studies showed significant improvement when combined with standard care, favoring recombinant human epidermal growth factor [38, 51].
- Shock Wave Therapy (ESWT): Promising trials demonstrated a > 50% reduction in wound volume in 12 weeks compared to standard care [39, 52].
- Stem Cell Therapy: Adult stem cells like BM-MSCs improve ankle-brachial index (ABI), angiogenesis, and blood flow, with decreased amputation rates. Combining UC-MSCs with angioplasty enhances outcomes [45–48, 53].

(b) Systemic and Local Antibiotics

Antibiotics are used for infected wounds defined by inflammation or purulence. Infections are categorized as mild, moderate, or severe. For moderate to severe infections, broad-spectrum parenteral antibiotics are recommended [52, 53].

(c) Negative Pressure Wound Therapy (NPWT)

NPWT uses vacuum pressure to stimulate healing by improving blood flow and removing excess extracellular fluid. Studies show better healing and lower amputation rates compared to standard therapy [54].

16.5.3 Invasive Treatment Strategies for DFI

(a) Debridement

Debridement is a cornerstone in the management of DFI as it prepares the wound for subsequent treatments by removing necrotic and nonviable tissue along with foreign debris. This step is critical for altering the wound's environment, which can significantly impede healing if left untreated. Although debridement alone may not ensure complete healing, it is an essential preparatory measure for other treatment modalities. Following debridement, the wound is carefully evaluated to determine the next course of action [55]. This approach is often combined with adjunctive therapies to optimize outcomes.

(b) Revascularization (Angioplasty)

Peripheral arterial disease (PAD) is a common comorbidity in patients with DFI, leading to delayed wound healing, higher complication rates, and an increased risk of amputation. For patients with both DFI and chronic limb ischemia, revascularization emerges as a vital treatment option. Studies have reported ulcer healing rates of 46–91% following revascularization, highlighting its efficacy compared to outcomes in PAD patients who do not undergo the procedure [56].

Revascularization techniques include stenting, surgical bypass, atherectomy, and advanced balloon-based therapies such as drug-coated balloons and cryoplasty, either alone or in combination with stenting. Despite its benefits, revascularization alone does not mitigate the mortality risk associated with PAD. Therefore, comprehensive therapy involving close monitoring of glucose, lipids, and blood pressure, as well as the use of antiplatelet agents, is crucial [57]. For example, combining endovascular therapy with supervised exercise training (SET) significantly improves walking distance, Ankle-Brachial Index (ABI), and reduces the risk of further interventions. Dual antiplatelet therapy with aspirin and clopidogrel or ticagrelor, along with statin therapy, is recommended post-procedure to prevent complications and stabilize plaques [58].

(c) Skin Grafting

When DFIs become severe, skin grafting offers a viable solution by replacing damaged or infected skin and promoting healing. Several grafting techniques are available, including autografts (from the patient), allografts (from another person), xenografts (from animals), and bioengineered or artificial skin. Randomized controlled trials (RCTs) revealed that combining skin grafting with standard treatment enhances healing rates and slightly lowers the risk of amputation. However, the long-term effectiveness of these techniques remains uncertain [59].

(d) Amputation

Amputation is considered a last resort in DFI management, reserved for chronic infections or deformities that render the foot non-functional. It is categorized as minor (e.g., toe or partial foot removal) or major (above or below a major joint like the knee). In a clinical trial, minor amputations accounted for 38.4% of cases, while major amputations occurred in 6.8% of patients with DFI [60]. While necessary in some cases, amputation highlights the importance of early detection and intervention in managing DFI.

16.6 Case Studies and Clinical Scenarios

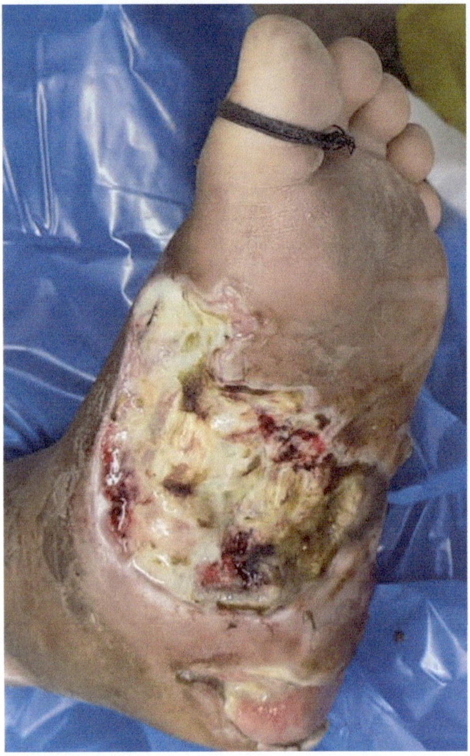

Fig. 16.1 A 60-year-old female patient presents with a left foot ulcer. She has a history of Type 2 Diabetes Mellitus (T2DM) for 20 years. The ulcer has been present for 2 months

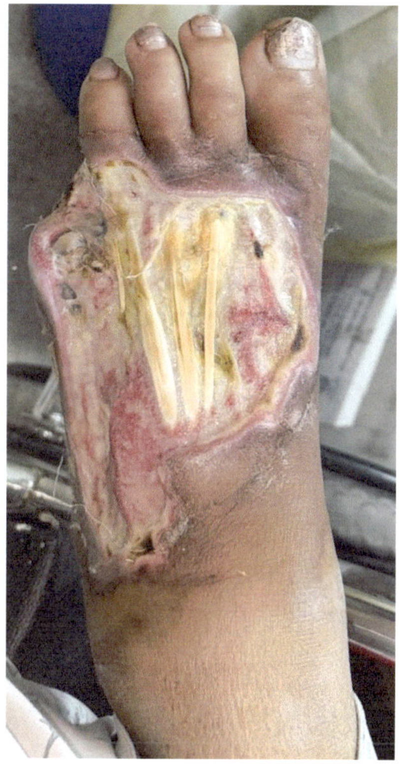

Fig. 16.2 A 58-year-old female patient presents with a left foot ulcer. She has a history of Type 2 Diabetes Mellitus (T2DM) for 12 years. The ulcer has been present for 1 month. Her HbA1c is 9.8%. The patient underwent amputation of the left fifth toe 1.5 months ago

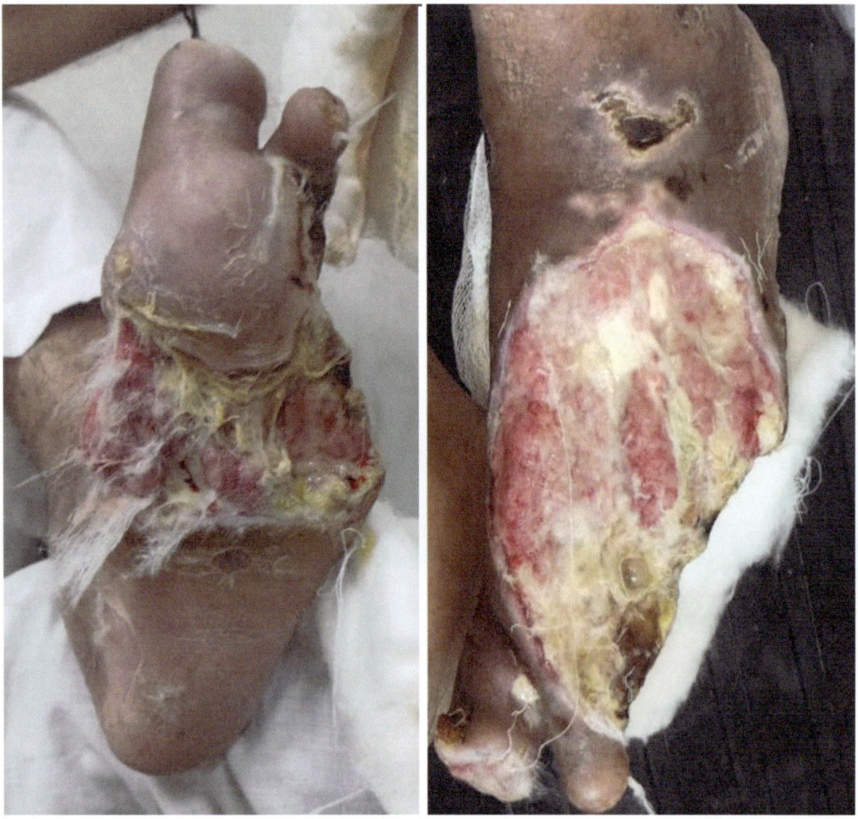

Fig. 16.3 A 62-year-old male patient presents with a left foot ulcer. He has a history of Type 2 Diabetes Mellitus (T2DM) for 25 years. The ulcer has been present for 6 months. The patient previously underwent amputation of the left third, fourth, and fifth toes

16.7 Conclusion

Diabetic foot infections (DFIs) significantly contribute to morbidity and mortality among individuals with diabetes, often resulting in prolonged hospital stays and escalating healthcare costs. Timely diagnosis and tailored management are crucial to addressing this common diabetes-related complication. Traditional treatments, including local and invasive care, combined with emerging therapies such as stem cell interventions, offer promising avenues to reduce morbidity, minimize the need for amputations, and lower mortality rates associated with DFIs. Advancing research into innovative treatment modalities can further enhance outcomes and alleviate the substantial healthcare burden posed by DFIs [61–65].

References

1. International Diabetes Federation. IDF Diabetes Atlas. 9th ed; 2019. Available online: http://www.diabetesatlas.org
2. Rathur HM, Boulton AJ. The diabetic foot. Clin Dermatol. 2007;25:109–20.
3. University of California San Francisco. Vascular & endovascular surgery – diabetic foot ulcers. [cited 22 October, 2022]. Available from: https://vascularsurgery.ucsf.edu/conditions–procedures/diabetic-foot-ulcers.aspx
4. Boulton AJ, Kirsner RS, Vileikyte L. Clinical practice. Neuropathic diabetic foot ulcers. N Engl J Med. 2004;351(1):48–55. https://doi.org/10.1056/NEJMcp032966.
5. Ramirez-Acuña JM, Cardenas-Cadena SA, Marquez-Salas PA, Garza-Veloz I, Perez-Favila A, Cid-Baez MA, et al. Diabetic foot ulcers: current advances in antimicrobial therapies and emerging treatments. Antibiotics (Basel). 2019;8(4):193. https://doi.org/10.3390/antibiotics8040193.
6. Brings S, Fleming T, Freichel M, Muckenthaler MU, Herzig S, Nawroth PP. Dicarbonyls and advanced glycation end-products in the development of diabetic complications and targets for intervention. Int J Mol Sci. 2017;18(5):984. https://doi.org/10.3390/ijms18050984.
7. Boyko EJ, Ahroni JH, Stensel V, Forsberg RC, Davignon DR, Smith DG. A prospective study of risk factors for diabetic foot ulcer. The Seattle diabetic foot study. Diabetes Care. 1999;22(7):1036–42. https://doi.org/10.2337/diacare.22.7.1036.
8. Tesfaye S. Recent advances in the management of diabetic distal symmetrical polyneuropathy. J Diabetes Investig. 2011;2(1):33–42. https://doi.org/10.1111/j.2040-1124.2010.00083.x.
9. Skopljak A, Sukalo A, Batic-Mujanovic O, Muftic M, Tiric-Campara M, Zunic L. Assessment of diabetic polyneuropathy and plantar pressure in patients with diabetes mellitus in prevention of diabetic foot. Med Arch. 2014;68(6):389–93. https://doi.org/10.5455/medarh.2014.68.389-393.
10. Falanga V. Wound healing and its impairment in the diabetic foot. Lancet. 2005;366(9498):1736–43. https://doi.org/10.1016/S0140-6736(05)67700-8.
11. Rubitschung K, Sherwood A, Crisologo AP, Bhavan K, Haley RW, Wukich DK, et al. Pathophysiology and molecular imaging of diabetic foot infections. Int J Mol Sci. 2021;22(21):11552. https://doi.org/10.3390/ijms222111552.
12. Brinkmann V, Reichard U, Goosmann C, Fauler B, Uhlemann Y, Weiss DS, et al. Neutrophil extracellular traps kill bacteria. Science. 2004;303(5663):1532–5. https://doi.org/10.1126/science.1092385.
13. Karima M, Kantarci A, Ohira T, Hasturk H, Jones VL, Nam BH, et al. Enhanced superoxide release and elevated protein kinase C activity in neutrophils from diabetic patients: association with periodontitis. J Leukoc Biol. 2005;78(4):862–70. https://doi.org/10.1189/jlb.1004583.
14. Menegazzo L, Ciciliot S, Poncina N, Mazzucato M, Persano M, Bonora B, et al. NETosis is induced by high glucose and associated with type 2 diabetes. Acta Diabetol. 2015;52(5):497–503. https://doi.org/10.1007/s00592-014-0676-x.
15. Byun K, Yoo Y, Son M, Lee J, Jeong GB, Park YM, et al. Advanced glycation end-products produced systemically and by macrophages: a common contributor to inflammation and degenerative diseases. Pharmacol Ther. 2017;177:44–55. https://doi.org/10.1016/j.pharmthera.2017.02.030.
16. Schmidt AM, Yan SD, Yan SF, Stern DM. The multiligand receptor RAGE as a progression factor amplifying immune and inflammatory responses. J Clin Invest. 2001;108(7):949–55. https://doi.org/10.1172/jci14002.
17. Mahali S, Raviprakash N, Raghavendra PB, Manna SK. Advanced glycation end products (AGEs) induce apoptosis via a novel pathway: involvement of Ca2+ mediated by interleukin-8 protein. J Biol Chem. 2011;286(40):34903–13. https://doi.org/10.1074/jbc.M111.279190.
18. Apte SS, Parks WC. Metalloproteinases: a parade of functions in matrix biology and an outlook for the future. Matrix Biol. 2015;44-46:1–6. https://doi.org/10.1016/j.matbio.2015.04.005.

19. Hopkinson I. Molecular components of the extracellular matrix. J Wound Care. 1992;1(1):52–4. https://doi.org/10.12968/jowc.1992.1.1.52.
20. Ferroni L, Gardin C, Dalla Paola L, Campo G, Cimaglia P, Bellin G, et al. Characterization of dermal stem cells of diabetic patients. Cells. 2019;8(7):729. https://doi.org/10.3390/cells8070729.
21. Alikhani Z, Alikhani M, Boyd CM, Nagao K, Trackman PC, Graves DT. Advanced glycation end products enhance expression of pro-apoptotic genes and stimulate fibroblast apoptosis through cytoplasmic and mitochondrial pathways. J Biol Chem. 2005;280(13):12087–95. https://doi.org/10.1074/jbc.M406313200.
22. Patel S, Srivastava S, Singh MR, Singh D. Mechanistic insight into diabetic wounds: pathogenesis, molecular targets and treatment strategies to pace wound healing. Biomed Pharmacother. 2019;112:108615. https://doi.org/10.1016/j.biopha.2019.108615.
23. Li J, Zhang YP, Kirsner RS. Angiogenesis in wound repair: angiogenic growth factors and the extracellular matrix. Microsc Res Tech. 2003;60(2):107–14. https://doi.org/10.1002/jemt.10249.
24. Kulwas A, Drela E, Jundziłł W, Góralczyk B, Ruszkowska-Ciastek B, Rość D. Circulating endothelial progenitor cells and angiogenic factors in diabetes complicated diabetic foot and without foot complications. J Diabetes Complicat. 2015;29(6):686–90. https://doi.org/10.1016/j.jdiacomp.2015.03.013.
25. Li X. The association between MCP-1, VEGF polymorphisms and their serum levels in patients with diabetic foot ulcer. Medicine (Baltimore). 2018;97(25) https://doi.org/10.1097/MD.0000000000010959.
26. Kajdaniuk D, Marek B, Borgiel-Marek H, Kos-Kudła B. Vascular endothelial growth factor (VEGF) – part 1: in physiology and pathophysiology. Endokrynol Pol. 2011;62(6):444–55.
27. Mizia-Malarz A, Sobol G, Woś H. Proangiogenic factors: vascular-endothelial growth factor (VEGF) and basic fibroblast growth factor–the characteristics and function. Przegl Lek. 2008;65(6):353–7.
28. Tecilazich F, Dinh T, Pradhan-Nabzdyk L, Leal E, Tellechea A, Kafanas A, et al. Role of endothelial progenitor cells and inflammatory cytokines in healing of diabetic foot ulcers. PLoS One. 2013;8(12) https://doi.org/10.1371/journal.pone.0083314.
29. Tepper OM, Galiano RD, Capla JM, Kalka C, Gagne PJ, Jacobowitz GR, et al. Human endothelial progenitor cells from type II diabetics exhibit impaired proliferation, adhesion, and incorporation into vascular structures. Circulation. 2002;106(22):2781–6. https://doi.org/10.1161/01.cir.0000039526.42991.93.
30. Chen MC, Sheu JJ, Wang PW, Chen CY, Kuo MC, Hsieh CJ, et al. Complications impaired endothelial progenitor cell function in type 2 diabetic patients with or without critical leg ischaemia: implication for impaired neovascularization in diabetes. Diabet Med. 2009;26(2):134–41. https://doi.org/10.1111/j.1464-5491.2008.02649.x.
31. Boström L, Linder LE, Bergström J. Influence of smoking on the outcome of periodontal surgery. A 5-year follow-up. J Clin Periodontol. 1998;25(3):194–201. https://doi.org/10.1111/j.1600-051x.1998.tb02428.x.
32. Wagner FW Jr. The dysvascular foot: a system for diagnosis and treatment. Foot Ankle. 1981;2:64122.
33. Oyibo SO, Jude EB, Tarawneh I, Nguyen HC, Harkless LB, Boulton AJ. A comparison of two diabetic foot ulcer classification systems: the Wagner and the University of Texas wound classification systems. Diabetes Care. 2001;24:848.
34. Lipsky BA, Berendt AR, Deery HG, Embil JM, Joseph WS, Karchmer AW, et al. Infectious Diseases Society of America. Diagnosis and treatment of diabetic foot infections. Clin Infect Dis. 2004;39:885910.
35. Armstrong DG, Lavery LA, Sariaya M, Ashry H. Leukocytosis is a poor indicator of acute osteomyelitis of the foot in diabetes mellitus. J Foot Ankle Surg. 1996;35:2803.
36. Crim B, Wukich DK. Osteomyelitis of the foot and ankle in the diabetic population: diagnosis and treatment. J Diab Foot Comp. 2010;1:2535.

37. Termaat MF, Raijmakers PG, Scholten HJ, Bakker FC, Patka P, Haarman HJ. The accuracy of diagnostic imaging for the assessment of chronic osteomyelitis: a systematic review and meta-analysis. J Bone Joint Surg Am. 2005;87:246471.
38. Schwegler B, Stumpe KD, Weishaupt D, Strobel K, Spinas GA, von Schulthess GK, et al. Unsuspected osteomyelitis is frequent in persistent diabetic foot ulcer and better diagnosed by MRI than by 18F-FDG PET or 99mTc-MOAB. J Intern Med. 2008;263:99106.
39. Palestro CJ, Mehta HH, Patel M, Freeman SJ, Harrington WN, Tomas MB, et al. Marrow versus infection in the Charcot joint: indium-111 leukocyte and technetium-99m sulfur colloid scintigraphy. J Nucl Med. 1998;39:34650.
40. Butalia S, Palda VA, Sargeant RJ, Detsky AS, Mourad O. Does this patient with diabetes have osteomyelitis of the lower extremity? JAMA. 2008;299:80613.
41. Fleischer AE, Wrobel JS, Leonards A, Berg S, Evans DP, Baron RL, et al. Post-treatment leukocytosis predicts an unfavourable clinical response in patients with moderate to severe diabetic foot infections. J Foot Ankle Surg. 2011;50:5416.
42. Akinci B, Yener S, Yesil S, Yapar N, Kucukyavas Y, Bayraktar F. Acute phase reactants predict the risk of amputation in diabetic foot infection. J Am Podiatr Med Assoc. 2011;101:16.
43. Dickhaut SC, DeLee JC, Page CP. Nutritional status: importance in predicting wound-healing after amputation. J Bone Joint Surg Am. 1984;66:715.
44. Lipsky BA, Armstrong DG, Citron DM, Tice AD, Morgenstern DE, Abramson MA. Ertapenem versus piperacillin/tazobactam for diabetic foot infections (SIDESTEP): prospective, randomised, controlled, double-blinded, multicentre trial. Lancet. 2005;366:1695703.
45. Lipsky BA. New developments in diagnosing and treating diabetic foot infections. Diabetes Metab Res Rev. 2008;24:S6671.
46. Diamantopoulos EJ, Haritos D, Yfandi G, Grigoriadou M, Margariti G, Paniara O, et al. Management and outcome of severe diabetic foot infections. Exp Clin Endocrinol Diabetes. 1998;106:34652.
47. Veves A, Falanga V, Armstrong DG, Sabolinski ML, Apligraf Diabetic Foot Ulcer Study. Graftskin, a human skin equivalent, is effective in the management of noninfected neuropathic diabetic foot ulcers: a prospective randomized multicenter clinical trial. Diabetes Care. 2001;24:290–5. [PMID: 11213881]. https://doi.org/10.2337/diacare.24.2.290.
48. Mueller MJ, Diamond JE, Sinacore DR, Delitto A, Blair VP 3rd, Drury DA, Rose SJ. Total contact casting in treatment of diabetic plantar ulcers. Controlled clinical trial. Diabetes Care. 1989;12:384–8. [PMID: 2659299]. https://doi.org/10.2337/diacare.12.6.384.
49. Roeckl-Wiedmann I, Bennett M, Kranke P. Systematic review of hyperbaric oxygen in the management of chronic wounds. Br J Surg. 2005;92:24–32. [PMID: 15635604 DOI: 10.1002/bjs.4863]
50. Mohd Zubir MZ, Holloway S, Mohd Noor N. Maggot therapy in wound healing: a systematic review. Int J Environ Res Public Health. 2020;17. [PMID: 32825736] https://doi.org/10.3390/ijerph17176103.
51. Sridharan K, Sivaramakrishnan G. Growth factors for diabetic foot ulcers: mixed treatment comparison analysis of randomized clinical trials. Br J Clin Pharmacol. 2018;84:434–44. [PMID: 29148070]. https://doi.org/10.1111/bcp.13470.
52. Galiano R, Snyder R, Mayer P, Rogers LC, Alvarez O, Sanuwave Trial Investigators. Focused shockwave therapy in diabetic foot ulcers: secondary endpoints of two multicentre randomised controlled trials. J Wound Care. 2019;28:383–95. [PMID: 31166864]. https://doi.org/10.12968/jowc.2019.28.6.383.
53. Chiang KJ, Chiu LC, Kang YN, Chen C. Autologous stem cell therapy for chronic lower extremity wounds: a meta-analysis of randomized controlled trials. Cells. 2021;10. [PMID: 34943815] https://doi.org/10.3390/cells10123307.
54. Wu Q, Lei X, Chen L, Zheng Y, Huang H, Qian C, Liang Z. Autologous platelet-rich gel combined with in vitro amplification of bone marrow mesenchymal stem cell transplantation to treat the diabetic foot ulcer: a case report. Ann Transl Med. 2018;6:307. [PMID: 30211195]. https://doi.org/10.21037/atm.2018.07.12.

55. Dash NR, Dash SN, Routray P, Mohapatra S, Mohapatra PC. Targeting nonhealing ulcers of lower extremity in human through autologous bone marrow-derived mesenchymal stem cells. Rejuvenation Res. 2009;12:359–66. [PMID: 19929258]. https://doi.org/10.1089/rej.2009.0872.
56. Qin HL, Zhu XH, Zhang B, Zhou L, Wang WY. Clinical evaluation of human umbilical cord mesenchymal stem cell transplantation after angioplasty for diabetic foot. Exp Clin Endocrinol Diabetes. 2016;124:497–503. [PMID: 27219884]. https://doi.org/10.1055/s-0042-103684.
57. Pinzur MS, Senneville E, Infectious Diseases Society of America. Infectious Diseases Society of America clinical practice guideline for the diagnosis and treatment of diabetic foot infections. Clin Infect Dis. 2012;54:e132–73. [PMID: 22619242]. https://doi.org/10.1093/cid/cis346.
58. Kwon KT, Armstrong DG. Microbiology and antimicrobial therapy for diabetic foot infections. Infect Chemother. 2018;50:11–20. [PMID: 29637748]. https://doi.org/10.3947/ic.2018.50.1.11.
59. Borys S, Hohendorff J, Frankfurter C, Kiec-Wilk B, Malecki MT. Negative pressure wound therapy use in diabetic foot syndrome-from mechanisms of action to clinical practice. Eur J Clin Invest. 2019;49:e13067. [PMID: 30600541]. https://doi.org/10.1111/eci.13067.
60. Lebrun E, Tomic-Canic M, Kirsner RS. The role of surgical debridement in healing of diabetic foot ulcers. Wound Repair Regen. 2010;18:433–8. [PMID: 20840517]. https://doi.org/10.1111/j.1524-475X.2010.00619.x.
61. Vouillarmet J, Bourron O, Gaudric J, Lermusiaux P, Millon A, Hartemann A. Lower-extremity arterial revascularization: is there any evidence for diabetic foot ulcer-healing? Diabetes Metab. 2016;42:4–15. [PMID: 26072053]. https://doi.org/10.1016/j.diabet.2015.05.004.
62. Tepe G, Brodmann M, Werner M, Bachinsky W, Holden A, Zeller T, Mangalmurti S, Nolte-Ernsting C, Bertolet B, Scheinert D, Gray WA, Disrupt PAD III Investigators. Intravascular lithotripsy for peripheral artery calcification: 30-day outcomes from the randomized Disrupt PAD III trial. JACC Cardiovasc Interv. 2021;14:1352–61. [PMID: 34167675]. https://doi.org/10.1016/j.jcin.2021.04.010.
63. Pandey A, Banerjee S, Ngo C, Mody P, Marso SP, Brilakis ES, Armstrong EJ, Giri J, Bonaca MP, Pradhan A, Bavry AA, Kumbhani DJ. Comparative efficacy of endovascular revascularization versus supervised exercise training in patients with intermittent claudication: meta-analysis of randomized controlled trials. JACC Cardiovasc Interv. 2017;10:712–24. [PMID: 28385410]. https://doi.org/10.1016/j.jcin.2017.01.027.
64. Santema TB, Poyck PP, Ubbink DT. Skin grafting and tissue replacement for treating foot ulcers in people with diabetes. Cochrane Database Syst Rev. 2016;2:CD011255. [PMID: 26866804]. https://doi.org/10.1002/14651858.CD011255.pub2.
65. Kim SY, Kim TH, Choi JY, Kwon YJ, Choi DH, Kim KC, Kim MJ, Hwang HK, Lee KB. Predictors for Amputation in Patients with Diabetic Foot Wound. Vasc Specialist Int. 2018;34:109–16. [PMID: 30671420]. https://doi.org/10.5758/vsi.2018.34.4.109.

Bone and Joint Tuberculosis

17

Arjit Bansal, Siddhartha Sharma, and Mandeep Singh Dhillon

Abstract

Tuberculosis (TB) of the musculoskeletal system remains a significant public health challenge, especially in developing countries. Despite being an ancient disease, it continues to present diagnostic and therapeutic difficulties due to its insidious onset, diverse manifestations, and overlapping features with other pathologies. This chapter provides an in-depth overview of bone and joint tuberculosis, encompassing historical perspectives, pathogenesis, clinical presentation, diagnostic modalities, and current management protocols. The disease primarily affects the spine, hip, and knee joints, with rare involvement of small bones, flat bones, and atypical sites such as the shoulder, elbow, and foot. Advances in imaging, microbiological diagnostics, and anti-tubercular therapy (ATT) have revolutionized treatment, allowing for high cure rates and functional recovery in most cases. However, delayed diagnosis, drug resistance, and immunosuppression continue to pose challenges. This chapter also explores regional variants of osteoarticular TB, the impact of HIV co-infection, and the indications for surgical intervention. Emphasis is placed on early recognition, prolonged multidrug therapy, and the judicious use of surgery to prevent long-term deformity and disability.

Keywords

Osteoarticular tuberculosis · Spinal TB · Tuberculous arthritis · Antitubercular therapy · Musculoskeletal infection

A. Bansal · S. Sharma (✉)
Department of Orthopedics, PGIMER, Chandigarh, India

M. S. Dhillon
Department of Orthopedics, Fortis Hospital, Mohali, India

P. Kumar et al. (eds.), *Textbook of Orthopedic Infections*,
https://doi.org/10.1007/978-981-95-5029-6_17

17.1 Introduction

Tuberculosis (TB) has been a persistent affliction throughout human history, with evidence of its presence in ancient civilizations documented in medical literature [1]. In 1779, Percival Pott described spinal tuberculosis, a severe form causing vertebral collapse and deformities [2]. While affluent countries once saw a decline in TB, many clinicians today lack experience in diagnosing spinal TB, leading to delays [3]. High-risk groups include immunosuppressed individuals, HIV patients, drug users, and the elderly [4]. Laennec, who discovered the TB lesion "tubercle," tragically succumbed to the disease at 45 [1]. Despite hopes of eradication due to improved socio-economic conditions and anti-TB drugs in the 1980s, the AIDS pandemic led to a resurgence [5]. TB now affects nearly 30 million people worldwide, with India housing one-fifth of the global cases [6]. Skeletal TB accounts for 1–3% of all TB cases, with the spine being the most affected site [7]. Even in the UK, where TB was nearly eradicated, studies have shown a significant proportion of chronic spinal infections to be of tuberculous origin [8].

Chemoprophylaxis with isoniazid or a combination of anti-TB drugs is recommended for high-risk individuals, including those in close contact with TB patients or with immunosuppressive conditions [9]. Selective BCG vaccination offers 80% protection and is advised for healthcare workers and vulnerable groups [10]. However, socio-economic improvements remain the most effective long-term measure in TB control [11]. With increased global travel and persistent poverty, even developed nations are not immune to TB's resurgence.

Osteoarticular tuberculosis is caused by the hematogenous spread of *Mycobacterium tuberculosis* from a primary visceral infection. The primary focus may be in the lungs, lymph nodes, kidneys, or other organs, and the bacteria travel through blood vessels, mainly arteries, or via Batson's plexus in the axial skeleton [12, 13]. The disease usually manifests in bones and joints 2–3 years after the primary infection. Spinal tuberculosis often involves adjacent vertebrae due to shared blood supply, and in some cases, multiple skeletal sites may be affected simultaneously [14]. Radiological studies indicate that 7% of spinal tuberculosis cases have "skipped lesions," while 12% show involvement of other bones and joints [14]. Advanced imaging techniques reveal subclinical lesions in 40% of cases [15].

Experimental studies have demonstrated that injecting tubercle bacilli into visceral organs can induce spinal tuberculosis, emphasizing the role of direct hematogenous spread [16]. Studies on guinea pigs have shown that chronic tuberculous lesions develop within weeks of inoculation, affecting multiple organs [16]. Local trauma alone, without prolonged bacterial exposure, does not lead to osteomyelitis [17]. In osteoarticular tuberculosis, bacilli reach the joints via the bloodstream or by spreading from epiphyseal bone lesions [18]. Articular cartilage remains relatively intact for months, allowing for better functional recovery if treated early [19]. The infection typically starts in the metaphysis in children and near the bone end in adults [20]. Radiological signs include bone destruction, demineralization, and reactive new bone formation [21]. The disease spreads from the metaphysis to the joint through the capsule or epiphyseal plate [22]. When the infection reaches the subchondral region, cartilage loses its attachment, potentially leading to joint deformities in children [18].

Patients with competent immunity often develop a slow-progressing synovitis [19]. Tuberculous granulation tissue invades subchondral bone, leading to "kissing lesions" and sequestra [20]. In chronic cases, "rice bodies" may form due to necrotic cartilage and fibrin deposits in the joint [21]. If growth centers are damaged in childhood, deformities such as shortening or angulation of bones may result [22] (Fig. 17.1).

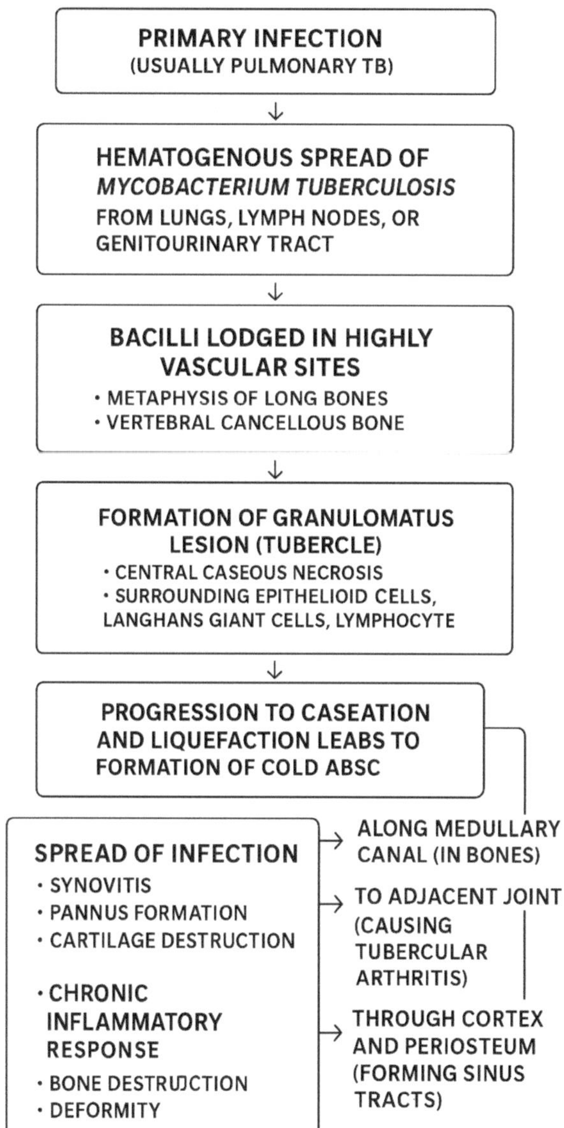

Fig. 17.1 Flowchart explaining the pathogenesis of tuberculosis of bone and joints

Spinal tuberculosis and other tuberculous infections are linked to immune system efficiency [23]. Only a small percentage of infected individuals develop an active disease, but immunosuppression (e.g., HIV) significantly increases susceptibility [24]. HIV weakens the immune system, making patients vulnerable to tuberculosis and drug-resistant strains [25]. The rise of HIV/AIDS has led to a resurgence of tuberculosis, particularly with atypical mycobacterial infections [5]. Poor wound healing in advanced HIV stages further complicates tuberculosis management [23].

Treatment-resistant tuberculosis may result from drug-resistant strains, atypical mycobacteria, or immune suppression [24]. Immunomodulation, including BCG vaccination and other therapies, has shown promise in improving immune response and treatment outcomes in multidrug-resistant cases [10]. Before pasteurization, bovine bacilli caused many skeletal tuberculosis cases in Western countries, especially in children [25]. In the Indian subcontinent, boiling milk likely prevented this [19]. Most skeletal tuberculosis cases are now due to human-type bacilli [26]. The disease is paucibacillary, making culture and diagnosis challenging [27]. Studies at Banaras Hindu University, India, found that 92% of cultures were *Mycobacterium tuberculosis*, while 8% were chromogenic acid-fast bacilli [19]. Drug resistance varies globally, with some strains resistant to multiple drugs [24]. Atypical mycobacteria, like *M. kansasii*, can also cause infections, especially in immunocompromised patients [28]. Ongoing research aims to understand mycobacterial metabolism and drug resistance [24].

17.2 Treatment of Tuberculosis (TB) of Bones, Joints, and Spine

The treatment of tuberculosis (TB) of bones, joints, and the spine has evolved significantly, divided into two key eras: the pre-antitubercular and post-antitubercular drug periods.

17.2.1 Pre-antitubercular Era

Before anti-TB drugs, treatment relied on conservative methods like immobilization, rest, and heliotherapy [29]. Ancient physicians attempted manual corrections of spinal deformities, but with little success [1]. Hospitalization for years was common, though mortality remained high [30]. Some surgeries, like drainage of abscesses, were attempted but often led to persistent infections and poor outcomes [31]. Spinal fusion techniques were later introduced to stabilize diseased areas, but paraplegic patients had limited recovery [32].

17.2.2 Post-antitubercular Era

With the introduction of streptomycin (1947), PAS (1949), and isoniazid (1952), treatment improved drastically [33]. Initially, surgery was widely used alongside drugs [34]. However, over time, chemotherapy alone became the preferred approach, with surgery reserved for complications [35]. Modern regimens focus on prolonged, uninterrupted multidrug therapy (12–18 months) to prevent drug resistance [9]. Healing rates improved significantly, and mortality dropped [36]. Drug therapy also helped resolve complications like sinus formation and ulcers without surgery [37]. Despite advancements, skeletal TB remains challenging, with occasional relapses requiring extended monitoring and treatment adjustments [38]. Today, systemic therapy and chemotherapy form the backbone of TB management, with surgery reserved for select cases [9].

17.3 Clinical Presentation and Diagnosis

Skeletal tuberculosis primarily affects individuals in their first three decades of life, though elderly populations in affluent societies are increasingly diagnosed [39]. The disease has a gradual onset and often presents with monoarticular or mono-osseous involvement, accompanied by constitutional symptoms like low-grade fever, weight loss, night sweats, and anemia [40]. Local symptoms include pain, muscle wasting, and joint immobility due to muscle spasms, which relax during sleep, leading to "night cries" in children [41].

Diagnosis in developing countries relies on clinical and radiological findings, but in affluent societies, where tuberculosis was once rare, confirmation often requires invasive procedures [42]. Risk factors include corticosteroid use, alcoholism, diabetes, and immunosuppressive therapy [43]. X-rays reveal localized osteoporosis, bone destruction, and joint deformities, while CT scans and MRIs help detect early stage lesions [44]. Laboratory tests, including PCR, histopathology, and acid-fast bacilli culture, aid confirmation [27]. Mantoux testing and blood tests, including ESR, are useful but not definitive [41].

Differentiating skeletal tuberculosis from conditions like brucellosis and rheumatoid arthritis is critical [42]. Modern imaging techniques, such as CT-guided biopsy, enhance diagnostic accuracy [46]. Despite technological advances, delays in diagnosis remain common, emphasizing the need for increased awareness and timely investigation [40]. The advent of modern antitubercular drugs (ATT) has transformed the prognosis of bone and joint tuberculosis, drastically reducing mortality and severe complications like meningitis, miliary TB, and paralysis [43]. Early diagnosis and aggressive treatment now enable healing without residual joint stiffness (ankylosis) [44]. Previously fatal or debilitating outcomes, such as amyloidosis or crippling deformities, are now rare [45]. Surgical interventions, even in active disease, are safer due to effective ATT, minimizing risks of infection spread or non-healing sinuses [47].

17.4 Disease Progression and Classification

Untreated osteoarticular TB progresses through five stages [44]:

1. *Synovitis*: Preserved joint motion (> 75%) with soft tissue swelling and osteoporosis.
2. *Early Arthritis*: Moderate motion loss (50–75%), joint space narrowing, and marginal bone erosions.
3. *Advanced Arthritis*: Severe motion loss (< 25%), marked joint destruction.
4. *Subluxation/Dislocation*: Joint deformity (e.g., "wandering acetabulum" in hips, triple knee deformity).
5. *Terminal Arthritis*: Ankylosis (fibrous or bony), degenerative changes, or painless fibrous union.

17.5 Management Principles

17.5.1 Systemic Treatment

ATT is paramount. Intensive phases (isoniazid, rifampicin, pyrazinamide, ethambutol) target replicating bacteria, followed by continuation phases (9–18 months) to eliminate dormant pathogens [9]. Prophylactic phases may extend therapy to 24 months in high-risk cases [43].

17.5.2 Rest and Mobilization

Joints are rested in functional positions using braces or traction [45]. Traction corrects deformities, reduces inflammation, and preserves joint space [19]. Gradual mobilization with assisted exercises prevents stiffness and promotes fibrocartilage repair [44].

17.5.3 Weight-Bearing

Introduced cautiously 3–6 months post-symptom resolution, guided by clinical progress [45].

17.5.4 Adjunctive Measures

- *Abscess/Sinus Management*: Aspiration with ATT instillation suffices in most cases; surgery is reserved for unresolved or secondary infections [19].
- *Surgical Interventions*: Synovectomy or debridement addresses refractory early disease [47]. Advanced cases may require excision arthroplasty (e.g.,

Girdlestone's procedure for hip mobility) or arthrodesis (joint fusion) for stability [44]. Corrective osteotomies fix healed deformities [45].
- *Drug Considerations*: Hepatotoxic drugs (e.g., rifampicin) require pre-surgical caution [9]. Multi-drug resistance (MDR-TB) necessitates tailored regimens (e.g., fluoroquinolones) [24].

17.6 Relapse and Compliance

Relapse rates (2–11%) are linked to poor compliance, malnutrition, immunosuppression (e.g., diabetes, HIV), or inadequate treatment duration [48]. Noncompliant patients (e.g., alcoholics) need supervised therapy [49]. Reactivation can occur decades later, emphasizing lifelong monitoring [38].

17.7 Healing Indicators

1. Resolution of systemic symptoms (fever, weight loss) [41].
2. Normalized inflammatory markers (e.g., ESR) [27].
3. Radiological remineralization, trabecular restoration, and reduced edema on MRI [46].

17.8 Tubercular Osteomyelitis

Tubercular osteomyelitis is a rare but significant manifestation of musculoskeletal tuberculosis. It represents approximately 2–3% of all osteoarticular tuberculosis cases [50]. Unlike articular tuberculosis, which affects the joints, tubercular osteomyelitis primarily involves the bone without necessarily extending into adjacent joints. This condition most commonly affects the long tubular bones, ribs, and flat bones such as the pelvis and vertebrae. Despite its rarity, a lack of clinical suspicion often leads to delayed diagnosis and treatment [19].

17.9 Pathological Characteristics

The initial tuberculous lesion is invariably localized within the bone [50]. In pediatric patients, the disease exhibits a distinct pattern, particularly in short tubular bones [51]. Due to the limited anastomotic network of osseous arteries in children, tuberculous-induced thrombosis may precipitate the sequestration of a substantial portion of the diaphysis [52]. The necrotic diaphysis, once infected, becomes enveloped by newly formed subperiosteal bone, resembling pyogenic chronic hematogenous osteomyelitis [19]. Notably, comprehensive histological and microbiological investigations in atypical cases of hematogenous osteomyelitis could reveal a higher prevalence of tuberculous etiology than previously recognized [50].

Tubercular osteomyelitis without contiguous joint involvement predominantly affects the ribs, metacarpals, metatarsals, calcaneum, femur, tibia, fibula, radius, humerus, sternum, facial bones, pelvis, and skull [19]. While any bone can be involved, tubercular osteomyelitis of long tubular bones is exceedingly rare, often leading to underdiagnosis [50]. The reported incidence of isolated tubercular osteomyelitis is approximately 2–3% of all osteoarticular tuberculosis cases [50], with multifocal involvement occurring in nearly 7% of cases [54]. The insidious nature of disease progression, coupled with mild and non-specific local symptoms, frequently results in delayed diagnosis [40]. A high index of suspicion is crucial, particularly in the presence of tuberculous sinuses, ulcers with undermined edges, or cold abscesses, which hold significant clinical relevance [19].

17.10 The Primary Clinical Manifestations Include

- Persistent bone pain and localized tenderness.
- Swelling with warmth over the affected site.
- Boggy soft tissue swelling, indicative of abscess formation.
- Chronic draining sinuses.
- Enlargement of regional lymph nodes.

17.11 Radiological Features

Radiographic findings vary with disease progression. Key features include:

- Irregular osteolytic cavities with minimal surrounding sclerosis, creating a honeycomb-like appearance [21].
- Soft feathery sequestra within the cavities [21].
- Subperiosteal new bone formation, resembling spina ventosa [51].

In cases complicated by secondary infection or sinus formation, there may be intense reactive sclerosis, cortical sequestration, and, in rare instances, pathological fractures [50]. In growing children, tuberculous lesions often straddle the epiphyseal cartilage plate, necessitating prompt therapeutic intervention to prevent growth disturbances [52].

17.12 Differential Diagnosis

The radiological and clinical features of tubercular osteomyelitis must be carefully differentiated from chronic pyogenic osteomyelitis, Brodie's abscess, neoplastic conditions, including bone tumors, and other granulomatous diseases, such as BCG osteomyelitis, which may exhibit a similar presentation [53]. Additionally, disseminated skeletal tuberculosis remains exceedingly rare, accounting for 5–10% of reported cases [54]. This condition predominantly affects malnourished individuals and is hypothesized to result from either simultaneous hematogenous dissemination or repeated bacterial seeding at different intervals [50].

17.13 Management and Prognosis

17.13.1 Medical Therapy

The primary treatment modality for tubercular osteomyelitis is prolonged ATT, which has demonstrated a high success rate [9]. Serial radiographic evaluation every 6 months is recommended to monitor disease resolution [55]. With early initiation of chemotherapy, sequestra often undergo revascularization and reincorporation, mimicking a bone graft, ultimately restoring near-normal osseous texture [56].

17.13.2 Surgical Intervention

While medical therapy remains the cornerstone of treatment, surgical intervention is warranted in select cases [47]. Indications for surgery include:

- Diagnostic uncertainty requiring biopsy.
- Large abscess formation necessitating drainage.
- Persistent sinuses or non-healing sequestra.
- Extensive bone destruction leading to functional impairment.

Surgical procedures, including curettage, sequestrectomy, and debridement, have demonstrated efficacy, though studies suggest that conservative chemotherapy alone yields comparable outcomes [57]. A subset of patients may develop secondary pyogenic infections, which delay healing [50]. In such cases, combined antitubercular and antimicrobial therapy, with or without surgical excision, is required for long-term disease control [19]. However, with early and appropriate treatment, most patients achieve complete disease resolution, thereby preventing long-term disability [44].

17.14 Regional Involvement and Tubercular Arthritis

1. *Tuberculosis of Hip*

Tuberculous hip disease is the second most common osteoarticular tuberculosis (15% of cases), after spinal involvement [7]. Initial lesions often arise in the acetabular roof, femoral epiphysis, metaphysis (*Babcock's triangle*), or greater trochanter, progressing to joint destruction ("osteoarticular" disease) [53]. Synovial involvement may present as transient synovitis [44]. Advanced cases feature cold abscesses

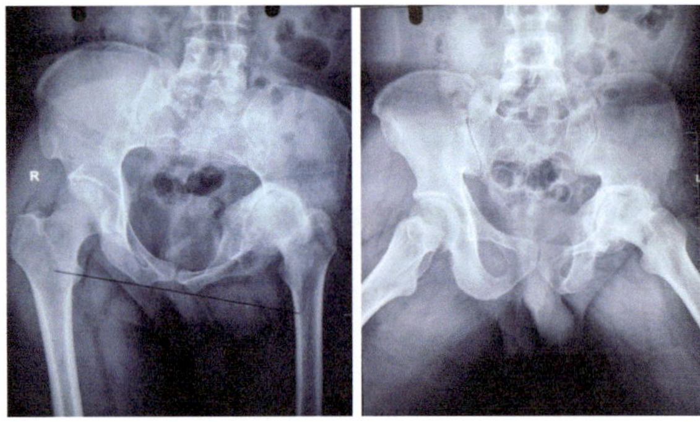

Fig. 17.2 Radiographs of patient suffering from tuberculosis of the left hip joint

tracking along neurovascular pathways, appearing in the femoral triangle, pelvis, or ischiorectal fossa [19]. Clinically, patients (typically <30 years) present with pain (radiating to the knee), antalgic gait, night cries (children), and flexion-adduction-internal rotation deformities [41]. Imaging reveals osteoporosis, erosions, and joint space loss (Fig. 17.2), with MRI aiding early detection [46]. Untreated cases risk pathological dislocation or protrusio acetabuli [53]. Differential diagnoses include Perthes' disease, pyogenic arthritis, and transient synovitis, necessitating biopsy for confirmation [42]. Early diagnosis prevents severe deformity and disability [44]. Treatment combines antitubercular therapy, traction, and joint preservation exercises; advanced cases may require surgery [45].

Four stages are recognized [53]:

- *Stage I* (synovitis: joint swelling, apparent lengthening).
- *Stage II* (early arthritis: true shortening, joint space narrowing).
- *Stage III* (advanced arthritis: bone destruction, fixed deformities).
- *Stage IV* (subluxation/dislocation: "wandering acetabulum," femoral head collapse).

17.15 Clinical Features

Patients typically present with a limp, pain radiating to the knee, and nighttime cries in children [41]. Cold abscess formation occurs in some cases, tracking along anatomical planes to present in unusual locations such as the ischiorectal fossa or femoral triangle [19]. In untreated cases, the hip adopts a characteristic triple deformity of flexion, adduction, and internal rotation [53].

17.16 Radiological Classification

Shanmugasundaram's classification describes various radiological patterns, including "traveling acetabulum," "Perthes-like type," and "protrusio acetabuli," which influence prognosis and treatment outcomes [53].

17.17 Treatment Approaches

Treatment is primarily medical, with anti-tubercular chemotherapy forming the cornerstone of management [9]. Conservative methods include traction and protected ambulation [45]. However, surgical intervention is required in selected cases [47]:

- Synovectomy and Joint Debridement—Performed in early arthritis when medical therapy fails.
- Excision Arthroplasty (Girdlestone Procedure)—Provides a pain-free mobile hip but results in shortening and instability.
- Arthrodesis (Fusion of the Hip Joint)—Recommended for advanced disease in patients who can adapt to a stiff hip.
- Total Hip Replacement (THR)—Considered in healed tuberculosis but carries a risk of disease reactivation.

Early detection and treatment with modern chemotherapy improve outcomes, often preserving joint function [44]. However, advanced arthritis generally results in ankylosis or significant deformity, requiring surgical correction [47]. Secondary osteoarthritis is a common long-term complication [19].

2. *Tuberculosis of Knee*

Tuberculosis of the knee joint is the third most common manifestation of osteoarticular tuberculosis, following spinal and hip involvement [7]. The disease predominantly affects children and young adults, presenting with insidious onset, progressive joint destruction, and eventual deformity [41].

17.18 Pathogenesis and Stages

Tuberculosis of the knee may arise from either the synovium or the bone [44]. In pediatric patients, the primary lesion typically originates in the metaphysis or epiphysis, leading to the formation of tuberculous abscesses [52]. As the infection progresses, granulomatous tissue infiltrates the joint, resulting in cartilage erosion and extensive joint damage [20]. A characteristic triple deformity may develop, marked by flexion, posterior subluxation, lateral rotation, and abduction of the tibia [44].

The disease progresses through four distinct stages [44]:

1. Synovitis (Stage I)—Characterized by synovial inflammation, joint effusion, and mild pain. Radiographs may reveal generalized osteoporosis and widening of the joint space due to fluid accumulation [21].
2. Early Arthritis (Stage II)—Cartilage destruction becomes evident, accompanied by localized osteolysis and marginal erosions [20].

3. Advanced Arthritis (Stages III & IV)—Significant bone loss, joint deformity, and fibrous or bony ankylosis develop [44]. In chronic cases, gross deformity leads to joint instability and pathological subluxation [53].

17.19 Clinical Presentation

Patients often present with progressive knee swelling, which is frequently the first observable symptom [41]. Swelling commonly occupies the parapatellar fossae and may extend into the suprapatellar pouch or popliteal fossa [19]. The joint is warm, with a characteristic boggy consistency, particularly palpable on the medial aspect [44]. As the disease advances, quadriceps wasting becomes prominent, often accompanied by regional lymphadenopathy [41].

Neglected cases typically result in severe flexion deformity, exacerbated by hamstring contractures [53]. In advanced disease, the triple deformity worsens, contributing to functional impairment and significant disability [44].

17.20 Diagnostic Modalities

Radiological findings vary according to disease stage [21]. Early-stage manifestations include osteoporosis and soft tissue swelling, while advanced disease is characterized by joint space narrowing, subchondral bone destruction, osteolytic cavities, and sequestra [20]. Magnetic resonance imaging (MRI) is particularly useful for detecting early synovial involvement [46]. Differential diagnoses include pyogenic arthritis, rheumatoid arthritis, and chronic traumatic synovitis [42].

17.21 Management Strategies

17.21.1 Conservative Treatment

- Antitubercular chemotherapy remains the cornerstone of management, typically administered for a duration of 12–18 months [9].
- Traction and bracing are employed to prevent deformity and maintain joint alignment [45].
- Intra-articular injections of streptomycin and isoniazid may be considered for cases of persistent synovitis [19].
- Physical therapy is introduced as inflammation subsides to restore mobility and prevent stiffness [44].

17.21.2 Surgical Intervention

- Synovectomy and debridement are indicated in cases of refractory synovitis or early arthritis [47].
- Arthrodesis (joint fusion) is considered for advanced disease associated with severe pain and instability [44].
- Corrective osteotomy may be performed to address deformities while preserving joint mobility [45].
- Total knee arthroplasty (TKA) is reserved for cases with end-stage arthritis and is recommended only after a disease-free period of at least 5–10 years to minimize the risk of reactivation [47].

With early diagnosis and appropriate antitubercular therapy, favorable functional outcomes can be achieved [44]. However, in advanced cases, significant joint damage and residual deformities may lead to long-term disability [19].

3. *Tuberculosis of the Shoulder*

TB of the shoulder is an uncommon but serious condition that primarily affects adults [51]. It often presents with progressive pain, stiffness, and restriction of movement, particularly in abduction and external rotation [41]. Over time, patients experience significant muscle wasting, particularly of the deltoid and supraspinatus muscles, leading to weakness and loss of function [44]. Unlike pyogenic infections, TB of the shoulder progresses slowly, with minimal systemic symptoms such as fever and weight loss [40]. In some cases, the disease may present as "caries sicca," a dry, atrophic form of arthritis characterized by joint destruction without significant effusion or abscess formation [19].

As the disease advances, radiographic imaging may reveal characteristic findings such as osteoporosis, narrowing of the joint space, erosion of the articular margins, and destruction of the humeral head and glenoid cavity [21]. In some cases, sequestrated bone fragments may be seen within the joint [20]. However, early stage disease may not show significant changes on X-ray, making advanced imaging techniques such as MRI and CT scans essential for diagnosis [46]. These modalities help assess the extent of bone and soft tissue involvement and guide the selection of appropriate biopsy sites for microbiological and histopathological confirmation [27].

The primary treatment for shoulder TB is anti-tuberculosis therapy (ATT), consisting of an intensive phase with four drugs—rifampicin, isoniazid, pyrazinamide, and ethambutol—followed by a continuation phase of two drugs for a total duration of 10–16 months [9]. In addition to pharmacological treatment, joint immobilization using a sling or brace is recommended during the acute phase to reduce pain and prevent further damage [45]. However, prolonged immobilization should be avoided as it can lead to secondary stiffness and loss of function [44].

Surgical intervention is required in cases with large abscess formation, extensive joint destruction, or painful fibrous ankylosis [47]. Procedures such as joint debridement, synovectomy, and abscess drainage can help reduce bacterial load and facilitate healing [19]. In patients with severe joint destruction, arthrodesis (joint fusion) may be performed to provide stability and pain relief [44]. In select cases with extensive joint involvement but good surrounding musculature, joint replacement may be considered after the infection has been completely eradicated [47].

4. *Tuberculosis of the Elbow*

TB of the elbow is another rare form of skeletal TB that can affect individuals of all age groups [51]. The disease typically develops gradually, with patients experiencing persistent pain, swelling, and progressive limitation of movement [41]. Unlike acute septic arthritis, TB of the elbow has a more indolent course, with minimal systemic symptoms in the early stages [40]. As the disease progresses, patients may develop significant muscle wasting in the arm and forearm, leading to weakness and functional impairment [44]. In advanced cases, pathological posterior dislocation of the elbow can occur, resulting in joint deformity and instability [53]. Cold abscess formation and sinus tract development are also common features of severe disease [19].

Radiographic imaging of the elbow may show lytic lesions in the olecranon, lower humerus, or upper radius, along with joint space narrowing and periosteal reaction [21]. In chronic cases, destruction of the trochlear notch and capitellum may be observed, leading to severe joint deformity [20]. MRI and CT scans provide a more detailed assessment of soft tissue involvement and help differentiate TB from other inflammatory or degenerative joint conditions [46]. In cases where the diagnosis remains uncertain, a synovial biopsy is often required to confirm the presence of TB bacilli [27].

Similar to shoulder TB, the cornerstone of treatment for elbow TB is a prolonged course of ATT [9]. Immobilization of the elbow in a plaster or brace for 4–6 weeks helps reduce pain and inflammation [45]. The elbow is typically positioned at 90 degrees of flexion with the forearm in a mid-prone position to optimize functional recovery [44]. Once the acute phase subsides, gradual mobilization through physiotherapy is encouraged to prevent stiffness and improve range of motion [45].

Surgical intervention is considered in cases with extensive joint destruction, persistent sinuses, or ankylosis [47]. Joint debridement and synovectomy are commonly performed to remove infected tissue and facilitate healing [19]. In patients with severe joint damage, excision arthroplasty may be considered to restore some degree of movement [44]. Arthrodesis is usually reserved for patients requiring high joint stability, such as manual laborers [47]. In rare cases, total elbow replacement may be an option for patients with advanced disease who have completed ATT and have no active infection [47].

5. *Tuberculosis of Foot and Ankle*

In the early stages, tuberculosis of the foot and ankle presents with mild pain, localized swelling, and difficulty in walking [41]. Systemic symptoms such as fever and weight loss are usually absent, making the diagnosis challenging [40]. As the disease progresses, joint stiffness, muscle wasting, and deformities become evident [44]. In some cases, the infection leads to the formation of cold abscesses and draining sinuses, further complicating the condition [19]. Patients may also develop pathological fractures due to extensive bony destruction, making weight-bearing increasingly painful [50]. Because TB progresses slowly, patients often present at an advanced stage, with significant joint and bone destruction already in place [55].

The ankle joint is most commonly affected in adults, with the infection usually beginning as a synovial lesion that gradually extends to the bones [55]. The distal tibia, talus, and malleoli are frequently involved, with the infection sometimes spreading from the calcaneus or the subtalar joint [52]. Affected individuals typically experience persistent swelling, tenderness, and progressive restriction of movement [41]. Radiographic imaging in the early stages may show only mild osteoporosis, while later stages reveal joint space narrowing, periarticular erosions, and bony destruction [21]. MRI and CT scans are crucial for assessing the full extent of disease involvement, particularly in cases where plain X-rays do not provide definitive findings [46]. If there is diagnostic uncertainty, a synovial or bone biopsy may be necessary to confirm the presence of *Mycobacterium tuberculosis* [27].

Tuberculosis of the foot is often localized to the calcaneus, talus, or mid-tarsal bones, though it can affect any part of the foot [55] (Figs. 17.3, 17.4, 17.5, and 17.6). The infection typically remains confined to a single tarsal or metatarsal bone for a prolonged period before spreading to adjacent structures [50]. The calcaneus is particularly vulnerable, and TB of this bone may cause a characteristic "heel-up limp" due to pain and tenderness over the heel [55]. When the infection extends to the intertarsal joints, rapid progression leads to widespread joint destruction, deformity, and disability [44]. The late stage disease is often accompanied by draining sinuses and secondary bacterial infections, further complicating treatment [19].

Treatment for TB of the foot and ankle is primarily medical, involving a prolonged course of anti-tuberculosis therapy (ATT) [9]. The standard regimen consists of an intensive phase of rifampicin, isoniazid, pyrazinamide, and ethambutol for

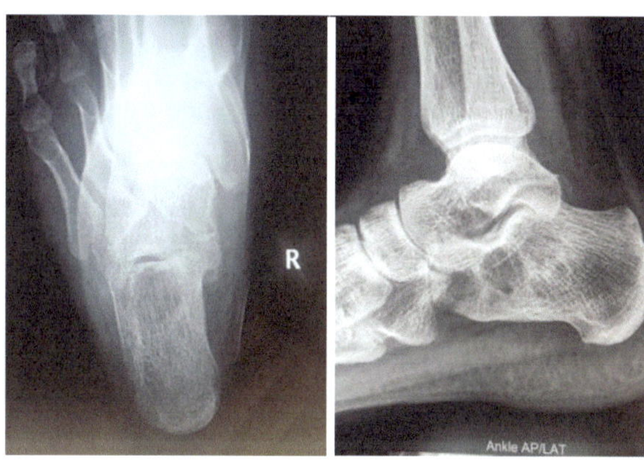

Fig. 17.3 Radiographs showing calcaneal TB in a 32-year-old female

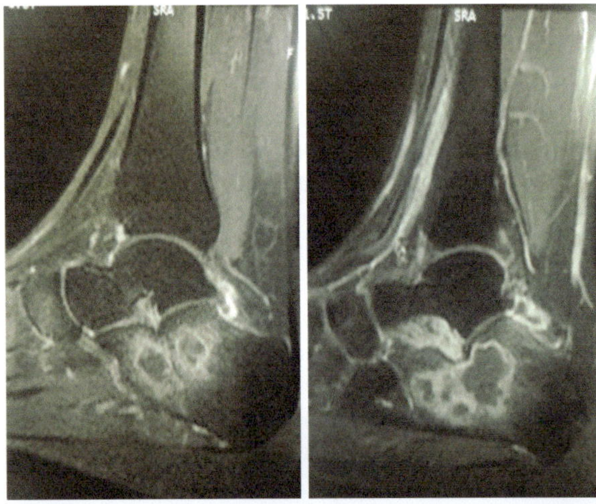

Fig. 17.4 MRI images of the same patient showing hyperintense lesions in the right calcaneum

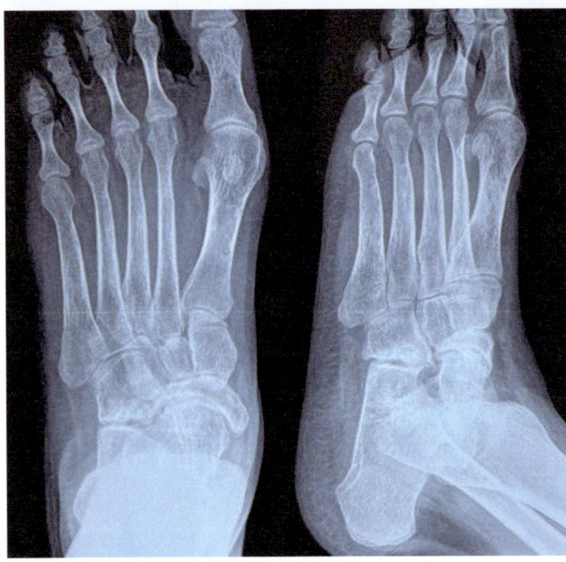

Fig. 17.5 Radiographs showing midfoot TB in a 30-year-old female involving the navicular bone

2 months, followed by a continuation phase of rifampicin and isoniazid for an additional 10–16 months [9]. Early initiation of ATT is essential to halt disease progression and prevent long-term complications [44]. In addition to pharmacological treatment, immobilization of the affected joint in a below-knee cast or ankle-foot orthosis is recommended during the initial phase [45]. This allows the joint to heal in a functional position while reducing pain and inflammation [44]. However, prolonged immobilization is discouraged as it may lead to joint stiffness and contractures [45].

Surgical intervention is necessary in cases with extensive joint destruction, large abscesses, or severe deformities that do not respond to medical treatment [47].

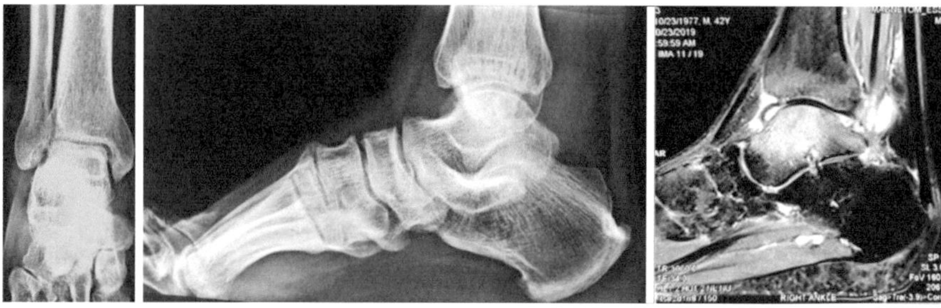

Fig. 17.6 Radiographs and MRI section of 42-year-old male diagnosed with TB of the subtalar joint

Procedures such as synovectomy and joint debridement help in removing infected tissue and reducing the bacterial load [19]. In cases where joint destruction is advanced, arthrodesis may be performed to stabilize the foot and ankle [44]. Triple arthrodesis, which involves fusion of the subtalar, talonavicular, and calcaneocuboid joints, may be required in patients with widespread midfoot involvement [55]. In rare cases where bone destruction is extensive and functional restoration is not possible, a below-knee amputation may be considered as a last resort [47].

The prognosis for TB of the foot and ankle depends largely on the stage at which treatment is initiated [55]. Approximately 80% of cases respond well to ATT and immobilization, with nearly half achieving full joint mobility and function [44]. However, around 30% of patients develop some degree of joint stiffness, while 20% progress to fibrous or bony ankylosis [55]. A pain-free, stable joint in a functional position is considered an acceptable outcome, even in cases where mobility is restricted [44].

6. *Tuberculosis of Other Small Bone and Flat Bones*

TB can also involve small and flat bones, leading to localized bone destruction, deformity, and chronic infection [50]. The small bones of the hands and feet, as well as flat bones such as the skull, scapula, sternum, clavicle, and pelvic bones, can be affected [19]. These forms of TB account for a small percentage of skeletal TB cases, making diagnosis and treatment challenging due to their rarity and the potential for misdiagnosis as pyogenic osteomyelitis, rheumatoid arthritis, or bone tumors [42].

TB of small bones, commonly referred to as tuberculous dactylitis, occurs most frequently in children [51]. It primarily affects the short tubular bones of the hands and feet, including the phalanges and metacarpals [50] (Fig. 17.7). The disease is characterized by spindle-shaped swelling of the affected digit, pain, and joint stiffness [41]. As the infection progresses, it causes extensive bone destruction, leading to characteristic radiographic findings such as cystic lesions and subperiosteal new bone formation, a condition known as spina ventosa [21]. Advanced cases may develop sinuses and soft tissue abscesses, which can lead to secondary bacterial

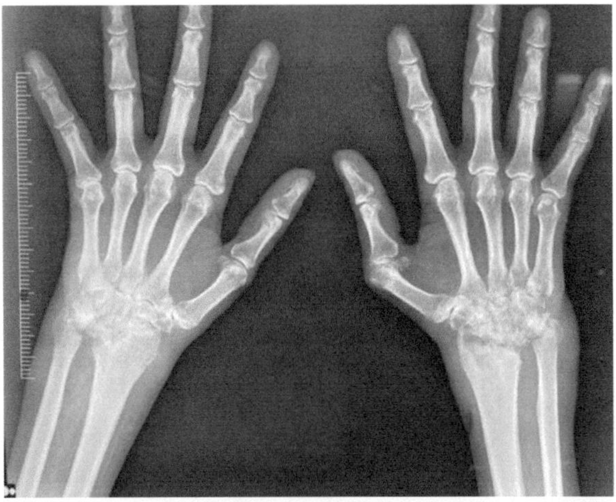

Fig. 17.7 Radiograph of a 27-year-old male patient suffering from bilateral tuberculosis of the wrist joint

infections [19]. Diagnosis is established through radiographs, MRI, and microbiological confirmation via biopsy [27]. Early initiation of anti-tuberculosis therapy (ATT) is essential to prevent deformity and functional impairment [9]. In cases with severe bone destruction, surgical intervention, including curettage or debridement, may be required to remove necrotic tissue [47].

Flat bones, such as those of the skull, scapula, ribs, clavicle, and sternum, are also rarely affected by TB [50]. The infection often originates from hematogenous spread and presents with localized swelling, pain, and, in some cases, the formation of draining sinuses [41]. TB of the skull and facial bones is particularly uncommon but can be highly destructive, often presenting as multiple discharging sinuses and adherent scars [19]. Radiological findings typically include irregular punched-out lytic lesions with little surrounding sclerosis [21]. TB of the sternum and ribs presents as tender, swollen masses that may eventually rupture, forming chronic draining sinuses [50]. The disease can mimic neoplastic conditions or chronic osteomyelitis, making histopathological confirmation necessary [27].

Tuberculosis of the clavicle is an extremely rare presentation and is often mistaken for a pyogenic infection or tumor [50]. It typically affects children and young adults, presenting with a painless swelling that may progress to abscess formation and sinus tract development [41]. X-rays often reveal diffuse thickening, honeycombing, and sequestration of bone [21]. In some cases, MRI or CT scans are required to assess the full extent of the disease [46]. ATT remains the primary treatment, though surgical excision may be necessary in refractory cases or when a large sequestrum is present [47].

Pelvic TB, particularly involving the symphysis pubis and ischial tuberosity, is another rare manifestation [50]. Patients may present with persistent pain in the hip or groin region, swelling, and occasionally discharging sinuses [41]. Radiological findings include irregular lytic lesions, sclerosis, and periosteal reaction [21]. In some cases, bone scans or MRI may be needed to detect early disease [46]. ATT remains the mainstay of treatment, with surgery indicated only in cases with significant sequestration or abscess formation [47].

The prognosis for TB of small and flat bones is generally favorable if diagnosed early and treated with a full course of ATT [44]. However, delayed diagnosis can lead to complications such as joint deformities, fibrous ankylosis, and chronic sinuses [19]. Surgical intervention is reserved for cases with extensive bone destruction, non-healing lesions, or secondary bacterial infections [47].

References

1. Daniel TM. The history of tuberculosis. Respir Med. 2006;100(11):1862–70.
2. Pott P. Remarks on that kind of palsy of the lower limbs. London: J. Johnson; 1779.
3. Pigrau-Serrallach C, Rodríguez-Pardo D. Bone and joint tuberculosis. Eur Spine J. 2013;22(Suppl 4):556–66.
4. Selwyn PA, Hartel D, Lewis VA, et al. A prospective study of the risk of tuberculosis among intravenous drug users with human immunodeficiency virus infection. N Engl J Med. 1989;320(9):545–50.
5. Narain JP, Raviglione MC, Kochi A. HIV-associated tuberculosis in developing countries: epidemiology and strategies for prevention. Tuber Lung Dis. 1992;73(6):311–21.
6. World Health Organization. Global tuberculosis report 2020. Geneva: World Health Organization; 2020.
7. Sharma SK, Mohan A. Extrapulmonary tuberculosis. Indian J Med Res. 2004;120(4):316–53.
8. Pertuiset E, Beaudreuil J, Lioté F, et al. Spinal tuberculosis in adults: a study of 103 cases in a developed country, 1980–1994. Medicine (Baltimore). 1999;78(5):309–20.
9. World Health Organization. Treatment of tuberculosis: guidelines. 4th ed. Geneva: World Health Organization; 2010.
10. Colditz GA, Brewer TF, Berkey CS, et al. Efficacy of BCG vaccine in the prevention of tuberculosis: meta-analysis of the published literature. JAMA. 1994;271(9):698–702.
11. Dye C, Lönnroth K, Jaramillo E, Williams BG, Raviglione M. Trends in tuberculosis incidence and their determinants in 134 countries. Bull World Health Organ. 2009;87(9):683–91.
12. Jain AK. Tuberculosis of the spine: a review. Clin Orthop Relat Res. 2010;468(7):1850–5.
13. Batson OV. The function of the vertebral veins and their role in the spread of metastases. Ann Surg. 1940;112(1):138–49.
14. Polley P, Dunn R. Noncontiguous spinal tuberculosis: incidence and management. Eur Spine J. 2009;18(8):1096–101.
15. De Vuyst D, Vanhoenacker F, Gielen J, Bernaerts A, De Schepper AM. Imaging features of musculoskeletal tuberculosis. Eur Radiol. 2003;13(8):1809–19.
16. Rich AR. The pathogenesis of tuberculosis. 2nd ed. Charles C Thomas; 1951.
17. Griffith JF, Kumta SM, Leung PC, et al. Imaging of musculoskeletal tuberculosis: a new look at an old disease. Clin Orthop Relat Res. 2002;398:32–9.
18. Watts HG, Lifeso RM. Tuberculosis of bones and joints. J Bone Joint Surg Am. 1996;78(2):288–98.
19. Tuli SM. Tuberculosis of the skeletal system. 5th ed. Jaypee Brothers Medical Publishers; 2016.
20. Ridley N, Shaikh MI, Remedios D, Mitchell R. Radiology of skeletal tuberculosis. Orthopedics. 1998;21(11):1213–20.
21. Rasool MN. Osseous manifestations of tuberculosis in children. J Pediatr Orthop. 2001;21(6):749–55.
22. Havlir DV, Barnes PF. Tuberculosis in patients with human immunodeficiency virus infection. N Engl J Med. 1999;340(5):367–73.

23. Kaplan JE, Benson C, Holmes KK, et al. Guidelines for prevention and treatment of opportunistic infections in HIV-infected adults and adolescents. MMWR Recomm Rep. 2009;58(RR-4):1–207.
24. Gandhi NR, Nunn P, Dheda K, et al. Multidrug-resistant and extensively drug-resistant tuberculosis: a threat to global control of tuberculosis. Lancet. 2010;375(9728):1830–43.
25. Keers RY. Pulmonary tuberculosis: a journey down the centuries. London: Bailliere Tindall; 1978.
26. Grosskopf I, David AB, Charach G, et al. Diagnostic difficulties in skeletal tuberculosis. J Infect Dis. 1994;169(5):1186–7.
27. Singh UB, Seth P. PCR diagnosis of tuberculosis—experience in India. Indian J Pediatr. 2002;69(Suppl 1):S20–4.
28. Griffith DE, Aksamit T, Brown-Elliott BA, et al. An official ATS/IDSA statement: diagnosis, treatment, and prevention of nontuberculous mycobacterial diseases. Am J Respir Crit Care Med. 2007;175(4):367–416.
29. Daniel TM. Captain of death: the story of tuberculosis. University of Rochester Press; 1997.
30. Davies PD. The history of surgical treatment of tuberculosis. J R Soc Med. 1991;84(12):758–60.
31. Konstam PG, Blesovsky A. The ambulant treatment of spinal tuberculosis. Br J Surg. 1962;50:26–38.
32. Hibbs RA. An operation for stiffening the spine in Pott's disease. NY Med J. 1911;93:1013–6.
33. Rajasekaran S, Soundarapandian S. Progression of kyphosis in tuberculosis of the spine treated by anterior arthrodesis. J Bone Joint Surg Am. 1989;71(9):1314–23.
34. Fox W, Ellard GA, Mitchison DA. Studies on the treatment of tuberculosis undertaken by the British Medical Research Council tuberculosis units, 1946-1986, with relevant subsequent publications. Int J Tuberc Lung Dis. 1999;3(10 Suppl 2):S231–79.
35. Medical Research Council. Streptomycin treatment of pulmonary tuberculosis: a Medical Research Council investigation. Br Med J. 1948;2(4582):769–82.
36. Tuli SM. Results of treatment of spinal tuberculosis by "middle-path" regime. J Bone Joint Surg Br. 1975;57(1):13–23.
37. Verver S, Warren RM, Beyers N, et al. Rate of reinfection tuberculosis after successful treatment is higher than rate of new tuberculosis. Am J Respir Crit Care Med. 2005;171(12):1430–5.
38. Held M, Hoppe S, Laubscher M, et al. Epidemiology of musculoskeletal tuberculosis in an area with high disease prevalence. Asian Spine J. 2017;11(3):405–11.
39. Leonard MK, Blumberg HM. Musculoskeletal tuberculosis. Microbiol Spectr. 2017;5(2)
40. Houshian S, Poulsen MB, Holm L. Delayed diagnosis of skeletal tuberculosis: a report of 5 cases. Acta Orthop Scand. 2000;71(6):637–40.
41. Yoon HJ, Song YG, Park WI, et al. Clinical manifestations and diagnosis of extrapulmonary tuberculosis. Yonsei Med J. 2004;45(3):453–61.
42. Colmenero JD, Ruiz-Mesa JD, Sanjuan-Jimenez R, et al. Establishing the diagnosis of tuberculous vertebral osteomyelitis. Eur Spine J. 2013;22(Suppl 4):579–86.
43. Blumberg HM, Leonard MK, Jasmer RM. Update on the treatment of tuberculosis and latent tuberculosis infection. JAMA. 2005;293(22):2776–84.
44. Shanmugasundaram TK. Bone and joint tuberculosis—guidelines for management. Indian J Orthop. 2005;39(5):266–75.
45. Dhillon MS, Tuli SM. Osteoarticular tuberculosis: principles of management. Indian J Orthop. 2001;35(3):147–53.
46. Sinan T, Al-Khawari H, Ismail M, et al. Spinal tuberculosis: CT and MRI features. Ann Saudi Med. 2004;24(6):437–41.
47. Benli IT, Acaroğlu E, Akalin S, et al. Anterior radical debridement and anterior instrumentation in tuberculosis spondylitis. Eur Spine J. 2003;12(4):424–31.
48. Weis SE, Slocum PC, Blais FX, et al. The effect of directly observed therapy on the rates of drug resistance and relapse in tuberculosis. N Engl J Med. 1994;330(17):1179–84.
49. Lambert ML, Hasker E, Van Deun A, et al. Recurrence in tuberculosis: relapse or reinfection? Lancet Infect Dis. 2003;3(5):282–7.
50. Tuli SM, Sinha GP. Skeletal tuberculosis: "Unusual" lesions. Indian J Orthop. 1969;3(2):5–18.

51. Martini M, Benkeddache Y, Medjani Y, Gottesman H. Tuberculosis of the upper limb joints. Int Orthop. 1986;10(1):17–23.
52. Ohtera K, Kura H, Yamashita T, et al. Tuberculosis of the ankle joint in children: a report of two cases. Foot Ankle Int. 2007;28(2):258–61.
53. Shanmugasundaram TK. A clinico-radiological classification of tuberculosis of the hip. Int Orthop. 1983;7(2):111–6.
54. Kumar K, Saxena MB. Multifocal osteoarticular tuberculosis. Int Orthop. 1988;12(2):135–8.
55. Dhillon MS, Nagi ON. Tuberculosis of the foot and ankle. Clin Orthop Relat Res. 2002;398:107–13.
56. Tuli SM. Tuberculosis of the spine: a historical review with special reference to chemotherapy. Indian J Orthop. 2002;36(3):147 52.
57. Lynder P. Conservative treatment of skeletal tuberculosis. Acta Orthop Scand. 1982;53(3):469–73.

Masquelet Technique

18

Dhruv Maini and Lalit Maini

Abstract

The Masquelet technique, or induced membrane technique, is a two-stage surgical approach for managing large segmental bone defects, particularly in the presence of infection or compromised soft tissue. Initially developed by Alain Masquelet, the method involves placing a polymethylmethacrylate (PMMA) cement spacer in the bone defect to induce a vascularized membrane, followed by delayed bone grafting within this biologically active chamber. This membrane promotes bone regeneration and prevents graft resorption. The technique is most commonly applied to post-traumatic lower limb defects, especially in the tibia, and is suitable for both adult and pediatric patients. Indications include post-infective defects, tumour resections, and complex nonunions. While there are no absolute contraindications, adequate soft tissue coverage and patient willingness to undergo a two-stage procedure are critical. The Masquelet technique continues to evolve as a reliable option in limb salvage and complex reconstructive orthopedic.

Keywords

Induced membrane technique · Segmental bone defects · Masquelet technique · Bone grafting · Limb reconstruction

D. Maini
Department of Orthopedics, VMMC & Safdarjung Hospital, New Delhi, India

L. Maini (✉)
Department of Orthopedics, Maulana Azad Medical College, New Delhi, India

P. Kumar et al. (eds.), *Textbook of Orthopedic Infections*,
https://doi.org/10.1007/978-981-95-5029-6_18

18.1 Introduction

The Masquelet technique, introduced by French plastic surgeon Alain Masquelet in the late 1970s, emerged serendipitously like many scientific discoveries [1]. Masquelet initially used bone cement spacers in metacarpal gap fractures to prevent the collapse of the dead space, ultimately allowing for future bone reconstruction. His success in multiple cases led him to recognize the potential of this method as an effective temporary solution for bone defects, particularly in the context of addressing soft tissue concerns first. Over time, this approach evolved into what is now known as the induced membrane technique, which relies on the formation of a periosteum-like membrane induced by bone cement placed in the bone defect. Masquelet's initial published work, a series of 35 cases, demonstrated a 100% success rate in healing bone defects between 5 and 20 cm [2, 3]. A key advantage of this technique is that the length of the bone defect is not a limiting factor, though it is important to note that the Masquelet technique is a two-stage procedure.

18.2 Principle

The Masquelet technique is based on the principle of using bone cement to induce the formation of a membrane that mimics the periosteum. This membrane forms in the space created by the bone defect, typically following the debridement of any infection or tumour present [4]. The membrane, a biological chamber, is highly vascular which helps healing when the bone graft is placed. Also, the membrane acts as a barrier to ingrowth of fibrous tissue in the bone defect area which is already occupied by bone cement. The induced membrane is highly vascular and contains pluripotent cells, as well as osteogenic factors such as BMP-2.6, and growth factors including VEGF, IL-6, IGF-1, and FGF, all of which promote bone healing. The membrane behaves as a closed chamber that surrounds the bone graft, helping to prevent its resorption while also promoting the formation of new bone and corticalization of the graft [5]. The bone cement in the defect provides stability, induces a foreign body reaction for the membrane to form and being a filler of dead space does not allow any granulation or fibrous tissue to form.

18.3 Indications [6, 7]

The Masquelet technique is primarily used to address bone defects, particularly those larger than 5 cm, as smaller defects can often be treated through single-stage procedures. Bone defects can arise from various causes, such as trauma, tumour resection, infections, or congenital conditions. The most common indication for the Masquelet technique is the management of bone gaps that are infected or at high risk of infection, typically in post-traumatic cases. The technique has seen more frequent application in the lower limbs, with tibial bone defects being the most common. Notably, the length of the bone gap does not impact healing time, although the typical healing period spans 8–10 months. The Masquelet technique has been used successfully in both paediatric and adult populations, though its use is less common in children due to challenges with obtaining adequate bone graft material. Although the classical Masquelet technique is designed to address bone defects rather than infections, antibiotic-laced bone cement is commonly used when infection is a concern [8]. Importantly, there is no detrimental effect of antibiotics on the properties or formation of the induced membrane.

18.4 Contraindications

While the Masquelet technique is versatile and applicable in many cases, its use must be evaluated based on individual patient circumstances. There are no absolute contraindications, but certain factors may render the technique less suitable or effective [9, 10]. One primary consideration is the adequacy of soft tissue coverage. If soft tissue is insufficient or of poor quality, the Masquelet technique may not be appropriate. Another crucial factor is bone stabilization; defects near joints or periarticular areas may pose challenges due to the difficulty in achieving proper stabilization. Furthermore, the technique requires at least two surgeries, which means that patient acceptance of a prolonged treatment process is essential. In some cases, the two-stage nature of the technique may be viewed as a disadvantage compared to other methods.

18.5 Technique

The Masquelet technique involves two distinct stages: Stage 1, in which the bone gap is created and a cement spacer is placed, followed by Stage 2, where the induced membrane is opened, the cement spacer is removed, and bone graft is inserted. Proper bone stabilization is essential throughout both stages.

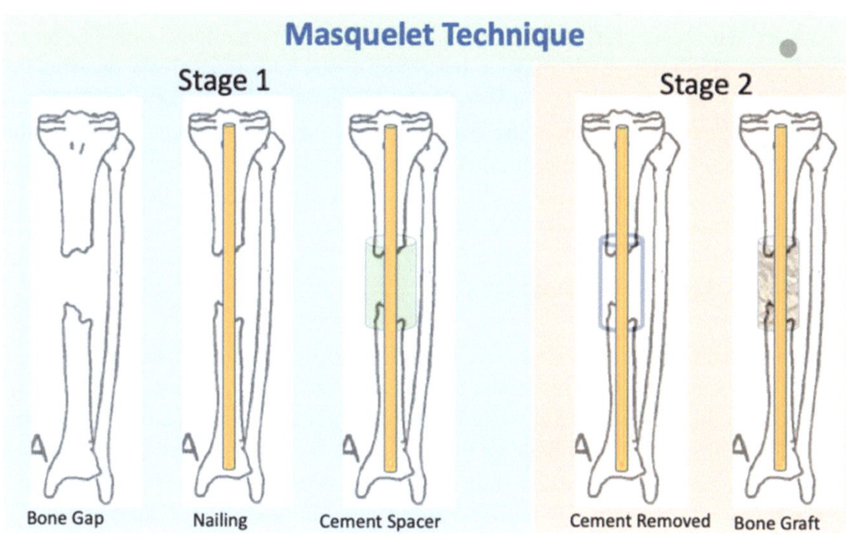

Stage 1: The first step in the Masquelet technique involves addressing the underlying cause of the bone defect, which could be due to infection, trauma, tumour resection, or congenital abnormalities. For infection-related defects, thorough debridement is critical. In cases of tumour resection, wide excision of the tumour is performed. Following the resection, the bone must be adequately stabilized, which can be achieved using nails, plates, or external fixation. External fixation is typically used for tibial defects, while internal fixation is preferred for most other bones. A bone cement spacer is placed into the defect, ensuring that it overlaps the host bone by approximately 1 cm at both ends. This overlap encourages the formation of the induced membrane beyond the resected bone ends, promoting better healing. In cases involving infection, antibiotic-impregnated bone cement is often preferred, although thorough debridement remains the most important factor for successful healing [11]. Once the cement spacer is in place, the wound is closed after meticulous haemostasis, and drains may or may not be used. If sufficient soft tissue coverage is not present, plastic surgery techniques are employed to achieve robust soft tissue coverage.

Stage 2: Stage 2 typically occurs 4–8 weeks after Stage 1, but the timing depends on various factors, such as wound healing and patient condition [12]. In some cases, the second stage may be delayed, especially in patients receiving chemotherapy following tumour resection. In the presence of infection, bone aspirates from both ends of the defect may be taken to rule out persistent infection before proceeding. If infection persists, Stage 1 may need to be repeated. During Stage 2, the surgical approach used in Stage 1 is followed. If a flap was raised for soft tissue coverage, it is elevated again to allow access to the cement spacer. The bone stabilization may remain the same or be adjusted as needed. The induced membrane is carefully exposed and opened in a linear fashion. The cement spacer is then removed, and the bone ends are freshened by removing any fibrous tissue. Cultures are taken from multiple sites to assess for infection. The defect is filled with bone graft material, usually autogenous cancellous bone. For larger defects, additional grafts may be harvested from both iliac crests or even the posterior crest. If necessary, a free fibula, allogenic bone, or bone graft substitutes can be used to augment the grafting. The bone graft is placed loosely in the defect, and the induced membrane is sutured back over the graft to prevent its resorption. The rest of the wound is closed according to the surgical plan.

18.5.1 Post-operative Protocol

The post-operative protocol depends on the stabilization method used. After Stage 1, with the cement spacer in place, the bone is stabilized, allowing for partial weight-bearing with the aid of walking support. Following Stage 2, weight-bearing is usually delayed until sufficient healing has occurred. Ideally, cultures from the bone should be negative before proceeding to Stage 2. After the second stage, patients should be monitored regularly with monthly follow-up visits for clinical and radiological assessments. Weight-bearing and activity levels are gradually increased based on clinical and radiological healing progress.

18.6 Precautions

- Before opting for the Masquelet technique, the treatment team and the patient should thoroughly discuss the plan, as the healing process generally takes 10 months. The following precautions are essential for the success of the technique:
- Adequate resection is vital for infection control and tumour removal.
- Proper bone stabilization is essential to create an environment conducive to healing.
- High-quality soft tissue coverage is crucial for the success of the procedure.
- Repeated aspiration and cultures should be performed at each stage to rule out infection.
- The cement spacer should overlap the host bone by 1 cm at both ends to encourage membrane formation.
- Adequate bone graft must be available to fill the defect.
- Induced membrane closure after packing the graft is essential to prevent resorption.

18.7 Common Errors to Avoid Include

- Failing to adequately debride the bone or control infection before proceeding to Stage 2.
- Placing cement too close to the neurovascular bundle can lead to complications.

18.8 Modifications of the Technique

Several modifications to the Masquelet technique have been introduced to address challenges associated with large bone defects, including the need for large volumes of bone graft and effective bone stabilization.

RIA (Reaming Irrigation Aspiration) Technique This technique uses a specialized instrument to ream the femur, collecting the material for bone grafting. While it provides a large volume of bone graft material, it requires costly equipment and can cause morbidity in the donor bone.

Vascularized Fibula A free or vascularized fibula graft can provide structural strength in addition to serving as a bone graft. This technique is particularly useful for defects larger than 9 cm, though it requires specialized expertise.

Bone Graft Substitutes These can be used to augment the volume of bone graft material.

Ilizarov External Fixator To address the long treatment duration and delayed weightbearing, the Ilizarov fixator can be used in combination with the Masquelet technique, particularly in the second stage for bone transport [12, 13].

Various other bone defect fillers have also been experimented with; however, in clinical practice, PMMA is still the most accepted. Many bio-inert and biodegradable materials like TCP, Poly lactate, and Polyamide have not demonstrated similar efficacy.

18.9 Outcome

The Masquelet technique is highly effective in treating complex bone defects, achieving a success rate of around 90% [14–18]. While alternative methods like distraction osteogenesis with Ilizarov may have higher healing rates, the extended use of external fixators can lead to increased morbidity.

18.10 Conclusion

The Masquelet technique has become an established method for treating large bone defects, particularly in cases involving infection. Although the healing process takes 10–12 months, the length of the bone defect does not significantly impact the outcome, making this technique a reliable option for complex bone reconstruction [19–22].

18.10.1 Case Examples

Case 1 Post-traumatic Bone Defect

This is a case of road traffic injury with an open fracture of the proximal femoral bone. There was a wound of about 12 cm on the anteromedial aspect of the upper leg with a bone fragment exposed out of it. The wound was badly contaminated with road dust, grass, and cloth. Figure 18.1 shows the clinical picture and the radiograph at presentation. The patient was managed with debridement and an external fixator as seen in Fig. 18.1

Patient was further managed on daily dressings but there was a need for another debridement. On the second debridement, free avascular bone had to be removed and also the distal fragment was freshened. The knee spanning fixator was replaced by an Ilizarov fixator since the proximal fragment was too small. The bone defect was filled up with gentamycin impregnated bone cement. In the follow-up, the wound gradually healed over the next 5 weeks (Fig. 18.2).

After wound healing core needle aspiration were taken from both bone ends to rule out infection. The blood parameters also settled by 5 weeks and the patient was taken up for second stage of Masquelet technique. In the second stage, the cement spacer was removed and iliac crest autograft was packed in the defect. Ilizarov fixator was retained as it was providing good stability. The patient was encouraged weight bearing with the Ilizarov fixator. Over the next 7 months the bone defect healed gradually. At 7 months the fixator was removed and PTB brace was continued for over the next 12 months (Fig. 18.3).

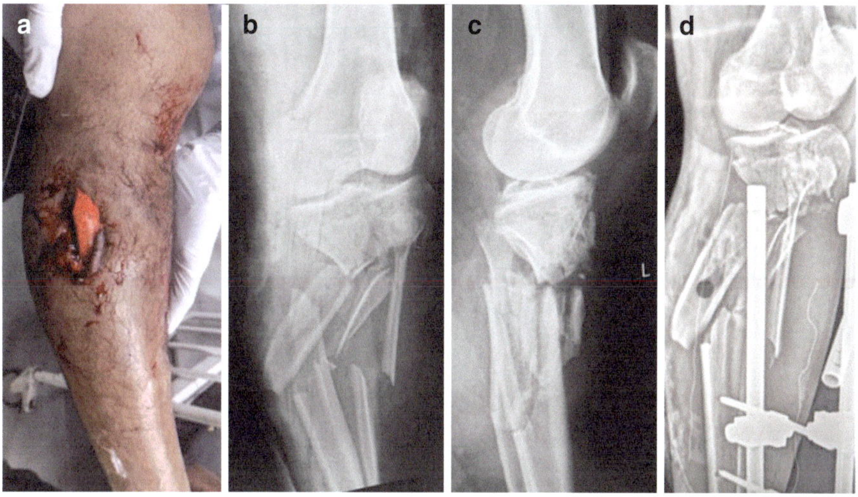

Fig. 18.1 (**a**) Clinical picture of injured limb (**b**) AP X-ray of the leg with knee showing a comminuted fracture of tibia and fibula (**c**) Lateral X-ray of Leg with knee (**d**) X-ray showing stabilisation of the fracture using a knee spanning external fixator

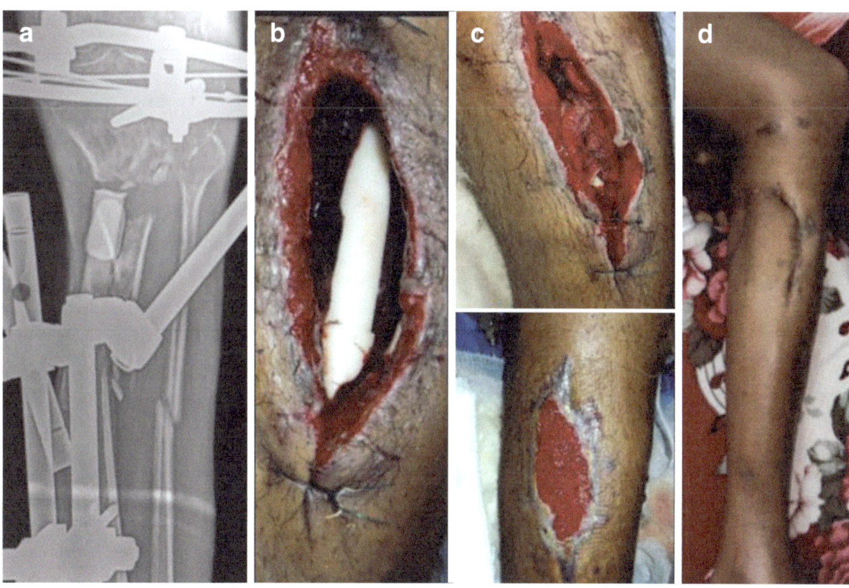

Fig. 18.2 (**a**) Fracture stabilised with Ilizarov fixator and bone defect filled with gentamycin impregnated cement spacer (**b**) Cement Spacer visible in the wound (**c**, **d**) Wound healing over next 5 weeks

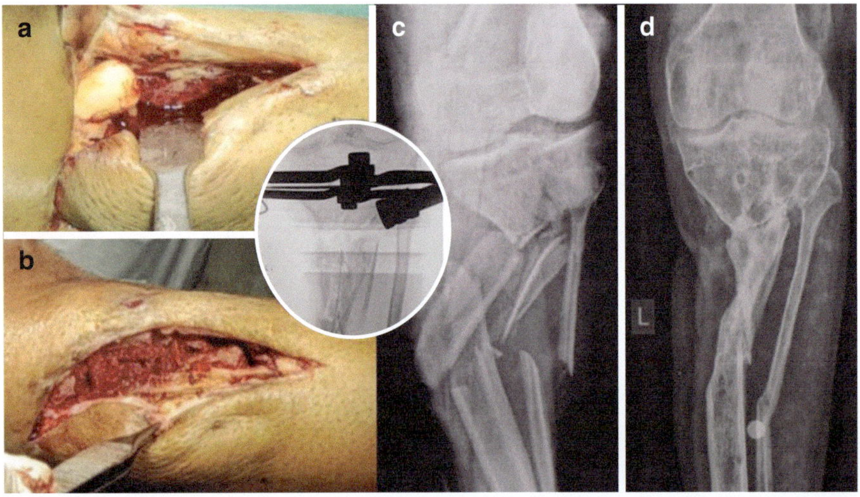

Fig. 18.3 (**a**) Induced membrane visible after removal of cement spacer (**b**) Iliac crest cancellous bone graft packed in the bone defect (**c**) Inset X-ray with Ilizarov fixator and bone graft (**d**) Post injury X-ray showing fracture pattern and follow-up AP X-ray showing healing

Case 2 Post-tumour Resection Bone Defect

This was a biopsy proven case of fungating Talengectatic Osteosarcoma. On staging there was no distant metastasis. CT scan of the leg confirmed breach only of anterior and medial cortex of tibia, with posterior and lateral cortex being intact. Advanced imaging (MRI) of the leg suggested only the tibia involvement with no involvement of the muscles. Culture swab from the fungating mass had staphylococcus (Fig. 18.4).

Patient was planned for wide resection and limb salvage. Pre-operative chemotherapy was not considered due to the fragile infected fungation. Reconstruction after the wide resection was a challenge due to the infected mass and large soft tissue defect due to the resection. Bone defect was managed with an antibiotic spacer mounted on a k nail. The spacer was covered with an ipsilateral Gastrocnemius soleus flap. Additional stability was needed to the large defect and care of muscle flap, for which an external fixator was added (Fig. 18.5).

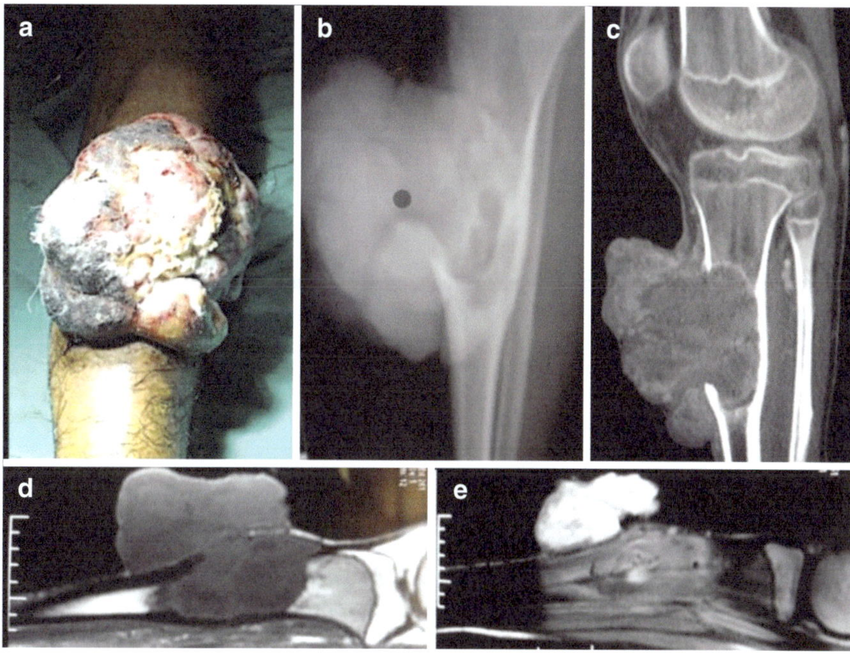

Fig. 18.4 (**a**) Clinical picture of fungating mass over the proximal tibia (**b**) X-ray lateral view of proximal tibia showing anterior soft tissue mass and cortical breach (**c**) CT scan confirming anterior breach and intact posterior cortex (**d**, **e**) MRI sagittal images showing extent of the tumour

Once the wound healed, the external fixator was removed and the limb was placed in an above-knee plaster. Patient then received chemotherapy for six months, with the ability to ambulate on a plaster non-weight-bearing. After completion of chemotherapy patient was taken up for bone grafting. Iliac crest cancellous bone, as well as a free fibular graft, were used to fill the bone defect. In addition, an Ilizarov fixator was applied to provide stability and allow weight bearing. The bone defect gradually healed, and the patient, at a 10-year follow-up, is self-employed (Fig. 18.6).

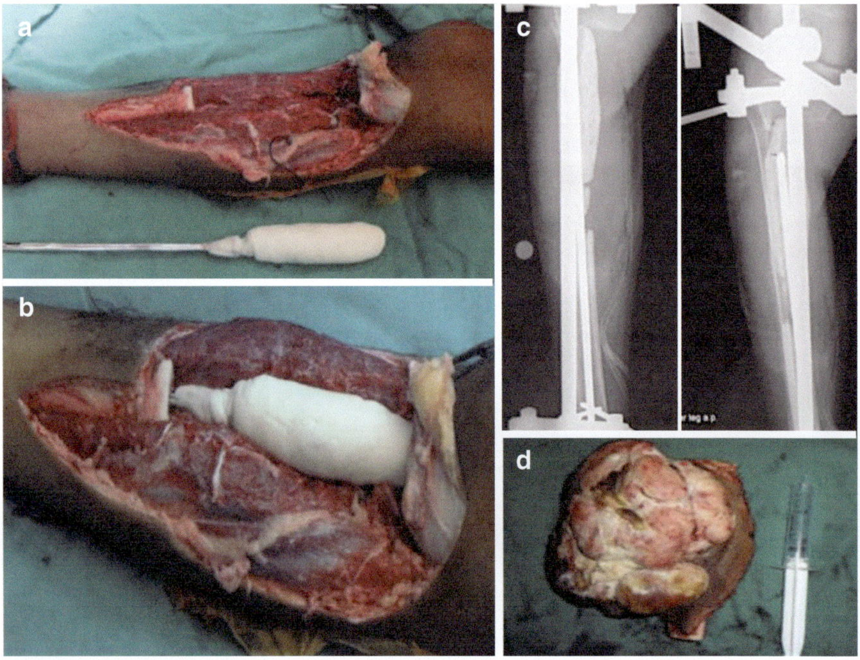

Fig. 18.5 (**a**) Wide resection of the tumour with creation of a nail-mounted cement spacer (**b**) Cement spacer placed in the bone defect (**c**) Post-operative X-ray showing additional external fixator for stability and wound care (**d**) Excised tumour specimen

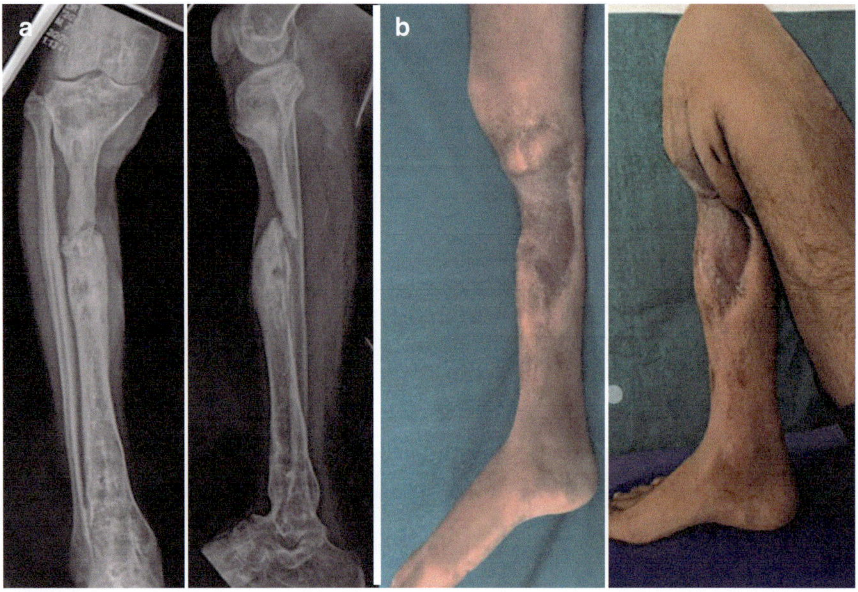

Fig. 18.6 (**a**) X ray AP & Lateral View at 10 year follow up (**b**) Clinical picture of leg with knee function at follow up

References

1. Alford AI, Nicolaou D, Hake M, McBride-Gagyi S. Masquelet's induced membrane technique: review of current concepts and future directions. J Orthop Res. 2021;39(4):707–18.
2. Mi M, Papakostidis C, Wu X, Giannoudis PV. Mixed results with the Masquelet technique: a fact or a myth? Injury. 2020;51(2):132–5.
3. Careri S, Vitiello R, Oliva MS, Ziranu A, Maccauro G, Perisano C. Masquelet technique and osteomyelitis: innovations and literature review. Eur Rev Med Pharmacol Sci. 2019;23(2 Suppl):210–6.
4. Morelli I, Drago L, George DA, Gallazzi E, Scarponi S, Romanò CL. Masquelet technique: myth or reality? A systematic review and meta-analysis. Injury. 2016;47(Suppl 6):S68–76.
5. Mauffrey C, Giannoudis PV, Conway JD, Hsu JR, Masquelet AC. Masquelet technique for the treatment of segmental bone loss have we made any progress? Injury. 2016;47(10):2051–2.
6. Masquelet AC. The induced membrane technique. Orthop Traumatol Surg Res. 2020;106(5):785–7.
7. Sharma A, Sharma A, Tomar S, Mishra A, Kashyap A, Maini L. Is Masquelet technique A successful viable treatment in reconstructing large tumor bone gaps in adolescent and adult? Arch Bone Jt Surg. 2023;11(5):348–55.
8. Allesina L, Alessio-Mazzola M, Belluati A, Mosca S, Placella G, Salini V. Surgical treatment of critical size bone defects with Masquelet technique versus bone transport: a systematic review and meta-analysis of comparative studies. Arch Orthop Trauma Surg. 2023;143(12):7081–96.
9. Griffin JT, Landy DC, Sneed CR, Liu B, Kavolus M, Pectol RW, Gitajn IL, Oh JK, Aneja A. Masquelet technique for the Tibia: a systematic review and meta-analysis of contemporary outcomes. J Orthop Trauma. 2023;37(1):e36–44.
10. Micev AJ, Kalainov DM, Soneru AP. Masquelet technique for treatment of segmental bone loss in the upper extremity. J Hand Surg Am. 2015;40(3):593–8.
11. Xie J, Wang W, Fan X, Li H, Wang H, Liao R, Hu Y, Zeng M. Masquelet technique: effects of vancomycin concentration on quality of the induced membrane. Injury. 2022;53(3):868–77.
12. Pruzansky ME, Lee Y, Pruzansky J. Masquelet technique for phalangeal reconstruction and osteomyelitis. Tech Hand Up Extrem Surg. 2020;25(1):52–5.
13. Liu K, Shi L, Liu Y, Yusufu A. Ilizarov bone transport versus Masquelet technique for the treatment of bone defects caused by infection: a meta analysis. Asian J Surg. 2023;46(12):6109–11.
14. Frese J, Schulz AP, Kowald B, Gerlach UJ, Frosch KH, Schoop R. Treatment outcome of the Masquelet technique in 195 infected bone defects-A single-center, retrospective case series. Injury. 2023;54(10):110923.
15. Hatashita S, Kawakami R, Ejiri S, Sasaki N, Toshiki N, Ito M, Konno SI, Hakozaki M. Acute Masquelet technique' for reconstructing bone defects of an open lower limb fracture. Eur J Trauma Emerg Surg. 2021;47(4):1153–62.
16. Singh S, Toci GR, Kapadia K, Colon A, Greenberg P, Iyer H, Katt B, Shah A. Vascularized bone grafting versus the 2-Stage Masquelet technique for upper-extremity bone reconstruction: a meta-analysis. J Hand Surg Am. 2023;48(10):984–92.
17. Gannamani S, Rachakonda KR, Tellakula Y, Takkalapally H, Maryada VR, Gurava Reddy AV. Combining non-vascularized fibula and cancellous graft in the masquelet technique: a promising approach to distal femur compound fracture management with large defects. Injury. 2024;55(2):111233.
18. Masquelet AC, Begue T. The concept of induced membrane for reconstruction of long bone defects. Orthop Clin North Am. 2010;41(1):27–37.
19. Klein C, Gindraux F, Masquelet AC, Mentaverri R, Gouron R. Questions about using the induced membrane technique to manage cases of congenital Tibial Pseudarthrosis. Cells. 2023;12(14):1918.
20. Ren C, Li M, Ma T, Li Z, Xu Y, Sun L, Lu Y, Wang Q, Xue H, Zhang K. A meta-analysis of the Masquelet technique and the Ilizarov bone transport method for the treatment of infected bone defects in the lower extremities. J Orthop Surg (Hong Kong). 2022;30(2):10225536221102685.

21. Masquelet A, Kanakaris NK, Obert L, Stafford P, Giannoudis PV. Bone repair using the Masquelet technique. J Bone Joint Surg Am. 2019;101(11):1024–36.
22. Cuvillier M, Meucci JF, Cazorla C, Carricajo A, Neri T, Boyer B. Masquelet's induced membrane technique associated with Reamer Irrigation Aspiration grafting and intramedullary Nailing (MaRIAN) for chronic diaphyseal osteomyelitis of the lower limb. Orthop Traumatol Surg Res. 2022;108(7):103395.

Necrotizing Soft Tissue Infections (NSTI) 19

Yashwant Raj Sakaray and Maninder Singh

Abstract

Necrotizing soft tissue infections (NSTIs), such as necrotizing fasciitis and myonecrosis, are swiftly progressive, life-threatening infections causing necrosis of skin, subcutaneous tissue, fascia, or muscle. Known since the fifth century, NSTIs have a mortality rate of 8–17% and pose diagnostic challenges due to nonspecific early symptoms (redness, warmth, pain) mimicking milder infections. Risk factors include obesity, diabetes, immunosuppression, and minor trauma, but healthy individuals can also be affected. The Laboratory Risk Indicator for Necrotizing Fasciitis (LRINEC) score and CT imaging aid diagnosis, with surgical exploration as the definitive step. Treatment involves aggressive surgical debridement, broad-spectrum antibiotics, and intensive care for sepsis. Adjunctive therapies like hyperbaric oxygen and other upcoming treatments, more studies are required. Wound care with negative pressure wound therapy and advanced tissue substitutes, plus tailored rehabilitation, are crucial for recovery. Early diagnosis and intervention are critical to improve outcomes.

Keywords

Necrotizing fasciitis · Myonecrosis · Fournier's gangrene · Meleney's synergistic gangrene · Flesh-eating disease · Rapidly progressive infection · Tissue necrosis · LRINEC score · Immunosuppression · Negative Pressure Wound Therapy (NPWT) · Hyperbaric oxygen therapy · Wound care · Hospital gangrene · Surgical debridement

Y. R. Sakaray (✉) · M. Singh
Post-Graduate Institute of Medical Science and Research, Chandigarh, India

P. Kumar et al. (eds.), *Textbook of Orthopedic Infections*,
https://doi.org/10.1007/978-981-95-5029-6_19

19.1 Introduction

As the name suggests NSTI, flesh-eating disease, is rapidly advancing infections of skin and soft tissue with necrosis of the dermis, subcutaneous tissue, superficial fascia, deep fascia, or muscle. It's called necrotizing fasciitis (NF) when it spreads through deep fascia and if it affects the muscles it's called myonecrosis.

In the fifth century, Hippocrates illustrated necrotizing fasciitis as a severe complication of "erysipelas," characterized by rapid spread from minor wounds, extensive tissue destruction, and high mortality. He detailed putrefaction distinct from pus and noted severe cases involving limb loss and genital infections, demonstrating that this condition was accurately observed long before modern medicine [1].

In the eighteenth and nineteenth centuries, surgeons from British navy termed NSTI as "hospital gangrene" and the first comprehensive validation of NSTI was done in 1871 by Dr. Joseph Jones, a Confederate army surgeon (on 2646 cases). His work emphasized the seriousness of the disease and the necessity of swift surgical action and better sanitation, paving the way for modern-day management strategies [2].

NSTI of perineum and genitalia is known as "Fournier's gangrene" after the name of French dermatologist Dr. Jean Alfred Fournier who first described it as the shameful exposure of testes [3], "Meleneys synergistic gangrene" is NSTI of abdominal wall which typically develops after abdominal surgeries and trauma, first described by an American surgeon Dr. Franklin H. Meleney [4].

Obesity, type 2 diabetes, and chronic immunosuppressive states are the frequently related risk factors whereas subclinical trauma, corticosteroids, and chronic alcohol consumption are some of the emerging risk factors. These risk factors suppresses the immune system and makes body vulnerable for NSTIs [5, 6]. Specifically chronic alcoholism can lead to deranged immune function and compromised skin integrity [7].

Though very rare but NSTI can occur in healthy adults and children also. Minor skin barrier loss or injury follows the infection by weeks; streptococci and clostridia spread swiftly (hours to days), on the other hand, Staphylococcus aureus, gram negative, and mixed flora progress slowly (days to weeks), and if untreated, mortality has been reported to range from 8–17% in recent studies (nearly 3800–5800 cases occuring annually in the United States) [8–10].

Atypical presentations of NSTI involving the thigh, perineum, and abdominal wall secondary to bowel perforations from various causes have also been documented. [11–14]

Irrespective of the different bacteria causing these infections in various parts of the body, it has typical characterising feature, that is, quick death of tissue, very prone to sepsis, and high fatalities.

19.1.1 Learning Points

Definitions

NSTI: rapidly progressing infection—necrosis of skin, subcutaneous tissue, fascia (necrotizing fasciitis) and muscle (myonecrosis).

Fournier's gangrene: NSTI of perineum and genitalia (Dr. Jean Alfred Fournier—French dermatologist)

Meleney's synergistic gangrene: NSTI of abdominal wall mostly secondary to abdominal trauma and surgeries (Dr. Franklin H. Meleney—American surgeon)

Historical Insights

Hippocrates earlier described it in fifth century as severe tissue infection.

British naval surgeons later termed it as "hospital gangrene" in 18th–19th centuries.

Dr. Joseph Jones—a confederate army surgeon—did comprehensive study on broad no. of people in 1871 called attention on high fatality and highlighted sanitation and early surgical intervention.

Risk Factors

Common: obesity, diabetes, and immunosuppressive conditions.

Emerging: Chronic alcoholism, corticosteroids, and subclinical trauma.

Etiopathogenesis

Trauma, poor sanitation

- Rapidly progressing infections by Streptococci and Clostridia (hours to days).
- Slow progressing infections by Staphylococcus aureus and mixed flora (days to weeks).

Atypical Presentations

Bowel perforation due to variable reasons may present as NSTI of abdomen, perineum, and lower extremities.

Clinical Feature

Rapid tissue necrosis is the hallmark feature.

Severe sepsis and mortality if not treated.

Mortality rate 8–17%.

19.2 Significance of Early Diagnosis and Timely Intervention

Difficulty in diagnosing NSTI promptly is the main reason for mortality. Early skin symptoms are slight, deceives clinician to underdiagnose the severity of the disease which is expanding deep into the subcutaneous tissue, necrotizing fasciitis (NF), and muscles. The most common symptoms are redness, warmth, and pain (in 90% cases) but these are also related to milder infection like cellulitis which leads to neglect of the accurate diagnosis of NSTI in initial phases. More specific signs are crepitus (a crackling sensation under the skin), necrotic skin, or the formation of bullae (blisters) (Fig. 19.1), but these are infrequent (less than 40%) and makes it unreliable for diagnosis [15]. When necrosis is visible, it signals the urgency of immediate intervention, but the absence of this shouldn't discourage further diagnostic efforts.

Along with above-mentioned signs and symptoms, systemic signs of infection shouldn't be ignored. As fever is likely to present in every kind of infection fall in blood pressure is an alarming signal should be spotted on time. Systemic signs of organ failure like acute kidney injury, respiratory failure, and laboratory examination along with local signs in the body raise the suspicion of NSTI.

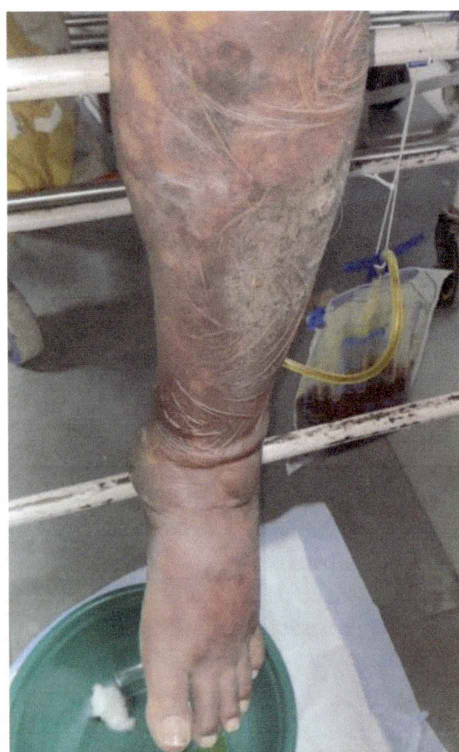

Fig. 19.1 Classical signs of necrotizing soft tissue infection

Table 19.1 The Laboratory Risk Indicator for Necrotizing LRINEC System Scoring

Parameters	Points
C-reactive protein	
< 150 mg/L,0	0
≥ 150 mg/L,4	4
White blood cell count	
< 15 × 10^9/L	0
15–25 × 10^9/L,1	1
> 25 × 10^9/L	2
Hemoglobin	
> 13.5 g/dL	0
11–13.5 g/dL	1
< 11 g/dL	2
Sodium	
≥ 135 mmol/L	0
< 135 mmol/L	2
Creatinine	
≤ 141 µmol/L (≤ 1.6 mg/dL)	0
> 141 µmol/L (> 1.6 mg/dL)	2
Glucose	
≤ 10 mmol/L (≤ 180 mg/dL)	0
> 10 mmol/L (> 180 mg/dL)	1

Six biochemical markers which are observed more likely to be deranged in NSTIs have been utilized to develop the laboratory risk indicator for necrotizing fasciitis (LRINEC) scoring system (Table 19.1). Variables used are C-reactive protein, white blood cell count, hemoglobin, Serum sodium, creatinine, and glucose levels.

19.2.1 Interpretation of LRINEC scoring system

- Score 0–5: Low risk for NSTI (< 50%).
- Score 6–7: Intermediate risk for NSTI (50–75%).
- Score ≥ 8: High risk for NSTI (> 75%).

This scoring system can help differentiate NSTIs from less severe infections by evaluating specific lab values that are typically abnormal in NSTIs. However, its predictive value is debated, with some studies suggesting limited utility. Still, any abnormal lab results, such as sudden high blood sugar, kidney issues, or low sodium levels, should prompt clinicians to rule out NSTI with further imaging or surgical exploration [16].

Signs and Symptoms
Earliest signs of inflammation, that is, pain, redness, and warmth—it resembles cellulitis often leads to delayed diagnosis.

Specific sign—bullae, necrotic skin, and crepitus though less frequent but pathognomic systemic sign—febrile episodes, hypotension, and signs of organ failure like acute kidney injury (AKI) and respiratory failure are red flags and shouldn't be ignored.

19.3 Diagnostic Modalities

As a dreaded infection and complexity in diagnosing NSTIs based on physical signs and symptoms alone, radiological imaging techniques are often used to aid in identifying the infection. X-rays, ultrasonography, magnetic resonance (MR), and computed tomography (CT) scans have all been explored as tools for diagnosis, but CT is the most commonly preferred option due to accessibility and convenient to interpretate. Most pivotal sign on CT imaging is the presence of gas in soft tissues along with other findings including multiple fluid pockets, lack of tissue enhancement following intravenous contrast, and significant inflammation around the fascia.

It has shown that CT scans can have high sensitivity (100%) and specificity (98%) [17]. In recent comparison on multiple MR and CT studies on NSTI imaging, it has shown T2 hyperintensity of deep fascia at MRI has sensitivity higher than CT and average specificity but presence of gas at CT has sensitivity lower and higher specificity [18].

When uncertainty remains after imaging, surgical exploration is often the next logical step. A small elliptical incision through the skin, fascia, and muscle (usually about 2 cm) is performed to assess for necrotizing infection. This can be done under local anesthesia at the bedside for extremities or in the operating room for areas like the groin. The surgeon looks for signs of necrosis, gray discoloration, or purulent fluid. If the tissue feels abnormally soft, indicating that infection has spread, further extensive surgical debridement is needed to remove all affected tissues. Adequate fluid samples and debrided tissue should be instantly sent for gram staining and cultures.

19.3.1 Learning Points

Diagnostic Tools
CT scan—preferred modality—accessible and easy to interpret. Findings include:

- Gas in soft tissues,
- Multiple fluid pockets,
- Lack of tissue enhancement, and
- Fascial inflammation.

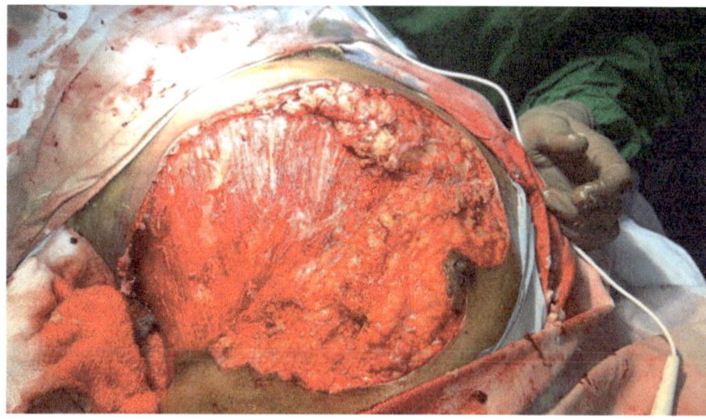

Fig. 19.2 Post-debridement wound of NSTI

MRI scan provides higher sensitivity but slightly lower specificity than CT.

In case of uncertainty, surgical exploration remains the gold standard. A small incision can confirm the diagnosis by assessing necrosis, gray discoloration, purulent fluid, or tissue softness.

The primary treatment for NSTIs is surgery, where all infected tissue is removed with at least a 1 cm margin of healthy tissue (Fig. 19.2). Surgeons use "push test" or "finger test," where they check if tissue separates easily under pressure, to guide how much tissue needs to be cut away. Bleeding isn't a liable sign of healthy tissue, as infections causes inflammation which leads to excessive bleeding. In critically ill patients, the use of tourniquets and careful control of bleeding is crucial.

As soon as NSTI is suspected, immediately broad spectrum antibiotics targeting anerobic, gram positive and gram negative organisms are deployed. Once the sepsis settles in, patient's condition stabilizes and treatment can be fine-tuned by de-escalating antibiotic cover as per culture sensitivity and institutional spectrum. Lately, studies have shown that hard-to-culture anaerobes play a silent but deadly role, demanding attention [19]. Clindamycin is the antibiotic of choice as a toxin-neutralizer, especially in streptococcal and clostridial infections. Newer agents, such as linezolid and daptomycin, are the go-to weapons against resistant foes like MRSA [20].

19.4 Intensive Care

Frequently, patients may develop hypotension secondary to sepsis and need fluid resuscitation by colloids and crystalloids or often need inotropes, further oxygenation, and even ventilatory support require intensive care or high-dependency care.

Some studies have also suggested the use of hyperbaric oxygen and IV immunoglobulins but outcome still warrants further researches. Emerging treatments, such as combinations of IV vitamin C, thiamine, and hydrocortisone, have shown promise in managing sepsis, though their role in NSTIs specifically is still under investigation [21].

19.4.1 Antibiotics

Broad spectrum antibiotics—targeting—gram positive, gram negative, and anaerobic organisms. Clindamycin—toxin neutralization—streptococcal and clostridial infections.

De-escalate antibiotics as per culture-sensitivity and as patient stabilizes.

19.4.2 Resuscitation

Septic shock to be managed with I/V fluids (colloids and crystalloids) if needed inotropes
Oxygenation and ventilatory support

Advanced Therapies

Hyperbaric oxygen
IV immunoglobulins
Vitamin C, Thiamine
Hydrocortisone

19.5 Wound Care

The surgical wound is left open initially and requires continuous monitoring. Although first judicious debridement is most important in controlling the infection but serial debridements might be needed in later stages. Daily wet dresses or irrigation with antibiotics to keep tissue wet for healing. Once the infection is controlled, vacuum-assisted closure (VAC) or negative pressure wound therapy (NPWT) helps in earlier and better wound closure. Recent advancement in traditional NPWT includes topical instillation which has shown better outcomes [22].

This large raw area after NPWT can be covered with skin grafts after two to four weeks. Advanced tissue substitutes, like acellular dermal matrices, biodegradable scaffolds, and bioengineered skin substitutes are also available which can enhance the recovery, encourages natural revival of the tissue. These advances though add financial burden to the patients but hold the capability to reduce rehabilitation times and improve quality of life for NSTI patients.

19.5.1 Rehabilitation

Patient-specific addressal of the issue like physical, psychological, and financial burden in an NSTI patient.

19.6 Point-Wound Care

Continuous monitoring
Serial debridements
Vacuum-assisted closure
Acellular dermal matrices or bioengineered skin

19.6.1 Learning Points-Rehabilitation

Patient-centric approach
Financial and psychological burdens

19.7 Conclusion

NSTI, a flesh-eating disease, is a rapidly spreading infection causing quick death of tissue and highly fatal if not treated on time and mortality rate of 8–17% in recent studies.

Initially described by Hippocrates in the fifth century, it was later widely known as "hospital gangrene" by British naval surgeons, but comprehensively studied by Dr. Joseph Jones, confederate army surgeon in 1871, in large population. NSTI of perineum is called "Fournier's gangrene" and of abdominal wall "Meleney's gangrene."

Common risk factors are obesity, diabetes, immunosuppression, alcoholism, and trauma. It can also occur in healthy individuals.

Early signs and symptoms (pain, redness, warmth) resemble cellulitis that may mislead the diagnosis and further delays treatment. Advanced signs include discoloration, necrosis, and systemic signs with further signs of systemic failure. LRINEC scoring which uses biochemical markers can be used for making diagnosis, radiological imaging (X-ray, ultrasound and CT/MRI) are helpful and when in doubt surgical exploration should be considered.

Management includes resuscitation with IV fluids, broad spectrum antibiotics initially followed by culture-specific antibiotics, intensive care and emerging supplements like vitamin C and supportive care like hyperbaric oxygen.

Prompt surgical intervention with serial debridement is the key. Subsequent frequent follow-up aided with NPWT, tissue substitutes, and skin grafts helps better recovery. Prognosis depends upon timely diagnosis and intervention.

Conclusion: NSTI is rapidly progressive life-threatening condition requiring early diagnosis, aggressive surgical intervention, and comprehensive multidisciplinary management.

Regardless of the advancement in the radiological imaging techniques, diagnosis is difficult. Timely recognition and immediate intervention are critical to improve outcomes and prevents mortality.

Ongoing research into diagnostic tools and therapies offers hope for better management and recovery in the future.

Key Takeaway

Early diagnosis, timely surgical intervention, and aggressive infection management is crucial in preventing deaths. Advanced wound care technologies improve outcomes and quality of life but may pose financial challenges for patients.

References

1. Descamps V, Aitken J, Lee M. Hippocrates on necrotising fasciitis. Lancet. 1994;344(8921):556.
2. Jones J. Investigation upon the nature, causes and treatment of hospital gangrene as it prevailed in the confederate armies 1861–1865. In: Surgical Memories of the War of Rebellion. New York: United States Sanitary Commission; 1871.
3. Beeson BB. Alfred Fournier, his life and works. Arch Dermatol Syphilol. 1924;10(3):297–303.
4. Meleney FL. Hemolytic streptococcus gangrene. Arch Surg. 1924;9(2):317–64.
5. Liu V, Escobar GJ, Greene JD, et al. Hospital deaths in patients with sepsis from 2 independent cohorts. JAMA. 2014;312:90–2.
6. Ban KA, Minei JP, Laronga C, et al. American College of Surgeons and Surgical Infection Society: surgical site infection guidelines, 2016 update. J Am Coll Surg. 2017;224:59–74.
7. Yeh DD, Velmahos G. Necrotizing soft tissue infections. In: Geriatric trauma and critical care; 2017. p. 187–200.
8. Audureau E, Hua C, De Prost N, Hemery F, Decousser JW, Bosc R, Lepeule R, Chosidow O, Sbidian E, Henri Mondor Hospital Necrotizing Fasciitis group. Mortality of necrotizing fasciitis: relative influence of individual and hospital-level factors, a nationwide multilevel study, France, 2007–12. Br J Dermatol. 2017;177(6):1575–82.
9. Psoinos CM, Flahive JM, Shaw JJ, Li Y, Ng SC, Tseng JF, Santry HP. Contemporary trends in necrotizing soft-tissue infections in the United States. Surgery. 2013;153(6):819–27.
10. Harbrecht BG, Nash NA. Necrotizing soft tissue infections: a review. Surg Infect. 2016;17(5):503–9.
11. Garg N, Singla K, Singh M, Singh M, Bansiwal RK, Sharma R. Bowel perforation presenting as necrotizing soft-tissue infection of thigh a rare presentation. Int Surg J. 2020;7(12):4206–8.
12. Kumar D, Cortés-Penfield NW, El-Haddad H, Musher DM. Bowel perforation resulting in necrotizing soft-tissue infection of the abdomen, flank, and lower extremities. Surg Infect. 2018;19(5):467–72.
13. Saldua NS, Fellars TA, Covey DC. Case report: bowel perforation presenting as subcutaneous emphysema of the thigh. Clin Orthop Relat Res. 2010;468(2):619–23.
14. Nijhof HW, Steenvoorde P, Bonsing BA, Hartgrink HH. Necrotizing soft tissue infection of the thigh: consider an abdominal cause. World J Surg. 2006;30:1836–42.
15. Wong CH, Chang HC, Pasupathy S, Khin LW, Tan JL, Low CO. Necrotizing fasciitis: clinical presentation, microbiology, and determinants of mortality. JBJS. 2003;85(8):1454–60.
16. Fernando SM, Tran A, Cheng W, Rochwerg B, Kyeremanteng K, Seely AJ, Inaba K, Perry JJ. Necrotizing soft tissue infection: diagnostic accuracy of physical examination, imaging, and LRINEC score: a systematic review and meta-analysis. Ann Surg. 2019;269(1):58–65.
17. Martinez M, Peponis T, Hage A, Yeh DD, Kaafarani HM, Fagenholz PJ, King DR, de Moya MA, Velmahos GC. The role of computed tomography in the diagnosis of necrotizing soft tissue infections. World J Surg. 2018 Jan;42(1):82–7.
18. Kwee RM, Kwee TC. Diagnostic performance of MRI and CT in diagnosing necrotizing soft tissue infection: a systematic review. Skeletal Radiol. 2022;51:727–36.

19. Zhao-Fleming H, Dissanaike S, Rumbaugh K. Are anaerobes a major, underappreciated cause of necrotizing infections? Anaerobe. 2017;45:65–70.
20. Goldstein EJC, Anaya DA, Dellinge EP. Necrotizing soft-tissue infection: diagnosis and management. Clin Infect Dis. 2007;44(5):705–10.
21. Marik PE, Khangoora V, Rivera R, Hooper MH, Catravas J. Hydrocortisone, vitamin C, and thiamine for the treatment of severe sepsis and septic shock: a retrospective before- after study. Chest. 2017;151(6):1229–38.
22. Afzal H, Dawson E, Fonseca R, Canas M, Diaz L, Filippis A, Mazuski J, Bochicchio KM, Bochicchio GV. Negative pressure wound therapy with and without instillation in necrotizing soft tissue infections. Surg Infect. 2024;25(3):199–205.

MIX
Papier aus verantwortungsvollen Quellen
Paper from responsible sources
FSC® C105338

If you have any concerns about our products,
you can contact us on
ProductSafety@springernature.com

In case Publisher is established outside the EU,
the EU authorized representative is:
Springer Nature Customer Service Center GmbH
Europaplatz 3, 69115 Heidelberg, Germany

Printed by Libri Plureos GmbH
in Hamburg, Germany